TOXIC CIRCLES

TOXIC CIRCLES

Environmental Hazards from the Workplace into the Community

HELEN E. SHEEHAN • RICHARD P. WEDEEN
Editors

Rutgers University Press • New Brunswick, New Jersey

Library of Congress Cataloging-in-Publication Data

Toxic circles : environmental hazards from the workplace into the
  community / Helen E. Sheehan, Richard P. Wedeen, editors.
     p.   cm.
  Includes bibliographical references and index.
  ISBN 0-8135-1990-X (cloth)
     1. Occupational diseases.   2. Occupational diseases—New Jersey.
  3. Environmental health.   4. Environmental health—New Jersey.
  I. Sheehan, Helen E., 1944–   . II. Wedeen, Richard P., 1934–   .
     [DNLM: 1. Environmental Exposure—adverse effects—New Jersey.
  2. Environmental Pollutants—adverse effects—New Jersey.
  3. Occupational Diseases—etiology—New Jersey.   4. Poisons—
adverse
  effects—New Jersey.   WA 400 T755]
  RC964.T65 1992
  363.11′2′0973—dc20
  DNLM/DLC
  for Library of Congress   92-48258
                                                                  CIP

British Cataloging-in-Publication information available

To Morris Saffron, M.D., Ph.D. (history), friend, collaborator, and teacher, whose leadership in studies of the history of medicine inspired the present endeavor. As prime mover in the creation of the Medical History Society of New Jersey in 1980, Dr. Saffron nurtured the view that medical education should reach beyond the cure of disease and into the realm of the humanities, ethics, and social values. This venture was undertaken at the behest of the Tenth Anniversary Committee of the Medical History Society of New Jersey (Estelle Brodman, Vincent Cirillo, Francis Chinard, and David Cowan) in homage to Dr. Saffron as the first teacher of medical history in New Jersey at the Seton Hall Medical School in 1958 and at its successor, the New Jersey Medical School in Newark. Sadly, Dr. Saffron passed away on April 28, 1993, aware that the book had been dedicated to him but before seeing the published text.

Contents

Acknowledgments

We gratefully acknowledge the assistance of Michael Gordon, Kelly Conklin, Arnold Cohen, Raimo Liias, Fred D. McKie, Andrew Wilner, and Ronald Ross, M.D., in identifying sites for photographic illustrations. The photographs by Lynn Butler were supported in part by New Jersey Historical Commission Minigrant WS91. Joan D. Lovero, head librarian, New Jersey Room, Jersey City Public Library, helped locate historical and contemporary sources on New Jersey government and industry.

We are deeply grateful to Irving J. Selikoff, M.D., who gave strong support for the creation of this book. Dr. Selikoff's death in 1992 deprived us of a great leader in occupational medicine and deprived the book of his promised contribution on the history of asbestos disease.

List of Contributors

Francis P. Chinard, M.D., Distinguished Research Professor and Professor of Medicine, Department of Medicine, University of Medicine and Dentistry of New Jersey—New Jersey Medical School, Newark, New Jersey.

Michael Gordon, Esq., Gordon & Gordon Law Firm, West Orange, New Jersey.

Lynn D. Kelly, Gordon & Gordon Law Firm, West Orange, New Jersey.

John G. Lione, M.D., Adjunct Associate Professor, Department of Environmental Sciences, School of Public Health, University of Texas, Austin, Texas.

David Michaels, Ph.D., M.P.H., Associate Professor, Department of Community Health and Social Medicine, The City of New York Medical School.

Christopher C. Sellers, M.D., Ph.D., Assistant Professor of History, Humanities Department, New Jersey Institute of Technology, Newark, New Jersey; Graduate Faculty in History, Rutgers University, Newark, New Jersey.

William D. Sharpe, M.D., Director, Laboratories, Cabrini Medical Center, New York, New York.

Helen E. Sheehan, Ph.D., Assistant Professor, Department of Sociology/Anthropology, St. John's University, Jamaica, New York.

Ellen K. Silbergeld, Ph.D., Professor, The University Program in Toxicology, University of Maryland, Baltimore, Maryland. Silbergeld was a recipient of a McArthur Fellowship in 1993.

Helene A. Stapinski, former columnist/reporter *The Jersey Journal*, currently News Director, KNOM, Nome, Alaska.

John J. Thorpe, M.D., Clinical Professor, Environmental and Occupational Medicine, University of Medicine and Dentistry of New Jersey—New Jersey Medical School, Newark, New Jersey.

Richard P. Wedeen, M.D., Associate Chief of Staff for Research and Development, Department of Veterans Affairs Medical Center,

East Orange, New Jersey; Professor, Department of Medicine and Department of Preventive Medicine and Community Health, University of Medicine and Dentistry of New Jersey—New Jersey Medical School, Newark, New Jersey.

TOXIC CIRCLES

• INTRODUCTION •

Sharing the Toxic Burden

RICHARD P. WEDEEN, M.D., and
HELEN E. SHEEHAN, Ph.D.

How many times must a man look up
Before he can see the sky?
Yes, 'n' how many ears must one man have
Before he can hear people cry?
Yes, 'n' how many deaths will it take till he knows
That too many people have died?
The answer, my friend, is blowin' in the wind,
The answer is blowin' in the wind.

"Blowin' in the Wind," Bob Dylan, 1962

In 1832, the Board of Health of Lansingburgh, New York, posted a broadside displaying regulations designed to reduce environmental pollution (Figure I.1). The order prohibited dumping "any offal, carcass, or putrefying substance, or other nuisance, into the Hudson River . . . unless such offal, carcass, or other nuisance, shall be sunk by weights, and confined below the surface of the water." By submerging the offending matter, the Board of Health hoped to protect the health and nostrils of its citizens and may also have protected people living downstream in New York and the eastern townships of northern New Jersey. Local pollution had a regional impact. Toxic wastes deposited at one location spread in many directions.

After flowing through northern New Jersey, the Passaic and Hackensack rivers meet in the Meadowlands as they enter Newark Bay, merging with the Raritan and Rahway rivers along the southern reaches of Staten Island. Designated the ninth most endangered river in the country, the Passaic has received wastes from industrial plants in New Jersey for a century. Since World War I,

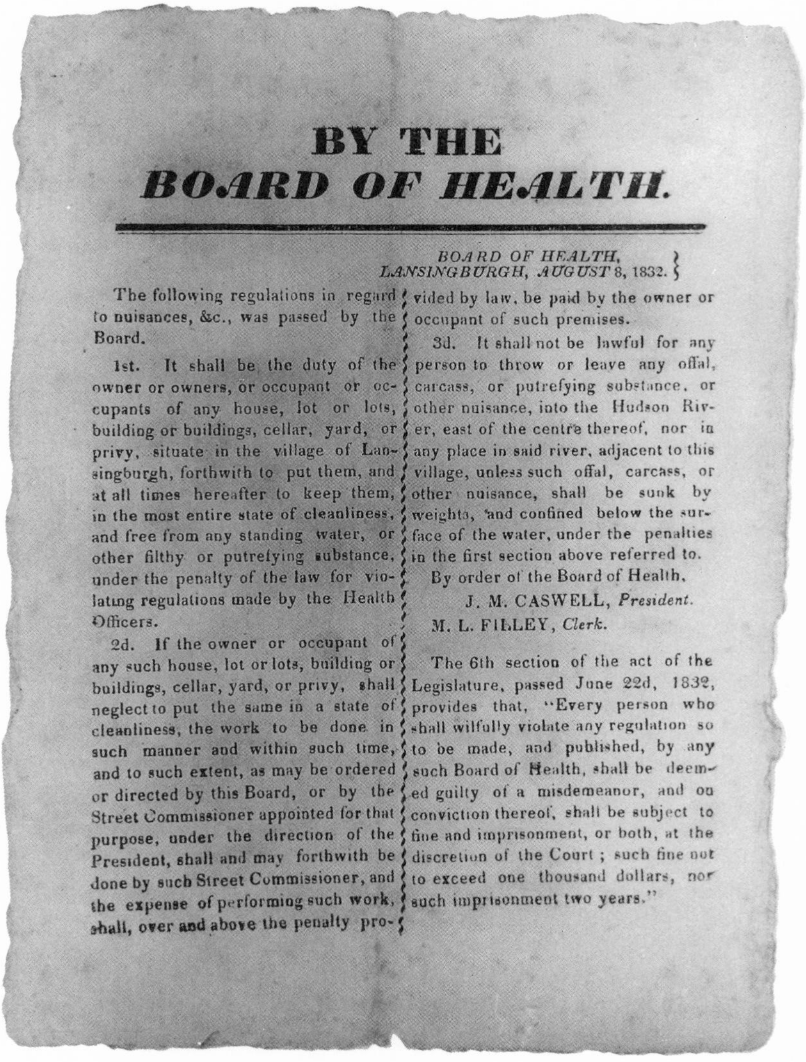

BY THE BOARD OF HEALTH.

BOARD OF HEALTH,
LANSINGBURGH, AUGUST 8, 1832.

The following regulations in regard to nuisances, &c., was passed by the Board.

1st. It shall be the duty of the owner or owners, or occupant or occupants of any house, lot or lots, building or buildings, cellar, yard, or privy, situate in the village of Lansingburgh, forthwith to put them, and at all times hereafter to keep them, in the most entire state of cleanliness, and free from any standing water, or other filthy or putrefying substance, under the penalty of the law for violating regulations made by the Health Officers.

2d. If the owner or occupant of any such house, lot or lots, building or buildings, cellar, yard, or privy, shall neglect to put the same in a state of cleanliness, the work to be done in such manner and within such time, and to such extent, as may be ordered or directed by this Board, or by the Street Commissioner appointed for that purpose, under the direction of the President, shall and may forthwith be done by such Street Commissioner, and the expense of performing such work, shall, over and above the penalty provided by law, be paid by the owner or occupant of such premises.

3d. It shall not be lawful for any person to throw or leave any offal, carcass, or putrefying substance, or other nuisance, into the Hudson River, east of the centre thereof, nor in any place in said river, adjacent to this village, unless such offal, carcass, or other nuisance, shall be sunk by weights, and confined below the surface of the water, under the penalties in the first section above referred to.

By order of the Board of Health,

J. M. CASWELL, *President.*

M. L. FILLEY, *Clerk.*

The 6th section of the act of the Legislature, passed June 22d, 1832, provides that, "Every person who shall wilfully violate any regulation so to be made, and published, by any such Board of Health, shall be deemed guilty of a misdemeanor, and on conviction thereof, shall be subject to fine and imprisonment, or both, at the discretion of the Court; such fine not to exceed one thousand dollars, nor such imprisonment two years."

FIGURE I.1. Broadside: "By the Board of Health, Lansingburgh, August 8, 1832." An early environmental law in the Hudson Valley. From the personal collection of Richard P. Wedeen, M.D.

Monsanto, Hoechst–Celanese, Diamond Shamrock, and Sherwin–Williams have led the field in fouling the river (Rosenfeld 1991c). The Hudson empties into Newark Bay at Kill van Kull, where Staten Island and several New Jersey towns discussed in this book face New York Harbor. From here, the accumulated wastes from the Hudson Valley and the western hills of New Jersey flow into the Atlantic Ocean.

The interconnections between New Jersey and New York were not, of course, limited to the confluence of rivers. Geography made New Jersey the transportation corridor and locus for supporting industries for the great East Coast cities. This supporting role also made New Jersey a prime site for major industrial pollution as well as the perennial butt of harsh humor. As the main thoroughfare between New York and Philadelphia, New Jersey has been traversed hastily for three centuries. The odors emanating from Exxon's Baywater Refinery, which straddles the New Jersey Turnpike in Linden, reminded the early twentieth-century traveler that the stench of rotten eggs hovered over someone else's back yard. Even after Exxon controlled the sulfurous emanations, ominous vapors rising from the refinery continue to greet the traveler in the shadow of the Statue of Liberty. The richest and most populous state in the Union long ago became inured to a monotonous litany of patronizing jokes.

Just north of Exxon's forest of smokestacks and storage tanks lies Jersey City, whose urban ills serve as a reminder of the toxic time bombs, the industrial fallout, that border New York City. Past its prime as an industrial center, Jersey City suffers from problems characteristic of America's older cities in the 1990s, compounded by the added burden of vast chromium landfills. On April 10, 1991, the struggling metropolis literally exploded. A toxic fire in an abandoned lot on Aetna Street, just a few hundred yards from the New Jersey Turnpike, was reminiscent of the massive 1916 explosion, allegedly set by German saboteurs, of a Jersey City munitions depot known as "Black Tom." Great plumes of black smoke once again billowed across the Hudson River, threatening residents of Manhattan, Brooklyn, and Staten Island.

The Aetna Street fire was ignited by homeless men attempting to scavenge copper from electrical wire stripped from nearby abandoned buildings. The salvage process requires burning off the wire's plastic coating. Fueled by automobile tires and 555-gallon metal drums filled with benzene, ethylbenzene, petroleum hydro-carbons, methylene chloride, and polychlorinated biphenyls, the acrid blaze raged out of control for eight hours (Rosenfeld 1991a:1). The New Jersey Department of Environmental Protection (DEP) had ordered Jersey City, owner of the sixteen-acre, rubbish-strewn lot, to clean up the illegal dump in 1987 (Rosenfeld 1991b:1). Anthony Cucci, mayor of Jersey City at the time, could not recall the DEP directive. Gerald McCann, mayor at the time of the fire, stated candidly, "The City doesn't have the resources to clean up such dumps," before pointing an accusing finger at Cucci, his predecessor and longtime political rival (Rosenfeld 1991b). New Jersey invaded New York with a cloud that extended for over fifty miles. Unable to control the blaze, Jersey City requested seven fire units from New York to assist its 140 firemen and twenty-three units. Seventy-two firemen from New Jersey and 3 from New York were taken to hospitals (Jamieson 1991:1). New Jersey's microcosm of environmental pollution became a macrocosm encompassing New York City and beyond. Photographed from Ellis Island, the cloud over Jersey City seemed impenetrable (Figure I.2), and the pall over New York hung heavy (Figure I.3). The abandoned lot in Jersey City served as a reminder of bureaucratic loopholes threatening the quality of life, and life itself, on a worldwide scale (Figure I.4). For a moment in time, attention was focused on the environment.

The explosive event symbolized the complex web of interests that communities share whether they wish to or not. The economic interdependence of New York and New Jersey was evident early in the nineteenth century as roads, canals, and rivers made New York City a convenient market for goods produced in the sparsely populated lands to the west. New Jersey made every effort to be hospitable to industry by minimizing government regulation. The laissez-faire philosophy guided industrial management as well as economic growth. Ample port facilities in Bayonne, Passaic, Edgewater, Camden, Hoboken, Elizabeth, and Jersey City invited industrial growth. Corporate taxes were kept low, and interlocking directorates, in which the same board members controlled many different corporations, were encouraged. Newark and the towns surrounding it became home to light industries producing beer, leather goods, carriages, silk, jewelry, and hats for sale to prosperous New Yorkers as well as for more distant markets. In southern New Jersey, glass manufacturing was the first successful growth industry. In Paterson, locomotives

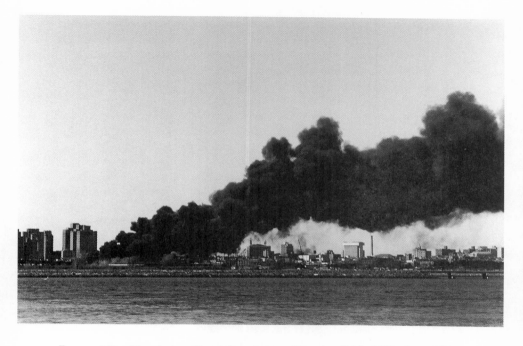

FIGURE I.2.   The Aetna Street fire, Jersey City, April 10, 1991, from Ellis Island. Photo by Lynn Butler.

were produced for the rapidly expanding railroads. Beginning in 1875, huge oil refineries were constructed in Bayonne and Port Elizabeth. By the twentieth century, the giants of the petrochemical industry—Standard Oil, I. E. duPont de Nemours, Allied Chemical, American Cyanamid, and Colgate–Palmolive—were headquartered in New Jersey.

New Jersey industries were thus central to the growth of the northeastern corridor, extending from Boston to Washington, D.C. Industrial toxins were produced in prodigious quantities in eastern New Jersey. The brooks, streams, and rivers of New Jersey were a convenient source of power as well as a handy waste disposal system. Factories discharged sewage and industrial effluents directly into the streams; toxins that even today spread over land and time to remind a wary public and nervous politicians of the price of "progress."

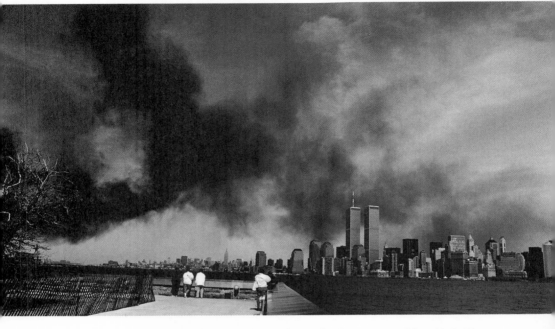

FIGURE I.3. Smoke from the Aetna Street fire hovers over New York City as seen from Ellis Island. Photo by Lynn Butler.

As the New Jersey towns surrounding New York City, including Newark, Jersey City, and Elizabeth, evolved into industrial centers, explosive growth brought urban problems along with prosperity. New Jersey relinquished its agricultural past reluctantly, remaining steadfastly pastoral in its southern and western regions. As the nineteenth century progressed, skilled artisans employed by small industries were displaced by unskilled labor as larger factories with automated machinery came to dominate the economic landscape. As the petrochemical and pharmaceutical industries found New Jersey increasingly hospitable, local communities could no longer cope with the pressures of industrialization by themselves. Protection of women and children from fire and traumatic injury in the workplace could not be left to local devices but required state government intervention.

New Jersey's conflict between economic growth and protection

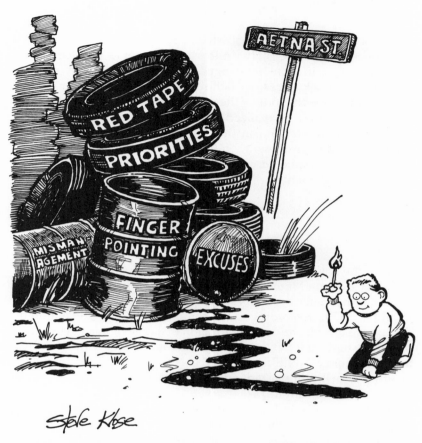

FIGURE I.4. The Aetna Street fire in Jersey City symbolizes universal frustrations. "Klose Encounters," *Jersey Journal*, April 19, 1991. With permission from Steve Klose.

of health was a byproduct of industrial development and paralleled dilemmas encountered throughout the nation—indeed, throughout the world. Environmental damage and occupational disease were of little interest to entrepreneurs preoccupied with productivity. A complex state bureaucracy was created in part to protect health, in part to encourage industrial expansion. Competing voices sounded; voices that echo in contemporary environmental controversies. A vast cadre of experts of progressively increasing specialization, but narrowing vision, developed to address the diverging goals of productivity and health. Rather than widening discourse, their expertise constricted it. Specialization created separate subcultures, ostensibly addressing the same problems, but communicating in different languages. Through a series of case histories this book traces the failure of communication among experts, in the hope that one of the nobler goals of historians, to learn from the past, may be realized. We examine the discord between the producers of wealth, on the one hand, and the protectors of health and the environment, on the other, that continues to reverberate across a planet now perceived to be quite vulnerable to human encroachment.

Public Health in New Jersey

In 1866, the New Jersey Sanitary Commission was established and advised Governor Marcus L. Ward that the state had a responsibility to protect the public health (New Jersey State Legislative Documents [NJSLD] 1887b). According to the commission, "The prevention of disease is a grander and nobler thing than its alleviation or cure; and one of the highest functions of government is to secure the health of its constituency" (NJSLD 1887b:31). New Jersey's role in public health was institutionalized a decade later with the creation of the state Board of Health in 1876 (Cowan 1961).

The Sanitary Commission's primary concern was to prevent the spread of contagious disease. In the second half of the nineteenth century, in the decades before the germ theory was established, contagionists advocating rigid isolation of exposed individuals vied with anticontagionists, who focused on environmental causes of disease but favored individual vigilance over community action. The anticontagionists identified filth, bad climate, and bad ventilation as major causes of disease. They believed miasma emanating from putrefying organic matter was the cause of epidemics. The contagionists advocated strong public health measures, including quarantine, while the anticontagionists felt individuals should assume responsibility for their own protection by avoiding bad air. The commission wisely avoided taking sides in the dispute, favoring community action as well as individual discretion. It proposed to stop the spread of epidemics by use of "sanitary antidotes," believing that disinfectants, hygiene, and a contingent of public health workers would stop the spread of infectious disease. The commission was confident it could subdue cholera, typhoid, and smallpox if given sufficient authority. But the Sanitary Commission saw beyond the need to control the spread of infections. It identified inmates of the almshouses as potential beneficiaries of preventive measures to stop "one generation of paupers providing the next" (NJSLD 1887b:38). The commission's report petitioned the legislature to enact laws to protect the health of laborers: "A great amount of sickness and death could be prevented, if a little intelligent humanity were exercised by proprietors. . . . It is for a wise legislation to work it to a proper conclusion" (NJSLD 1887b:39).

The commission's humanitarian impulses were reinforced by the practical need for a healthy workforce "to secure that prevalent, vigorous vitality conducive to prosperity and wealth, and to unimpeded labor" (NJSLD 1887b:40). The recommendation that the state collect data on occupational disease upon which preventive legislation could be based resulted in the creation of the New Jersey Bureau of Statistics of Labor and Industries in 1878, the sixth state labor bureau in the nation (Kober 1921). The bureaucratic apparatus to monitor safety in the workplace was thereby established, but accountability remained elusive. Fragmentation of responsibility for health and safety in the workplace and the separation of these functions from medical services introduced problems in implementation. Labor statistics were indeed collected, but effective legislation to prevent occupational disease was not enacted until a hundred years later, with the creation of the federal Occupational Safety and Health Administration (OSHA) in the 1970s. By 1933, eight bureaus had been established under the New Jersey Department of Labor, with activities ranging from protecting the minimum wage to overseeing industrial hygiene (Newman 1943). Fragmented responsibility assured ineffective administration.

The philosophy of the New Jersey Bureau of Statistics of Labor and Industries was influenced by European debates on working conditions and American ambivalence toward immigrant laborers. Cheap labor was valued by employers but deeply resented by displaced native workers. From the outset, the bureau seemed to have a philosophical bent not evident after World War II, when statistical tabulations displaced the discussion of ideas in government reports. Earlier, the purpose of government, to protect the working population, was always evident. Later, these ideological goals were obscured by a sea of abstract numbers. The 1884 report of the Bureau of Statistics bemoaned the fate of a valued research library collection of six hundred volumes on political economy, social science, and statistics, many in French and German, that had been lost in an office fire (New Jersey, Bureau of Statistics [NJBOS] 1884; NJSLD 1885). The Bureau of Statistics annual reports revealed a progressive refinement in the presentation of data, which included numbers and types of workshops, age, sex, worker's country of origin, wages, corporate earnings, and production quantities. The "diseases of occupation" were recorded by diagnosis, industry, worker characteristics, and work activity. Since the submission of data by employers was voluntary, determining the fraction of the workforce for which statistics were actually reported, the total population from which the reported sample was drawn, or the validity of the information was impossible. The rationale for the attention to worker health was nevertheless explicitly stated in a cost–benefit analysis.

> The State being prosperous in direct ratio to its productive forces, it is to the interest of the State to prolong the productive period of the life of the worker to the fullest extent. . . . The means conducive to that end come legitimately within the sphere of legislation. (NJBOS 1889:6; NJSLD 1890)

Consequently, the bureau looked into "the 'effect of occupations on the health and duration of the trade life of workmen.' A beginning has been made with three of our most important industries, namely, glass, hatting, and pottery" (NJSLD 1890:3).

In 1897, stimulated by the passage of a workers' compensation act in England, the New Jersey Bureau of Statistics of Labor and Industries focused attention on employer liability (NJBOS 1910; NJSLD 1911). The goal was to require that plant owners share some of the burden of injury traditionally borne entirely by the worker. Effective legislation to end "the cruel injustice of saddling both the physical suffering and financial loss on the victims" (xi) was passed by the New Jersey legislature in 1911, under the urging of Governor Woodrow Wilson. Montana and New York had created similar social insurance two years earlier. Nine other states also passed workers' compensation laws in 1911.

New Jersey's Workmen's Compensation Law was not intended to compensate the victims of chronic occupational disease. Rather, its intent was limited to having the employer pay the costs of immediate medical care and lost wages resulting from traumatic injury. The New Jersey legislation, nevertheless, proved to be important because, as interpreted by the courts, it removed "several defenses often used by defendant employers. These were: (1) that the employee had voluntarily 'assumed the risk,' (2) that his own negligence, or (3) that of a fellow employee had contributed to the accident" (Newman 1943:108). New Jersey thus challenged the traditional master–servant relationship inherited from British common law, a tradition that unabashedly favored property rights over the rights of the worker. But while shifting some of the costs of medical care to the employer, the law protected the employer and insurance carriers from far larger liability arising from civil suits outside of the compensation law system: tort litigation. Employers' responsibility for physical injury and accidents came under legal scrutiny. The law provided little incentive, however, to prevent exposure to toxic materials in the workplace and beyond. Chronic diseases arising from industrial exposure remained the responsibility of the worker. The employee was expected to assume this risk in return for employment.

Gradually, chronic diseases came under consideration by the workers' compensation courts. In 1924, amendments to the 1911 law brought ten chronic industrial diseases under workers' compensation: those due to anthrax, lead, mercury, arsenic, wood alcohol, chrome, phosphorous, high-pressure submersion (Caisson disease), benzene, and mesothorium (radium). In 1944, asbestos and silica were added to the list, apparently in an effort to reduce corporate vulnerability to tort litigation (Gelman 1988). Asbestos had been listed as a hazardous industrial material in the New Jersey Department of Labor Report of 1914 but was not covered by workers' compensation for many decades (New Jersey. Department of Labor [NJDOL] 1915:9). In 1951, the New Jersey legislature eliminated restrictions regarding which diseases were to be compensated, so that, at least in theory, any disease resulting from work could be brought before the workers' compensation court.

The lengthening shadow of environmental contamination caused by industrial use of toxic chemicals came to public attention in the case of asbestos. Evidence of the dangers of asbestos to workers was sufficient by the 1920s to warrant extreme caution in the asbestos industry. But industry ignored the early warnings, called for more proof, and succeeded in deferring protective measures for half a century. This policy of obstruction was breached by Irving J. Selikoff and his associates in the 1960s. Working in New Jersey union halls with a borrowed X-ray machine, the Mt. Sinai Hospital team screened hundreds of New Jersey workers for asbestos-induced lung disease (asbestosis). They gathered compelling statistical evidence that lung cancer was far more common in asbestos workers than in the general population. They also showed that a rare cancer of the lining of the lung, mesothelioma, represented the distinctive fingerprint of occupational exposure to asbestos (Enterline 1991). The industry continued to ignore the warnings, arguing that there was not enough information, until the courts forced the Johns–Manville Corporation into bankruptcy.

Selikoff next identified asbestos disease in users as well as in producers of asbestos products—the "second wave." A third wave of asbestos disease was then found in those who lived or worked in the presence of deteriorating asbestos. A fourth wave, of potential pulmonary disease was identified in 1991 among children of former asbestos workers from Paterson, New Jersey. Their fathers had brought fibers home from the workplace on their clothing forty-five years before. Chest X-rays of the children four decades later showed that the next generation also has pulmonary scars, indicating the potential for mesothelioma. Asbestos is not biodegradable; in industrial health circles, it is notorious for its stability in the environment. The recycling of the indestructible fibers from workplace to community has become all too common.

It is difficult to overstate the impact of the asbestos controversy on contemporary attitudes toward the relationship of environment to health. Had the asbestos industry heeded the early warnings, the fiscal catastrophe it confronted in the 1980s might have been avoided. Corporate responsibility for alerting employees to dangers in the workplace emerged as a general principle extending well beyond the asbestos industry. Who knew what, and when, became central to tort liability litigation. Past knowledge became present evidence. Medical history moved from dusty files into the courtroom. The acquiescence of scientists, funded by industry, in the suppression of asbestos information highlights the dangers of science failing to inform policy. By controlling the experts, industry controlled public policy on asbestos for five decades. To some observers, the systematic removal of asbestos from public buildings represents a costly overreaction to the loss of credibility of the federal monitoring agencies that permitted industry's dictation of asbestos policy for generations. To Selikoff, on the other hand, follow-up studies in New Jersey over four decades revealed that even the lowest levels of asbestos exposure represent an unacceptable risk of mesothelioma.

In the final analysis, ignoring the asbestos hazard jeopardized wealth as well as health. But the appeal of simply denying the causal relationship of asbestosis to pulmonary fibrosis and cancer, buttressed by greed and noble-sounding cries for more research, is powerful. Currently, industry spokespersons earnestly debate the relative lethality of different forms of the mineral. Canada's continued export of asbestos to underdeveloped countries is sure to reap a new harvest of regret and recriminations in the not-so-distant future.

The Professional Contribution of Physicians

Since the nineteenth century, physicians have been reluctant to grant public health the legitimacy assigned to scientific endeavors. The separation between curative medicine and public policy has a long tradition, as does the struggle of a few physicians to bring public health into the realm of medical practitioners. In 1876, when Britain's chief medical officer, the influential John Simon, proposed adding public health and hygiene to medical school curricula, the newly empowered General Medical Council thwarted him (Smith 1979:382). The council, responsible for public health and sanitation in Victorian England, exerted a powerful influence on medical education from 1858 until the turn of the century. In the crowded urban centers of Britain, community hygiene was seen as the business of government and the sanitary police, not of physicians. The working poor could not pay the fees expected by a practicing physician, and the unemployed sick were beyond the practitioner's responsibility. The evolution of the terminology used to describe public health activities reflects the forces competing for control of the resources. By the end of the nineteenth century, the terms "medical police," "personal hygiene," "public hygiene," "sanitation," and "sanitary science" each had found their own proponents. In the twentieth century, the phrases "social medicine," "preventive medicine," "public health," and "community medicine" replaced the earlier terminology (Leavitt 1980). By 1900, the technology of sanitary engineering had overwhelmed the medical aspects of public health except for infectious disease, which held its own as the germ theory gained acceptance. The new concepts of microbiology made infectious diseases the cornerstone of scientific medicine. Engineers gained control of urban hygiene and tended to exclude physicians from public health activities. Physicians remained primarily concerned with bedside care of individual patients.

The Protestant ethic had little tolerance for failure. Sickness among the destitute was widely attributed to dissolute behavior; workers were blamed for injury and disease they sustained in the workplace. The able-bodied poor were deemed unworthy of assistance because they exhibited "too little self-help and too much immorality" (Smith 1979:366). While holding paupers responsible for their own behavior did not necessarily exclude correcting contributing social factors, in practice, those unwilling or apparently unable to help themselves were often perceived as unworthy of the effort required for social reform.

Holding the worker responsible for injuries sustained in the workplace was typical in Victorian England. But Edwin Chadwick, the leader of poor-law reform, tempered contempt for the unclean habits of the working poor with an awareness of socioeconomic realities. In his seminal *Report on the Sanitary Condition of the Labouring Population of Great Britain* of 1842, Chadwick noted the social consequences of industrial injuries.

> The prevalent impression upon such instances would be expressed by such phrases as, 'If men will be so careless, there is no help for it; they must take the consequences:' but they only take part of the consequences—the sickness; the main part of the consequences are taken by others, especially if they are married, when the premature widowhood and orphanage are sustained by the wife and children, who are maintained at the expense of relations or the public. The recklessness is however the result of neglected education, of which the workmen are the victims, and for measures of beneficence such workmen are regarded and to be treated as children, for they are children in intellect. (Chadwick [1842] 1965:320)

Like his contemporaries, Chadwick considered the worker to be largely responsible for injuries suffered in the workplace. He saw, however, that an incapacitated breadwinner left an insurmountable burden on family dependents, a burden that, one way or another, society as a whole would have to shoulder. Despite the patronizing tone of his argument, Chadwick used this logic to thrust responsibility for a clean workplace on the employer.

The sanitary reform movement in Britain was slow to find proponents in the United States. In 1837, Benjamin W. McCready, published an obscure monograph entitled *On the Influence of Trades, Professions, and Occupations in the United States, in the Production of Disease* (McCready [1837] 1972). The paper followed the work on diseases of occupations by John Turner Thackrah, published in Britain in 1831. McCready was concerned that many Americans "are subjected to the deleterious influence of dust or effluvia, caused by the nature of their employment; and to these evils are added others occasioned by ignorance, negligence, or custom" (McCready [1837] 1972:33). He urged the use of good ventilation to reduce tuberculosis and dust exposure and provided a detailed description of industrial lead poisoning that preceded the much-acclaimed monograph on lead by Tanquerel des Planches, published in France in 1838 (Wedeen 1984).

In an 1845 monograph entitled *The Sanitary Condition of the Laboring Population of New York*, John H. Griscom, city inspector and attending physician at New York Hospital, shared Chadwick's view of the dependence of morals and productivity on the good health of the working class (Chadwick [1842] 1965). "When individuals of the pauper class are ill," Griscom noted, "their entire support, and perchance that of the whole family, falls upon the community" (Griscom 1845:1). Griscom saw a need to control epidemic infections, if not also toxic and traumatic hazards in the workplace. "Ventilate, ventilate," he urged, hoping to protect factory workers from dust and contagion. Griscom did not, however, neglect the need for sewage systems, temperance, and cleanliness to protect the health and morals of the poor crowded into New York's tenements (Griscom 1845:56). In his concern for the urban poor, Griscom reflected more his Quaker upbringing than the less sympathetic attitudes of his fellow physicians (Rosenberg and Smith-Rosenberg 1978).

Griscom believed that the conflict between health and wealth could be resolved by "a medical education in an Officer of Health" (Griscom 1845:50). He made a bid for the primacy of physicians in the field of public health. "On the one hand, the public health is to be protected at whatever cost, on the other, private property must not unnecessarily be destroyed," he cautioned, and then asked rhetorically:

> Can it be supposed that a decision of this frequently intricate question by an officer who has little or no knowledge of chemistry, nor

physiology, nor the laws of miasma, nor any other science bearing on it, will be satisfactory to the public, or to the holder of the property destroyed by his order? (Griscom 1845:50)

Griscom's plea for physician involvement in public health policy went unheeded. Public health issues, including occupational and environmental medicine, became progressively less interesting to practicing physicians as scientific medicine came into its own in the twentieth century. Laboratory science displaced sanitary science, culminating in massive government support for biomedical research through the National Institutes of Health (NIH) beginning in the 1950s (Leavitt 1980).

Conservationism to Environmentalism

Protecting the earth from the ravages of development is less controversial than protecting people from toxic wastes. "Earth Day" now has broad appeal. But in the nineteenth century, gold, silver, copper, lead, and zinc were gouged from the American West with little concern for posterity. For decades, the shortsightedness of unbridled commercialism disturbed few (Smith 1987). In the race to strike it rich, the squandering of the seemingly limitless land went virtually unnoticed. The cumulative effects of deforestation and pollution of the rivers were largely invisible to America's pioneers.

Conservation meant maximizing profits by increasing the efficiency of mineral extraction. The consequences downstream, and to the future, seemed irrelevant. To politicians, the new bacteriology fostered inventive interpretations of chemical pollution. According to the traditional theory of miasma as the cause of contagious disease, strong inorganic acids prevent the spread of infection. Some imaginative political leaders therefore decided that toxic industrial effluents would kill harmful bacteria. In 1894, confronting the pollution of streams by the hatting industry, the Board of Health of West Orange Township, New Jersey, envisaged a sanitizing effect from industrial pollutants in a township that lacked a sewer system: "The factories discharge a large amount of sulfuric acid, sulphate of copper, sulphate of iron and other disinfectants into the brooks, which greatly improves the streams" (New Jersey. Board of Health [NJBOH] 1894:159; NJSLD 1895).

Through the United States Geological Survey and, after 1910, the Bureau of Mines, the federal government championed unrestrained exploitation of the nation's mineral resources. In 1992, the Arkansas River is yellow-green as it flows from the Leadville, Colorado, mining district near the Continental Divide past the elegant ski resort in Vail, Colorado. The Arkansas has the same hue as the Hackensack River and rain puddles in Jersey City. In Colorado, the eerie color comes from iron tailings in long-ago flooded mine tunnels, whereas in Jersey City, chromium slag used as landfill since the 1950s colors the streams.

Assaults on the land during the California gold rush of 1849 and the Pike's Peak rush of 1859 were slow to elicit public reaction. By the last decade of the nineteenth century, however, the impact of smelters on health became a source of anxiety in Butte, Montana. The town's irate citizens found little reassurance in the smelter owners' contention that the fumes belching from the smokestacks purified the air by killing bacteria (Smith 1987). This dispute foreshadows modern environmental controversies; the smelter smoke was unacceptable to the citizens of Butte despite the profits and wages it represented.

The price of exploiting the land began to be perceived toward the end of the nineteenth century. Protecting wilderness gained respectability; the mountains of the West won eloquent spokespersons. As visual pollution became inescapable, John Muir raised his voice to protect the scenery and protested the loss of wilderness to posterity. As for sickness arising from work, present and future generations were left to their own devices. No voice was raised to protect miners from pneumoconiosis. Preserving the landscape became fashionable, but the promise of profit outweighed the danger of chemical pollution. The connection between occupational disease and environmental hazards remained remote. Activists were more comfortable righting planetary ills than human afflictions. Only in the last decades of the present century has government been expected to protect the land, the worker, and the community from industrial pollution with equal commitment.

The contemporary public, frightened beyond reason by traces of substances that could not have been measured only a few decades ago, looks to bureaucrats and political activists for expertise. Physicians, having demonstrated consistent indifference to such public health issues and having relegated prevention to public health officials, are bypassed. Environmental toxicology is not the province of medical practice. Occupational disease is the business of employers. Neither medical practitioners nor academicians are willing to redirect research priorities to mundane and recalcitrant issues of pollution. The public's quest for scientific answers to questions concerning industrial waste disposal is frustrated. Public anxiety grows and expertise is co-opted by politicians. The uncertainty of the medical profession elicits public distrust.

The Victorian Legacy

In the nineteenth century, medical indifference to the social context of disease left the lower classes to shoulder their own misfortunes. In Victorian England, doctors were not alone in their ambivalence toward charity cases. "As the big workhouses were built and rebuilt," F. B. Smith notes, "they increasingly became unknown to the outside world, while the outside world of novelists, journalists and social critics was content not to know" (Smith 1979:396). According to the medical model of "cases," the healthy unemployed were the unworthy poor; not people in need of help but misfits and deviants in need of discipline. Compassion was tempered by the potential for "pauperization"—the perpetuation of sloth, immorality, and poverty as a consequence of help received. Today we would term this unfortunate result of helping the poor "creating dependency."

American attitudes toward the working poor derived from these European traditions. But in the United States, private philanthropy met some of the needs of the poor that government was unwilling or unable to confront. Toward the end of the nineteenth century, religious and ethnic groups founded hospitals to serve specific groups of immigrants. Over time, these institutions expanded their functions to serve the wider community and became the major nondenominational medical institutions of the twentieth century. Diversity evolved from parochialism despite the narrow intentions of the philanthropic founders (Rosenberg 1987).

Ambivalence toward the poor in need of medical assistance nevertheless remains pervasive in contemporary America. In the voluntary hospitals of the antebellum South, when indigent patients' ingratitude led to confrontation with hospital benefactors, offending patients were punished with jail, reduced rations, or cold showers (Rosenberg 1987). In return for benevolence, the indigent were expected to conform to societal norms. Recipients of public largesses were expected to exhibit gratitude, conformity, and thrift (Smith 1979). Stinginess was justified as deterrence; humiliation moderated unrestrained charity and thus averted pauperization. Social responsibility was manifested by encouraging independence despite the provision of assistance. The worthy poor, reduced to dependence by illness or old age, were consequently largely ignored. The infirm, widowed, senile, mentally incompetent, insane, deaf, blind, and dying were sequestered, preferably out of sight, in alien institutions.

"Pauperism is a social evil and a sign of moral weakness," stated the New Jersey Bureau of Statistics in its annual report of 1883 (NJBOS 1883:373; NJSLD 1884). "The suppression of pauperism can be accomplished only by preventing what are held to be its chief causes: the neglect of destitute and pauper children, the improper administration of our alms-houses, and indiscriminate charity" (418). While reflecting a conventional view of poverty, the bureau also recognized a connection between wages and pauperism: "Insufficient compensation for labor brings on poverty" the report noted with nonjudgmental clarity (419). Nevertheless, the Essex County poorhouses estimated that "ninety per cent. of the pauperism was caused by intoxicants; ten per cent. is the result of the infirmities of old age" (385). Local political appointees chose not to delve too deeply into the root causes of poverty. Government provision of social support began later in the United States than in Britain in part because of the dominant role of private assistance organizations and a deep, not unwarranted, suspicion of political patronage and corruption (Orloff and Skopcol 1984).

The rudiments of the American welfare state can be found in programs devised to assist Civil War veterans. The main contribution of the federal government was the provision of pensions, a financial support system that was to create political tensions for decades to come. Following the tradition of providing half salaries to soldiers wounded in the revolutionary war, New Jersey opened the first state-supported medical facility for veterans in 1866. The New Jersey Home for Disabled Soldiers, as it was originally called, has been in continuous operation since that time. On his last day in office as president of the United States, Woodrow Wilson authorized an appropriation for hospitals for World War I veterans—a unique federal workers' compensation program, and possibly the largest ever created (Stevens 1991). Shifting views regarding which veterans should be served by public largesse continue to surface in the form of repeatedly revised "eligibility" criteria for veterans benefits, mirroring changing social policies toward other groups who find themselves in need of public assistance.

Occupational Medicine

Occupational diseases lie outside the mainstream of medical practice. Yet it is in the workplace that the heavy toxic exposure occurs that provides the scientific base for environmental medicine. The clinical manifestations of industrial disease afford a first approximation of the more subtle adverse effects resulting from lower exposure to environmental pollutants. Occupational disease in the few, exposed heavily at work, is a model for understanding environmental disease in the many, exposed to low concentrations but continuously, and in vast numbers.

Curative medicine focuses on individual patients; however, it is often impossible to determine the cause of environmentally induced chronic diseases from examination of a single patient. Epidemiologic methods can demonstrate an association between exposure and adverse affects in large populations. By determining the frequency of specific diseases, a causal relationship may be suggested. Causal relationships may also be revealed by converging lines of evidence from biochemistry, in vitro studies, animal experimentation, and intensive (and expensive) diagnostic testing. Epidemiologic techniques supplement the one-on-one physician–patient encounter and the traditional clinical investigation in which intensive diagnostic evaluations are performed for relatively few patients. Since most physicians earn their livelihood from curative medicine, implementation of the public health imperatives derived from epidemiologic findings is often left to public health officials.

In 1988, the Institute of Medicine of the National Academy of Medicine deplored the virtual absence of occupational and environmental medicine from the world of practicing physicians. In a monograph entitled *The Role of the Primary Care Physician in Occupational and Environmental Medicine,* the institute urged integration of these subjects into medical school and residency education (Warren 1988). Enumerating the manifold disincentives to physicians venturing into occupational medicine—low income, low prestige, conflicts of interest, legal harassment, and fragmented government responsibility, the report also noted that those hoping to revise medical curricula face formidable obstacles, including "institutional inertia, vested interests and competition among academic units" (Warren 1988:50). The financial viability of medical schools is tied to excellence, which is defined as scientific contribution and measured in research funds. Social responsibility, public policy, teaching, and even patient care do not fuel the fires of academe. "The average primary care physician," the report concludes, "does not consider occupational or environmental medicine part of the mainstream of medicine. Occupational medicine is considered a rather arcane subspecialty" (Warren 1988:72). Preventive medicine, which includes occupational and environmental medicine, lacks a strong professional constituency.

In 1990, the American College of Physicians echoed the concerns of the Institute of Medicine. Urging physicians to become responsive to the public perception of environmental degradation, the college advised internists to gain competence in risk assessment and the interpretation of epidemiologic data (American College of Physicians 1990). An accompanying paper exhorted the profession to insure "the academic viability of those specialists [occupational health physicians] in our medical schools" (Castorina and Rosenstock 1990). It would be remarkable if such pleas, unsupported by an economic driving force, could alter professional priorities. A major revision of physicians' aspirations would have to occur. But no inexorable pressure for such change is apparent. No equivalent of the germ theory or genetic engineering is on the horizon to raise academic prestige and economic incentives for preventive medicine. Nor will National Institutes of Health peer review panels soon be persuaded that scientific sophistication includes social responsibility. Occupational medicine remains an unwanted stepchild of preventive medicine, a status it is likely to retain until industrial pollution produces a crisis comparable to the epidemics of centuries past. The devastation produced by industrial pollution in Eastern Europe and Mexico may yet prove to be such crucibles for change. The promise of OSHA to reduce toxic exposure and environmental pollution in the workplace remains deferred. In the 1980s, OSHA employed but one physician, and enforcement remained a legal chess game.

The separation of occupational medicine from medical practice thus has strong economic and cultural roots. The pioneer contributions of Alice Hamilton at the turn of the century initially found few followers in the field of occupational medicine. The long-delayed appearance and multifactorial nature of chronic disease rendered etiology problematic. Industry capitalized on this uncertainty by perennially supporting research rather than prevention in the workplace. The medical investigator's insatiable quest for research funds presents a natural alliance with industry's demand for etiologic certainty. Decisions on worker protection can be deferred indefinitely under the guise of seeking scientific truth.

As a result of the states' compensation laws, by the second quarter of the twentieth century industry found a need to hire physicians to defend against false claims (Sellers 1991). Company physicians were also needed to prevent the hiring of workers with prior illness or handicaps. Physical condition was ascertained by preemployment physical examinations said to be for the benefit of the workers. These examinations and the obvious divided loyalties of company physicians created for occupational medicine a climate of distrust that has yet to be dissipated.

Tension between production and protection, between material and environmental well-being, is unavoidable in modern civilization. The conflicts created by industrial productivity are illustrated by seven chapters in this book, each devoted to a specific toxic material used or manufactured in New Jersey: mercury, dioxin, aniline dyes, paraffin, radium, lead, and chromium. Several scenarios involving the same corporate giants and "spin control" of scientific information repeat themselves even within this small group of substances. Lead, radium, and asbestos are stored for decades in tbe body. These stores provide continuous internal exposure, contributing to the long latency before the symptoms of disease are evident. The long-term storage in the body can also provide evidence of past exposure and, therefore, evidence of the cause of the occupational disease. Chromium- and radium-contaminated soils were used for landfill, spreading the long-term hazard within the state. The fact that supervisors and executives, as well as laborers, absorbed the toxins in the workplace and suffered occupational disease as a result was considered by appologists to be evidence that the dangers from these substances were unknown; exposure to mercury, radium, asbestos, chromium, and aniline dyes was considered harmless because it was universal in the industries involved in production. In retrospect, the risk taken by the managers who should have known better seems more like self-delusion inspired by greed.

The debate over who is responsible for the toxic residues of industry began over one hundred years ago. The following chapters describe key historical episodes that began as industrial hazards in New Jersey but evolved into broad community issues of environmental contamination, with both national and international implications for government policies. The dangers of lead and mercury in the workplace were described by Ezra Hunt in 1886 in his report to the New Jersey legislature (NJSLD 1887b). Lawrence T. Fell added chromium and aniline dyes to the list of dangerous substances in his first report as inspector of factories in 1887 (NJSLD 1887a). In 1924, radium was included among compensable diseases. The cause of scrotal cancers in wax pressmen was identified in the 1930s through a unique, circumscribed local episode in Bayonne, New Jersey. Dioxin became a political issue after the exposure of soldiers and Vietnamese civilians to Agent Orange during the Vietnam War: it remains a subject of controversy. As toxic pollution spread throughout the environment induces illness and the fear of illness in an ever-increasing population, the questions of who will share the burden and at what cost cannot be avoided.

References

American College of Physicians. 1990. "Occupational and Environmental Medicine: The Internist's Role." Position paper. *Annals of Internal Medicine* 113:974–982.

Castorina, J. S., and Rosenstock, L. 1990. "Physician Shortage in Occupational and Environmental Medicine." *Annals of Internal Medicine* 113: 983–986.

Chadwick, E. [1842] 1965. *Report on the Sanitary Condition of the Labouring Population of Gt. Britain.* Ed. M. W. Flynn. Edinburgh: University Press.

Cowan, D. L. 1961. *Medicine and Health in New Jersey: A History.* New Jersey Historical Series, vol. 16. Princeton, N.J.: Van Nostrand.

Enterline, P. E. 1991. "Changing Attitudes and Opinions Regarding Asbestos and Cancer 1934–1965." *American Journal of Occupational Medicine* 20:685–700.

Gelman, J. L. 1988. "Workers' Compensation Law." In *New Jersey Practice,* vol. 38. St. Paul, Minn.: West.

Griscom, J. H. 1845. *The Sanitary Condition of the Laboring Population of New York. With Suggestions for Its Improvement. A Discourse (with Additions) Delivered on the 30th December, 1844, at the Repository of the American Institute.* New York: Harper and Brothers.

Jamieson, W. 1991. "State Probing Toxic Blaze, Criminal Charges Possible." *Jersey Journal,* April 12, pp. 1, 7.

Kober, G. M. 1921. "History of Industrial Hygiene and Its Effect on Public Health." In *A Half Century of Public Health,* ed. M. P. Ravenel, 361–411. New York: American Public Health Association.

Leavitt, J. W. 1980. "Public Health and Preventive Medicine." In *The Education of American Physicians: Historical Essays,* ed. R. L. Numbers, 258–272. Berkeley: University of California Press.

McCready, B. W. [1837] 1972. *On the Influence of Trades, Professions, and Occupations in the United States, in the Production of Disease.* Reprint. New York: Arno Press and the New York Times.

New Jersey. Department of Labor. 1915. *Annual Report.* Document no. 35.

New Jersey State Legislative Documents. 1884. *Annual Report of the Bureau of Statistics of Labor and Industries (1883).* Vol. 1, document nos. 1–14. Pt. 4, "Pauperism," 371–444.

———. 1885. *Annual Report of the Bureau of Statistics of Labor and Industries. (1884).* Vol. 1, document no. 12. Introduction, xv–xxv.

———. 1887a. *Report of the Inspector of Factories and Workshops.* By L. T. Fell. Vol. 1, 28–49.

———. 1887b. *Report of the State Sanitary Commission to the Governor of New Jersey (1886).* By E. M. Hunt, S. B. Coleman, R. N. Cooper, T. Ryerson, and I. A. Nichols. Vol. 3, 31–40, 157–200.

———. 1890. *Annual Report of the Bureau of Statistics of Labor and Industries (1889).* Vol. 2, document nos. 11–23. Pt. 1, "The Effect of Occupation on the Health and Duration of Trade Life of the Workman," 3–43.

———. 1895. *Annual Report of the Board of Health (1894).* Vol. 1, Report of the Board of Health, Local Boards of Health, Essex County, West Orange Township, 158–159.

———. 1911. *Annual Report of the Bureau of Statistics of Labor and Industries (1910).* Vol. 3, document no. 18.

Newman, P. C. 1943. *The Labor Legislation of New Jersey.* Washington, D.C.: American Journal of Public Affairs.

Orloff, A. S., and Skopcol, T. 1984. "Why Not Equal Protection? Explaining the Politics of Public Social Spending in Britain, 1900–1911, and the United States, 1880–1920." *American Sociological Review* 49:726–750.

Rosenberg, C. E. 1987. *The Care of Strangers: The Rise of America's Hospital System.* New York: Basic Books.

Rosenberg, C. E., and Smith-Rosenberg, C. 1978. "Pietism and the Origins of the American Public Health Movement: A Note on John H. Griscom and Robert M. Hartley." In *Sickness and Health in America,* ed. J. W. Leavitt and R. L. Numbers, 345–349. Madison: University of Wisconsin Press.

Rosenfeld, D. 1991a. "Aetna Street Fire Site Still a Hazard." *Jersey Journal,* April 20, pp. 1, 4.

———. 1991b. "Lot a Low Priority for City and State." *Jersey Journal,* April 12, pp. 1, 7.

———. 1991c. "Passaic River Flood Tunnel Plan Called Threat." *Jersey Journal,* April 17, p. 3.

Sellers, C. 1991. "The Public Health Service's Office of Industrial Hygiene and the Transformation of Industrial Medicine." *Bulletin of the History of Medicine* 65:42–73.

Smith, D. A. 1987. *Mining America: The Industry and the Environment, 1800–1980.* Lawrence: University Press of Kansas.

Smith, F. B. 1979. *The People's Health 1830–1910.* New York: Holmes and Meier.

Stevens, R. 1991. "Can the Government Govern? Lessons from the Formation of the Veterans Administration." *Journal of Health Politics, Policy and Law* 16:281–303.

Warren, J., ed. 1988. *The Role of the Primary Care Physician in Occupational and Environmental Medicine.* Washington, D.C.: Institute of Medicine, National Academy of Medicine.

Wedeen, R. P. 1984. *Poison in the Pot: The Legacy of Lead.* Carbondale: Southern Illinois University Press.

• CHAPTER 1 •

Hatters' Shakes

HELEN E. SHEEHAN, Ph.D., and
RICHARD P. WEDEEN, M.D.

This chapter evolved from an earlier look at the subject by Richard P. Wedeen entitled "Were the Hatters of New Jersey 'Mad'?" The earlier paper used mercury poisoning as a case study of the failure of physicians, workers, and community alike to control a preventable occupational disease. In the present chapter, a broader view of the social and historical context of hat manufacturing shows that the evolution of the industry from artisans' workshops to modern mechanized factories increased, rather than decreased, the prevalence of mercurialism. The replacement of skilled craftsmen with unskilled machine operators, an increase in the number of employees, and loss of control of the working conditions by the hatters all led to an increase in mercury poisoning despite medical knowledge of the simple measures needed for prevention. And no one had the responsibility or the authority to stop it. Occupational hazards were considered normal, a price paid in exchange for employment.

This chapter focuses on the hatting industry in Newark and the Oranges in New Jersey. Other important hatting centers were situated in Philadelphia; Danbury, Connecticut; and New York City. Richard Greenwald (1990) narrates the experience of the Danbury hatters, where mercurialism was known as the "Danbury shakes." In Danbury, as in New Jersey, the hatters lived in communities with close ties to fellow hatters and their families. Throughout the nineteenth century, the craft was characterized by a high level of mobility among its workers, who traveled about and secured work at "fair" hatting shops, based on proof of union membership and introductions by fellow journeymen. Shops and workers not adhering to standards and wages established by hatters' unions were identified as "foul" (Bensman 1985).

The connections among hatters, strengthened by shared skills and a long union tradition, enabled them to unite in sufficient numbers to further their objectives. The hatters were leaders among workers in the nineteenth century in advancing union objectives and solidarity. Among the contributions they made were the introduction of the ten-hour day, the institution of the union label, and the right to strike to prevent employment of nonunion labor (Green 1944).

In contrast to the organized efforts hatters used to achieve work benefits and rights, they often dealt with the health problems covered by mercury by taking days off or during periods of seasonal layoff caused by slowdowns or stoppages in production. In Greenwald's view, "Taking time off was a characteristic of hatters' artisanal culture directly related to their health concerns" (Greenwald 1990:10). In Danbury, employers blacklisted hatters seeking treatment for mercury poisoning, thus reinforcing the workers' silence about the problem (Greenwald 1990:15).

The intricate history of occupational mercury poisoning, hat workers, physicians, state health and labor bureaucracies, and lay reformers comes together here. Mercury, however, remains environmental news. It has recently been found in excessive quantities in latex house paints (Aronow et al. 1990). In 1990, the New York State Court of Appeals held that the owners of a mercury thermometer plant were liable to criminal prosecution for exposing their employees to mercury vapor (Glaberson 1990). The possibility that corporate executives might go to jail for toxic exposure in the workplace contrasts with the position of the hatters' employers, who were protected against liability until the early twentieth century. Beginning in 1911, mercury poisoning in industry came under the workers' compensation laws in New Jersey, providing a legal barrier to liability suits and thus perpetuating employers' indifference to toxic exposure in the workplace while providing the hatters with the possibility of obtaining reimbursement for medical expenses.

● ● ●

A certain amount of mercurialism is inseparable from this calling, and can be eliminated only when a substitute is found for mercury. The most perfect machinery is imperfect; heat will be hot, steam wet; receptacles are never completely impervious to their inclosed dust; mercury will vaporize, fur will fly, and breathing will draw the atmosphere into the lungs. (Bates 1912:54)

I N these compelling phrases, Mrs. Lindon W. Bates, an investigator affiliated with the National Civic Federation, an organization dedicated to fostering cooperation between labor and management,[1] summarized the endemic problem of mercury poisoning among hat workers in her 1912 report *Mercury Poisoning in the Industries of New York City and Vicinity.* Mercury poisoning produces both acute and chronic disease effects, especially on the central nervous system, causing tremors of the limbs. "Hatters' shakes," or mercurialism, piqued interest as a medical problem and as a challenge to industrial engineering, particularly in New Jersey, where hats were crafted as early as the eighteenth century.

During the mid nineteenth century and into the early twentieth century, New Jersey was a center of the felt-hatting industry. As such, the state's physicians, as well as its health and labor agencies, played a significant role in the discovery of mercurialism and in efforts to ameliorate its effects among felt-hat workers. Bates's observation highlights how the situation of the New Jersey workers is representative of the problem: "The Newark–Orange cases can be fairly accepted as revealing the facts of mercury poisoning in hat manufacture" (Bates 1912:11).

Following her insight, this review of mercury poisoning in the hat industry focuses on the trade's settlement in the Orange Valley, near waterways that were subsequently despoiled by the industry; the trade's organization of work and work processes as they relate to the spread of mercurialism; the landmark medical studies on mercurialism; and the complex organizational and philosophical evolution of state agencies that attempted to address the problems of this occupational disease.

In the history of workers' health, the significance of hatters' shakes lies in showing the failure of knowledge and good intentions to effect change in the face of the industrial imperative to produce goods quickly and cheaply for the marketplace. For the hatters, the struggle for wages and control of their craft absorbed their energy, leaving none to devote to securing health in the workplace.

The lack of an authoritative and consistent policy backed by a comprehensive legislative approach allowed the hatters' work environment to be tinkered with, but never fully corrected, until World War II. From 1860 to 1940, physicians, as well as health and labor experts in New Jersey and elsewhere, counted cases and published recommendations. Effecting social change was not on the medical agenda, however, and the bureaucracies, by and large, were powerless to enforce their recommendations. Medical, scientific, and engineering findings, although embedded in government and social reports, were quite separate from the economic, social, and political agendas in the hatting industry. World War II and the declaration of mercury as a valued resource for the war effort, particularly in the production of detonators, was the political act that ended the use of mercury in the hatting industry (Felton et al. 1972). The purpose of this chapter is to understand how mercury use was sustained for over a century, despite a broad understanding of the health hazard it presented.

The Hatting Centers: Newark and the Oranges

Historians have established that innumerable hat craftsworkers situated in towns all over New Jersey from the eighteenth century onward (Weiss and Weiss 1961). By the mid-nineteenth century, Newark and the nearby towns of the Oranges were the established centers of the state's hatting industry, largely because of the invention of hat-making machinery. Hat blocks, flanges, frames, hat-forming machines, irons, tools, and hatters' supplies were manufactured in the area (see *Newark Business Directory* for 1893–94, 1903–04, 1913, 1923 and *The Directory of The Oranges* 1908). Charles H. Green, an officer of the United Hatters, Cap and Millinery Workers International Union and author of the union's official history, claimed that the introduction of hat-forming machines in Newark and Millburn between the years 1846 and 1859 made the Essex County towns "the great hat making centers for the manufacture of fur felt hat bodies" (Green n.d., b:24).[2] These machines increased production capacity in a craft noted for the many steps requiring the manual skills of its workers; they multiplied production thirty times ("Garment Trades" 1929:75). To meet market needs, workshops expanded to a factorylike scale, introducing both efficient production and greater profits (Hirsch 1978:16). By 1875, hatting was the leading industry in Orange. Forty factories, of varying size, produced one thousand hats a day in good times (Green n.d., c:3).

In the colonial period, a man's beaver fur hat might be expected to last a lifetime (Weiss and Weiss 1961). By the mid nineteenth century, however, hats for middle-class men, women, and children were items of fashion as well as necessity, with seasonal styles advertised by Newark's department stores. Corey and Stewart, Hatters, in an 1873 advertisement for its Broad Street store, boasted that its hats were noted for "variety, quality and price surpassing any other establishment in the Union." The company advised it had "a full assortment of youths' and children's hats and caps," that "ladies" could find "bonnets and round hats," and that "furs and straw goods" were available "in their seasons" (Corey and Stewart 1873). Hats were markers of class status and of occupation. During the Civil War, the Ferry Hat Company of Newark began to make hats for the Union Army and continued through World War I as a supplier of military headwear, making over three million "doughboy" hats ("Garment Trades" 1929:75).

Waterways capable of providing power were another significant incentive in the establishment of hat factories throughout the Orange Valley. After 1844, Newark and Essex County "were alive with industry," with even small streams providing power (Hirsch 1978:19).

According to Stephen Wickes, New Jersey's first medical historian, one of the most famous of these streams in the Oranges was

> Parrow Brook. . . . [in the early 1800s] On its east side was a large flat rock. To this rock all the hatters of the vicinity repaired, to wash the stock which had gone through their dye tubs. As the years advanced, the business increased, till all the running streams of the Orange region were discolored with hat dyes. (Wickes 1892:281)

Ezra M. Hunt, secretary of the state Board of Health, held yet another viewpoint on why certain industries were established in New Jersey: "From year to year there is an increasing tendency to locate such establishments in this State, in many cases because New York and Philadelphia authorities will not allow them within city limits" (New Jersey. Board of Health [NJBOH] 1882:19; New Jersey State Legislative Documents [NJSLD] 1883).

New Jersey actively encouraged the location of these industries in its own manufacturing centers. Hunt's primary concern was the possibility that certain industries, while beneficial from the business standpoint, might produce nuisances like smoke and odors that could prove dangerous not only to the workers' health but also to that of the community (NJBOH 1882:19; NJSLD 1883).

Reports of water pollution caused by hat factories appeared in state Board of Health reports. The Orange Valley streams, used by hat factories for power and as repositories for wastes, flowed into the Elizabeth, Rahway, and Passaic rivers, thereby polluting these waters as well.

As Hunt had feared, the hatting industry, attracted by Essex's abundant waterways, contributed to the crisis of river pollution. The economic imperative that put the hatters' health second to profit contributed to environmental destruction as well. The twin dilemmas of workers' health and environmental contamination became entwined in the ever-multiplying bureaucracies, themselves hampered by conflicting local and state jurisdiction. The 1906 report of the state Sewage Commission illustrates these limitations.

> A recent complaint was made by the health officer of South Orange against the pollution of the Rahway River by the city of Orange, a most just complaint. . . . The Commission was compelled to reply that it had ordered the pollution to cease, but that it could not enforce the order because its authority was limited by the exclusive grant of the power of initiative to another Commission. (New Jersey. *Sewage Commission 1906:4–5*; NJSLD 1907)

Despite its susceptibility to the vagaries of the economy and fashion, the hat-making industry remained viable in Newark until the 1930s. In 1925, hatting was the third largest of the garment industries in Newark, with fifteen fur- and felt-hat-making firms, employing 1,124 workers, producing products valued at $5,792,785 ("Garment Trades" 1929:75). In the Oranges, the industry had diminished by this time. Labor troubles led to the relocation of one of the best-known firms, the Berg Hat Company, to Danbury, Connecticut, an important hat-making city whose struggle with mercury disease is recounted by Greenwald (1990).

As far as the degradation of the waterways was concerned, immediate public health concerns about infectious disease were alleviated by reservoirs created in northwestern New Jersey's hilly areas for cities like Newark. The threat chemicals in the waters posed to aquatic life and the food chain was not realized until the 1950s, long after the hat factories' dyes and mercury had settled into the mud and silt of the waterways.

"Secretage":
Mercury and The Making of Hats

Mercury began to be used in hat making in France as early as the seventeenth century (D'Itri and D'Itri 1977:130). As beaver, the preferred fur for hat making, became more costly and difficult to obtain, European hatters turned to cheaper furs like rabbit and hare. These furs, however, did not felt, that is, pack into a dense, watertight fabric, as well as beaver (Sonenscher 1987:63). A preparation, initially made of water and nitric or sulphuric acid, was necessary for "carroting," the procedure that made the fur malleable, causing it to felt. In the 1770s, mercury nitrate was added to the mixture to make the fur malleable; shortly thereafter, its effect on hatters' health became apparent (Sonenscher 1987:63–80). Known as "eau de composition," "secret," or "secretage," this composition and its ill effects quickly became a source of struggle between French hat craftsworkers and manufacturers. Concerned about the mysterious ailment sickening hatters, the Academie Royale des Sciences of Paris announced "a competition to determine the nature and causes of the illnesses suffered by workers employed in the manufacture of hats" (Sonenscher 1987:28). In 1785, a doctor from Geneva named Gosse won the award for his essay on mercury poisoning.

In the United States, two reports published in 1915 confirmed the widespread risk of mercurialism in the hat industry. The Department of Health of the City of New York issued *A Clinical and Sanitary Study of the Fur and Hatters' Fur Trade* (City of New York 1915) and the New Jersey Department of Labor published *Sanitary Standards for the Felt Hatting Industry*. Both reports indicated that the hazards of mercury began with the fur-cutting and processing stage, which included carroting.

> With the carrotting process enters the hazard of mercury poisoning; a menace to health which must be guarded against from now on until the finish of the hat. . . . No further argument is needed for ventilating hoods above the carrotting tables than the blackened teeth, salivated gums, and occasional 'shakes' of many of those who now work day in and day out in a poisoned atmosphere (New Jersey. Department of Labor [NJDOL] 1915:13, 16)

Fur workers encountered mercury and dust from the carroted furs in drying, brushing, cutting, sorting, sacking, and storage. The sorting process was carried out by young girls and women (NJDOL 1915:19). In the final steps, the fur, placed in five-pound sacks according to grade, was sent to the hat factories. Storage of these sacks, either at the fur-cutting or hatting establishments, created a danger because of the mercury fumes. The report recommended good ventilation and advised that storerooms be of concrete or brick and shelving of metal, as wood absorbs fumes (19).

Once the processed fur arrived at the hat manufacturers, it was mixed and refined. In the early days, furs were mixed by hand or with a fork. "As this throws a cloud of poisonous fur and dust into the air, the method has been condemned as an unnecessary health hazard to the mixer" (24). The report noted that this work is now largely done by immigrants "who are too shifting to furnish reliable data as to occupational disease" (24). Despite the inability of the inspectors to obtain information from the workers, the report noted that "reference to hospital and dispensary records, however, give [sic] authentic cases of mercury poisoning, 'the shakes,' partial paralysis and suicidal melancholia among mixers" (24). On January 23, 1896, Clara Maass Hospital in Newark admitted a hatter who, according to the admission record,

> complains of tremor and ataxia involving chiefly the upper extremities. Also some pain in the course of the nerves. Reflexes about normal. Some stomatitis present.
> Diagnosis: Mercurial tremor (neuritis)
> Treatment: Kal Iod increasing doses.
>   Strychninia the same.
> Discharge well May 1st. (Newark German Hospital)

Some shops used a machine mixer, "the Devil," but dust laden with mercury remained a hazard unless the machine was adequately enclosed. The teeth and steel pickers of the machine also endangered fingers, hands, and arms; sparks from the machine could cause fires (NJDOL 1915:24–26).

After mixing, the horrors of hat making continued, with the blowing room posing serious dangers: mercury poisoning, consumption, fire, and excess heat and humidity. After the blowing process, the fur was fed into the hat-forming machine. The New Jersey Department of Labor report identified all feeders as women workers. Standing on elevated platforms, behind the forming machines,

> their heads so near the ceiling . . . that they are subjected to great heat . . . are forced to breathe contaminated air (owing to the preva-

lence of mercurialized fur dust); and are further exposed to mechanical hazard from the high-speed belts and driving wheels on the
machine . . . should they faint and fall from the platforms as sometimes happens. (33)

Next, the hat was formed on copper cones. The "coners" watched
the enclosed machine through "windows," but often they left
these open, thereby exposing all in the room to mercurialized
dust (33–36).

After the hat was formed, it was passed to a hardener, whose
task it was "to compact this body, and insure sufficient felting of
the fur-fibres to permit the sizing (or shrinking) operations" (36). In
hardening, two hazards affected the worker—eyestrain and "mercury poisoning by skin absorption through the hands" (36).

During the next procedures, "the wet processes," the hat was
shaped, the brim fashioned, and the hat dyed. These activities
were carried out in the "plank-shop," so named "because the workers stand on sloping planks around an open kettle, exactly like
those in use two centuries ago" (39) (Figure 1.1). Water, steam, and
excessive heat were major hazards. In referring to the hat-dying
process, the report stated, "The introduction of aniline dyes has
revolutionized what was formerly one of the most secret processes
of the trade; and has also lessened the health hazards" (42). The
hazards of aniline dyes were not evident for several decades after
exposure (see Chapter 3). The immediate horrors of the plank-
shops overrode other concerns.

> For those outside the trade, no adequate conception of the discom-
> forts of the typical Plank-shop can be conveyed by the mere state-
> ment that—from starting to blocking—the makers work over kettles
> of water kept at the boiling point. For the greater part of the year . . .
> the average sizing and dye rooms are filled with an impenetrable
> fog. (42, 44)

Next, the hat was sent to the drying room and the finishing
room, where it was dried, steamed, ironed, and finished. In these
processes, new dangers lurked for the skilled hat finisher: "The
wine shellac (owing to the highly poisonous and explosive character of wood alcohol fumes) constitutes a double menace to the
worker, who may experience headaches, eye trouble and mild
'jags' " (66). In ironing the crown and the brim, workers were
exposed to natural gas and carbon monoxide, because the pressing

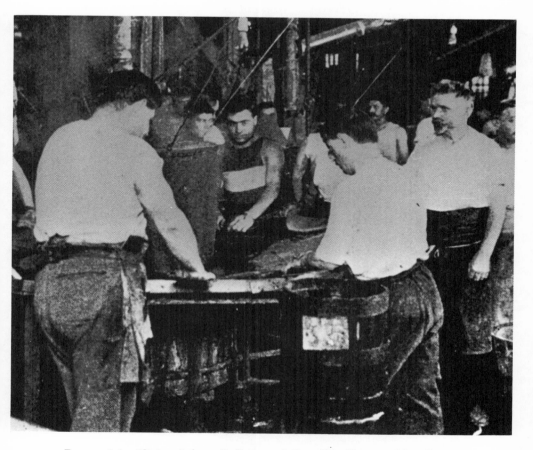

FIGURE 1.1 "Sizing," from F. Berg and Co., East Orange, New Jersey. Fiftieth anniversary advertisement (1914). Photo: Newark Public Library.

shells were heated by gas. Fire was a possibility. In addition to bad air and heat, dust was a problem, in part caused by "the practice of 'powdering' the cheaper grades of felts" (71).

The 1915 report by the New Jersey Department of Labor revealed, as no earlier reports on hatting had, that the hat-making processes endangered every worker in every segment of the industry. The hazards were not limited to mercury, and the mercury affected not only hat finishers but every category of worker.

As the report showed, all workers must be taken into account when measuring adverse effects of employment. Working conditions must be made conducive to the health of all, using the most vulnerable workers as the standard.

> The fact that a few "physically immune" workers are able to resist for years the effects of poison or lung-irritating dusts, is no argument for the continuance of unsanitary practices. It is not the occasional employee, with ten or fifteen years to his credit, who should fix the hygienic standards of this or of the hatting trade; but rather the ten or fifteen bread-winners who have been wrecked by unnecessary exposure to conditions they were constitutionally unable to combat, and whom the factory has thrown upon the community either infected with induced consumption, or helpless from the effects of acute or chronic mercurialism. (22)

In the 1887 annual report of the Board of Health, in the series on occupational disease, David Warman had observed, "Who do medical men find to resist best the unfavorable conditions of his employment and generally live the longest? Why, the man who is prudent and temperate in all things" (NJBOH 1887:106; NJSLD 1888). The 1915 report on the hatting industry stated that the view that a worker's constitution and habits accounted for resistance to disease was no longer supportable. Dismissing susceptible employees and "blaming the victim" were deemed dubious practices.

Mercury and the Physicians

New Jersey physicians were among the first physicians in the world to recognize mercury poisoning caused by the production of felt hats. The pioneering physicians of occupational medicine, Bernardino Ramazzini (1713), Charles Turner Thackrah (1832), Edwin Chadwick (1842), and John Simon (1887), appear to have been unaware of mercurialism in hatters. As mentioned, in 1785 the French rewarded Gosse for his essay on mercury's effects in the hatting trade. The first mention of occupational mercury poisoning in gilders has been attributed to Ulrich Ellenbog in 1524 (Goldwater 1964). But this obscure early treatise on occupational diseases was until recently known only to a few antiquarians. Mercurial ointments have been used in folk remedies for skin conditions from time immemorial. In the sixteenth century, preparations of mercury were popularized for internal use as well by the mystical physician–alchemist Paracelsus. Medical administration of mercurous chloride (calomel) was widespread in nineteenth-century America under the influence of Benjamin Rush, physician–signatory of the U.S. Constitution (Wedeen 1989).

While there is no scientific evidence that mercury ever cured any disease, mercury poisoning was the deliberate endpoint of such therapy. The dose of mercury was routinely increased until toxic side effects were present. Consequently, mercurialism was known to all practitioners: tremors, salivation, staggering gait, loose teeth, and a tendency to shyness and blushing that came to be known as erethism. Mercurialism was perhaps too familiar to elicit a sense of urgency or alarm when it appeared in hatters. Physicians saw mercury poisoning as potentially disabling but rarely fatal (Taylor 1901). In 1861, Adolf Kussmaul wrote the classic medical monograph on mercurialism; his treatise focused on mercurialism arising from elemental mercury in the mirror-manufacturing industry in Germany.

When a comparison is made with the devastating effects of tuberculosis, the relegation of mercurialism's threat to secondary importance is understandable. Pulmonary consumption, rampant among factory workers in the nineteenth century, remained the major cause of death among hatters well into the twentieth century. In 1908, 55 percent of the deaths in hatters (ages twenty-five to thirty-four) were attributed to tuberculosis, almost double the rate found in other American males of the same age (Hamilton 1922). The life insurance companies calculated the risk of death for journeymen hatters (ages thirty-five to thirty-nine) to be twice that for other American males (Association of Life Insurance Medical Directors 1913:58). As the bacterial cause of tuberculosis gained acceptance, public health efforts were directed toward alleviating the overcrowded, under-ventilated, and unsanitary conditions prevailing in factories.

In 1860, a young New Jersey physician, J. Addison Freeman, a graduate of Princeton and the New York Medical School, published the first comprehensive description of mercury poisoning in hatters, "Mercurial Disease Among Hatters." Freeman identified the disease among hatters in Orange, Newark, Bloomfield, and Millburn in the winter of 1858–59:

> The usual symptoms were ulceration of the gums, loosening of the teeth, foetor of the breath, abnormal flow of saliva, tremors of the

> upper extremities, or a shaking palsy . . . the result of inhaling air
> impregnated with mercurial vapor. . . . The persons affected would
> usually stop working for a while, and then gradually recover, often
> without treatment, though the various remedies for mercurial saliva-
> tion were found serviceable, especially, Iod. potassium. (Freeman
> 1860:62)

Freeman observed that those affected were hat finishers. The
source of the mercury was traced to the "carating" [sic] process;
mercury was being used in greater quantities than usual to carrot
cheap and shoddy goods at a Newark shop (63). According to Freeman, volatilized mercury caused the acute disease that led the hat
finishers to seek medical attention. The physician's remedy was
large, well-ventilated rooms; he observed that with the warmer
weather, when the doors and windows were open, "the disease
quite rapidly disappeared" (64).

Thus, Freeman identified the craft division in hatting (hat finishers), the type of workrooms (hot, poorly ventilated), the seasonal variation (worse in cold weather), and the type of materials
("old hats and clothing" poorly prepared with mercury), and reported how these four factors related to mercurialism (63). According to his report, while other workers were affected, none were
affected to the same degree as the hat finishers.

Hence, a formula for discussing mercurialism was established,
along with a method of remediation. Over time, as knowledge of the
causes and effects of mercury poisoning grew, new engineering
remedies and medical recommendations were developed and old
ones discarded. Social changes, in particular the entry of new immigrant groups into hat manufacturing and hat making, provided new
sources of speculation on the causes of mercurial disease. Alcohol
and tobacco use were singled out but then discredited as potential
contributors (NJSLD 1878). Unhygienic habits of the new immigrant
workers, uninformed of mercury's dangers, were also identified as
possibly contributing to mercurialism (Bates 1912:66–67).

Sometime after Freeman's 1860 report, a committee chaired by
Wickes, the medical historian, confirmed Freeman's findings that
improperly treated imported furs caused the cases of mercurialism.
According to Laban Dennis, who wrote about the Wickes' committee's activities in his own 1878 report on hatting, the committee
recommended to the state medical society that the facts about mercury poisoning be brought to the attention of the state's congressional representatives to the federal government, so "that such

prohibitory laws may be enacted, as shall secure the importation of proper and healthy materials" (NJBOH 1878:68; NJSLD 1878).

Dennis headed the Newark Bureau of Associated Charities (*New Jersey Review of Charities and Corrections* 1904:100) and was an original member of the state Board of Health. His report, "Hatting as Affecting the Health of Operatives," appeared in the annual report of the Board of Health (1878) (NJSLD 1878). The Board of Health (1876) and the Bureau of Statistics of Labor and Industries (1878) (hereafter, the Bureau of Statistics) were established with mandates outlining their responsibilities. Over time, these directives changed as it became evident that new types of legislation were required if these bureaus were to be effective. Workers' safety and health gradually became the responsibility of the Bureau of Statistics, especially with the institution of the chief of factory inspection in 1882, a position held by a hatter turned hat manufacturer, Lawrence Fell. In 1892, Fell became the mayor of East Orange, elected by the overwhelming support of the hatter citizens of the town (Bensman 1985).

State and local health bureaus interacted as the Board of Health published reports on workers' health, which initially were prepared for local boards of health by community physicians. In turn, these health reports proved of interest to the Bureau of Statistics. Reports like Dennis's (1878) and J. W. Stickler's (1886), both published in the state Board of Health Annual Reports (NJSLD 1887), were favorably commented upon in the Bureau of Statistics annual report (1889) because they were prepared "by physicians in active practice, among workers" (NJBOS 1889:14; NJSLD 1890).

Dennis's report was cited by Alice Hamilton in her 1922 transnational review article on mercury, "Industrial Diseases of Fur Cutters and Hatters," as a significant achievement in medical case studies of mercury (Hamilton 1922:228). Bates identified Dennis's investigation as a model for studying the problem (Bates 1912:74). Dennis identified economic competition as a major reason for mercurialism. One hat manufacturer informed Dennis that "the competition is so close, . . . the margin of profit so small, . . . that employers are calling for a stock that will felt rapidly and . . . reduce the time and expense of production" (NJBOH 1878:72; NJSLD 1878). In researching his report for the state, Dennis inspected twenty-five hat factories in Newark and its vicinity as well as two fur suppliers, one in Danbury and one in New York City.

Dennis reviewed the hat-making process, identifying the health dangers in each stage. He focused on three categories of disease: respiratory disease, caused by fur dust; mercurialism (shakes and sore mouth), caused by mercury; and rheumatism, caused by the "wet processes" of hat making and damp workrooms. Like Freeman, Dennis found the finishers most vulnerable to mercurialism. In fact, Dennis identified finishers of black hats as more prone to mercury's effects than finishers of white hats. Changes in the style of finishing black hats, requiring more dry-ironing, caused the mercury to be more freely volatilized (NJBOH 1878:80; NJSLD 1878). According to Dennis, the conditions favoring mercurial disease remained similar to those identified by Freeman: finishers were most affected, season of the year caused variation in the effects, and ventilation was a critical preventive measure. Dennis pointed to instances of excessive use of mercury as bringing about so many acute cases of poisoning that business was harmed. "Several furriers who are said to have used large quantities of mercury, in 'carroting' the stock, have gone out of business," he pointed out (80). Thus, again, the marginal conditions in the hat industry, which Freeman had noted led to the use of shoddy goods that needed excess mercury treatment, persisted nearly twenty years later. Bates in her 1912 report confirms the observations of Freeman and Dennis: "All through the early history of the hat trade one reads of the struggle with the narrow margin of profit and the endeavour—generally through the use of cheaper material—to protect against loss" (Bates 1912:70).

Dennis recognized that respiratory disease was the major threat to the health and lives of the hatters. He recommended use of a fan to remove the fine dust and of "close-fitting respirators of cotton wool" (NJBOH 1878:75; NJSLD 1878). Dennis found hat makers, those who did the initial shaping of the hats from the felted wool, to be least affected by mercurial disease. He attributed this to better-ventilated rooms, the active nature of their work, and "the addition of the sulphuric acid and the supply of an abundance of water effect . . . on the salts of mercury" (78). Workers in the trimming, flanging, and packing departments did not exhibit disease resulting from the hat-making process (81).

Dennis also addressed the question of the role of heredity and of tobacco and alcohol use in mercurial disease. He found the data insufficient to connect these to the disease, although he did state, "To the human body in a state of health, both stimulants [alcohol] and tobacco are not only worthless but positively detrimental" (85).

In 1886, Stickler visited the hat shops in person, as Dennis had done eight years before. Under the direction of the local board of health, Stickler, a physician from Orange, undertook a factory inspection, investigating working conditions and eliciting reports from the workers themselves and, in some instances, from employers. His 1886 Board of Health report, "Diseases of Hatters," was also reprinted with excerpts on pulmonary disease as "Hatters' Consumption," in the *New York Medical Journal* (1886). Like Freeman and Dennis, Stickler presented an extensive review of the hat-making process, pointing out how each stage contributes to the development of disease in workers. In keeping with the findings of his two fellow physicians, Stickler identified the hat finishers as facing the most detrimental working conditions because of the volatilized mercury. Stickler observed, however: "But I have not discovered that mercurial poisoning is common at the present day, on the other hand, it is uncommon, such as my observation instructs me. It seems to be the fine fur dust which does most permanent harm" (NJBOH 1886:184; NJSLD 1887).

Despite Stickler's statement that he found mercurialism to be uncommon, the report indicates that he found workers in every division in the factories suffering from the shakes, mercurial sore mouth, muscular tremors, and wasting muscles of the forearm (172–186). He found hatters' shakes in 15 to 50 percent of the men in the factories he inspected. Stickler concluded that tuberculosis was the most devastating disease among hatters, stating, "The most frequent cause of death among hatters is phthisis pulmonalis" (186).

To explain the association between pulmonary disease and mercurialism in hatters, one Dr. P., a physician interviewed by Bates, hypothesized that mercury poisoning made the hatters susceptible to pulmonary diseases: "It is difficult to measure the extent of trouble due to mercury. The poisoning destroys the tissues, leaving the victim susceptible to disease in any form, and either retards recovery or makes it impossible" (Bates 1912:5). Bates made the following observation regarding mercury's pervasive effects: "The fact that mercury so predisposes to other diseases leads to its own non-recognition and its submergence in the larger count, but no mention is made of the occupational poison, the contributory or superinducing cause in the secondary malady which it has begot" (10).

As mechanization of hat manufacturing progressed, factories increased in size, exposing more and more workers to contagious diseases, including tuberculosis. The role of mercurialism in increasing susceptibility to tuberculosis has never been established.

The perplexing, multifaceted nature of mercury poisoning, identified by the medical experts, formed the essence of the quandary faced by the health and labor bureaus over the years as they attempted to isolate the effects of the disease and resolve the engineering problems it created.

The Bureaucracies
and the Mercury Problem

The New Jersey physicians' chronicles on hatters' shakes, consumption, and rheumatism, coupled with their recommendations for changes in the workplace, are extraordinary in their detail. The physicians' reports showed a personal knowledge gained from investigations of the hatters' home and work conditions. These practitioners' reports contributed to the efforts of the Board of Health and the Bureau of Statistics to quantify occupational disease to better understand public health needs. The individual physicians and the government bureaus were conscious of their roles in making public health policy.

In 1880, the annual report of the Board of Health noted:

> The study of health questions is becoming organized into a system. From many of our cities and from some country and village localities, we have evidence of a comprehension of the necessities of a close watchfulness over the causes of disease, with a view to their prevention or abatement. It is no longer viewed as merely a professional matter, but as one which concerns the industrial welfare of the people. (NJBOH 1880:6; NJSLD 1881)

The nineteenth-century reports of the Orange Valley physicians—Freeman, Dennis, and Stickler—reveal the depth of knowledge they had regarding workers' health and work conditions. The 1915 New Jersey state report on felt hatting, "one of the most notable achievements in the history of American Trade Sanitation" (NJDOL 1915:27), synthesized the medical and engineering knowledge of the era. Over a period of fifty-five years (1860–1915), the need for regulations with enforcement powers to correct hazardous work conditions had become recognized. The formalized procedures of inspection, engineering changes, brochures, education, and medical supervision imposed by the responsible bureaucracies created an aura of completion, of a problem identified and remedied. Yet the 1915 report on felt hatting, definitive as it was, was followed by a report by the Department of Labor in 1929 on the discovery of mercurial poisoning in several factories.

> Of the plants visited where mercury was used four were hat factories, one was chemical plant, one a thermometer plant and one a storage battery plant. Despite the fact that chronic mercurial poisoning was considered a thing of the past in hat factories it was quite evident that many of the workers were still suffering from the disease. Tremors (shakes) were common in a large proportion of the men seen in these shops. A program of medical supervision for these plants has been developed and offered to the plant management as well as to the industrial worker. (NJDOL 1929:13)

Years earlier, in 1908, the Orange City Board of Health sent a report for the state Board of Health annual report. Although laudable for its educational goal, the report conveys an air of bureaucratic distance from the problem, leaving its resolution to the workers and manufacturers.

> With regard to tuberculosis . . . we are making arrangements with the Hatters Union and Hat Manufacturers Association to be given hearings before their bodies in order to point out to them the extreme prevalence of this disease among the hatters, and indicate simple methods of prevention. . . . A special circular is being prepared for distribution to the hatters. (NJBOH 1908:466; NJSLD 1909)

Along with other categories of workers, the hatters served as a focus of concern and of investigation for these New Jersey bureaucracies, as well as a justification for their existence and growth. But mercurial disease persisted. Despite knowledge of the hatters' disease and despite regulations for prevention and plans for education, changes wrought by bureaucratic procedures were not adequate to correct the problem.

By understanding the overall objectives of these bureaus, we can see the context for the studies they undertook of hatters and mercurialism. The 1889 report of the New Jersey Bureau of Statistics spelled out its intent to use the rational and scientific methods of the developing field of statistics in combination with investigative reports by physicians. Officials of the bureau were staking out their power and jurisdiction over employers and workers. With the worker identified as an economic asset, the state claimed its legal interest in the worker's health. The bureau's report of that year was noteworthy for its insight into the problem of occupational disease, its effort to develop a sophisticated longitudinal study of the problem, and its direct statement on the effects of industrial chemicals on workers.

After reviewing European and American studies of workers' health, the bureau stated, "The influence of occupation upon the health and trade-life of workmen never has been sufficiently investigated" (New Jersey Bureau of Statistics [NJBOS] 1889:xiii; NJSLD 1890). It determined

> to pursue a different but largely experimental line of inquiry in the investigation . . . into the "effect of occupation on the health and duration of the trade life of workmen." A beginning has been made with three of our most important industries, namely, glass, hatting and pottery. The effort was primarily directed to obtaining from journeymen, of twenty-one years and upwards, a sufficiently full history of their trade life for a correct estimation of its duration. . . .
>
> In connection with and as introductory to these original data, is given an account of the results of the more general observations of medical experts, based on private professional experience of the official inspection of workshops and mills. (xiv)

The bureau identified the health of the worker as dependent on occupation and measured the productive span of the worker in a particular occupation by establishing the age at which health began to fail. In industries that posed a danger to the workers' health and longevity, legislation was viewed as the proper remedy for correcting work conditions.

The bureau developed a set of "blanks" or questionnaires that it sent separately to employers and to workers beginning in 1878. The purpose of the questionnaires was to obtain information on aspects of industry and work deemed important to the bureau's functions. At the end of each blank, several questions related to health conditions were asked.

Initial inquiries conducted through these early questionnaires were expanded into the series of investigations into the health and diseases of occupation in key state industries, with the diseases of hatters forming a significant part of the series. The findings of medical experts, especially investigations such as those Dennis and

Stickler conducted on mercurialism for the Board of Health, were included in the reports.

As the account of the bureaucracies reveals, the last quarter of the nineteenth century was a period of exceptionally creative undertakings on the part of the developing state labor and health bureaus in an effort to understand the origin, development, and consequences of occupational disease. State-of-the-art statistics, labor studies, and public health methods were combined to present a comprehensive picture of occupational diseases in New Jersey.

Twelve years after the 1889 report, the bureau's 1901 report, while reiterating its earlier philosophy, also conveyed evidence of xenophobia, reflecting the ambivalence that existed regarding the arrival of immigrants, especially from eastern and southern Europe. In this report, in the series "Diseases and Disease Tendencies of Occupations," continuation of the bureau's objectives is noted, although now the concern for workers' health as affected by occupation is characterized, in part, as "sentimental":

> Although it has its material basis also . . . all modern factory legislation is based on the conviction that every possible protection to the working man against accidents and things injurious to health that are peculiar to his workday life is a public duty. (NJBOS 1901:347; NJSLD 1902)

Data were collected in a fashion similar to the methods of earlier reports.

> The information was furnished by owners or managers . . . also by physicians who practice largely among the workmen engaged in these industries and have thus become familiar with such disease tendencies as may be peculiar to them. The workmen's own version of how his health is affected by the conditions surrounding his labor is given. (348)

In this report, in a section entitled "The Health Conditions of the Hatting Industry," a series of questions rooted in the social and political concerns of the era appeared. These concerns included the character and habits of immigrant or foreign workers and the drinking habits of the lower socioeconomic classes. Replies from workers were sparsely reported.

The 1901 discussion on the hatting industry concludes that larger hatting factories are better, safer, and cleaner. In contrast, smaller ones have less machinery, the work is done by hand, the buildings are old. Moreover, these factories are usually owned by foreigners and filled with workers of their own race ("Hebrews, Polacks or Italians") (365). Summarizing replies from the hatting industry, the report stated:

> The nationalities of those employed in the hatting industry appear from the reports to embrace almost all those of Continental Europe. Only one firm [of eleven] reports the proportion of American workmen in his factory force as about one-third. The others say that at least 90 per cent. of the employes [sic] are foreigners, Russian and Polish Hebrews and Italians greatly outnumbering all the other nationalities combined. (353)

All the reports on hatters, from Freeman's in 1860 to the United States Public Health Service (USPHS) surveys of the 1930s (Neal and Jones 1937, 1938; Neal et al. 1941) discuss social organization of the workplace and the community. As the comments in the 1901 Bureau of Statistics report indicate, ethnicity of the new immigrants became integral to the effort to understand the sanitary and health conditions in the hat shops. In the remaining sections of this Chapter, the sociological phenomena of work organization, gender, and ethnicity among the hatters are examined, along with their union organizations.

Mercury and Social Conditions in the Hatting Workplace

The portrait of the hatters' workplace and community presented in medical and government reports enables us to see how mercury remained the nemesis of the hatters for decades. By 1886, the year of Stickler's report, the hatting trades in the Orange Valley and Newark had expanded; new technology had been introduced; craft skills had diminished; and the recruitment of less skilled laborers, namely, boys, women, and girls, was increasing rapidly (Bensman 1985). The expansion of the industry in terms of numbers and types of workshops, the number of workers employed in them as a result of an increased division of labor, the types of materials used—all can be identified as factors interacting with the mercury problem in the workplace. In prosperous times for the hat industry, "commission shops," set up in shedlike arrangements with a few workers, assisted larger hat shops with production (Green n.d., c:4).

The number of individuals likely to be exposed to mercury increased as the introduction of new machinery and the effort to divide tasks brought more unskilled, lower-paid workers into the industry. The establishment of shops in Newark, whose owners and employees were immigrants, largely from eastern and southern Europe, was identified by the hatters themselves (Bensman 1985), by a government report (NJBOS 1901; NJSLD 1902), and by Bates (1912:34, 66–67) as contributing to the deleterious conditions found in the hatting trade.

As a result of these conditions, several insurance companies refused to insure fur cutters, makers, starters, and sizers at all. Workers in other hat factory departments were charged high premiums (Bates 1912:8; NJDOL 1915). Philip Foner, historian of the furriers' union, wrote: "Life insurance companies refused to issue policies to fur workers. A common saying among the workers was: 'Furriers must pay with their health for the privilege of working' " (Foner 1950:41).

From New Jersey government and lay reports, like that of Bates, we learn details of the organization of the craft, the types of workers and their tasks, the departments in which women worked, and the facilities workers had for meals and sanitary needs. Historically, in Europe and in the United States, hatters decided among themselves where they would work. Many hatters were mobile, moving from town to town and factory to factory, as well as from department to department within a workshop (Bensman 1985). In some cases, these changes took place as a way of alleviating excess exposure to mercury. According to Bates, "A section like Newark–Orange, where there are many factories and shops, gives a man a chance to change environment if he becomes ill in his special factory, and change is generally the first remedy tried" (Bates 1912:11). The various reports indicate that workers affected by mercury always had improved health after a layoff, strike, or change to another department, or when the weather was warmer and open windows allowed the mercury fumes to be vented.

By the time Bates conducted her research, women worked in many departments—feeding, sorting, packing, and trimming. As the 1915 New Jersey Department of Labor report stated, with confirmation by the USPHS reports in the 1930s, the presence of mercurialized fur everywhere in the factory assured that volatilized mercury was always in the air, exposing all workers to danger (Neal and Jones 1938:337). Bates found that women often stayed in their jobs for shorter periods than men did, leaving to marry (Bates 1912:32). Physicians advised her that, nonetheless, despite the shorter exposure, women did suffer effects from mercury. "The tremor stage of mercurialism in women is often accompanied by menstrual suppression and miscarriage, and children born are apt to be scrofulous, ricketic and mentally defective" (Bates 1912:22). Bates, who in her report relied on physician and hospital data, speculated that the dearth of information on mercury's effect on women might be accounted for by their reluctance to enter the hospital rather than their lack of exposure (33). In her factory visits, Bates found that where women were employed, some better amenities were available, such as separate toilet and washing facilities for men and women. Women employees, at least, were allowed to quit work ten to fifteen minutes early to wash and change clothing (64–65).

Since meals were eaten in workrooms, food became contaminated by mercury. Sending out for pails of beer was common practice among hatters; Bates identified these pails as a source of contamination, since they were set down in the workrooms. Although many observers deplored the hatters' drinking habits, in the sweltering conditions of the hat factory, drinking beer for water replacement was understandable; in Bates's view especially since she saw no fit drinking water supplies in any of her inspections (33). Among her criticisms of hat factory organization, Bates noted that not one had signs posted informing workers of the processes used or any signs recommending hygienic measures (29). In addition, many non-English-speaking foreigners were employed in the factories, and they were totally unaware of the dangers involved in the hat-making process (29–30).

Hat Craftsmen
and the Hatters' Union

Studies of French hatters (Sonenscher 1987) and of American hatters (Bensman 1985, Greenwald 1990) describe them as skilled artisans determined to exert control over their work conditions. The contradiction in the New Jersey hatters' story is the inability of these craftsworkers and their union to protect hat workers against mercurialism, a major threat to their health and livelihood.

During the nineteenth century, the hatters engaged in significant struggles that led, by the end of the century, to changes in their culture of work, transforming them from "artisans" to "workers" (Bensman 1985). A distinction critical to understanding hatting as a craft and, in turn, as an industry is that the word, "hatters," both in Bensman's study and in the early medical studies of hatters' shakes, usually refers to the most skilled craftsworkers in hatting— the hat finishers. The oldest hatting union in the United States, founded in Newark in 1847, was the Hat-Finishers Association. Until the formation of the United Hatters' Union in the late nineteenth century, the hat finishers had struggled to preserve craft skills, to decide who was hired, and to assure an equal division of work among themselves. In the end, technological innovation in the shape of machines designed to carry out hat forming, curling, and other skilled tasks, both deskilled the craft and increased the division of labor. Economic hard times in the post–Civil War period forced the hat finishers to realize that unity, first with their fellow hat makers and, eventually, with all types of workers engaged in hat production, was the only means of preserving their jobs.

The very divisions among hatting workers, struggles over the introduction of technological innovations, and severe economic downswings in the late nineteenth century drove the hatters— finishers and others alike—to devote their energies to keeping their industry viable. Often they were forced to make concessions to the factory owners to maintain their jobs. Occupational disease was to be endured. Securing a living wage and maintaining craft traditions in the workplace were the primary concerns.

Handwritten minutes, dating from 1853, of the Hat-Finishers' Association of the City of Newark, are extant (Hot-Finishers' Association 1853–70). These minutes substantiate Green's observation that the hatters, engaged as they were in assuring fair wages, protecting craft secrets and practices, and preventing prison laborers and children from producing hats, never collectively raised the issue of work induced disease until after World War I. In an unpublished manuscript, "Adverse Business Conditions Have Their Effect (1916–1933)," Green discusses mercurialism and the lack of union knowledge or interest in the problem (Green n.d., a:110–115) According to Green, medical experts knew of mercurialism as a hatters' disease since 1860 but

> as far as can be gathered from the printed records, mercury poisoning was not mentioned in any report to the Union or at any of its conferences or conventions prior to 1914. In that year Michael Greene, then secretary of the Orange Makers, reported at a meeting of the Board of Directors about a "peculiar disease" of which workers were suffering and which was caused by mercury poisoning. (Green n.d., a:107)

In 1921, the Ninth International Congress of Hat Makers recommended that

> national organisations . . . make enquiries in their respective countries concerning the frequency of mercury poisoning, and to submit the results of these enquiries into mercury poisoning in the hat industry in various countries, especially with a view to ascertaining what steps have been taken in order to reduce this danger to a minimum. (International Federation of Hat Makers 1921:9)

At the 1914 meeting of the United Hatters' Union, referred to above, Greene, later to become general secretary and then president of the United Hatters, Cap and Millinery Workers International Union, reported that New Jersey labor organizations, especially the United Hatters' locals, were attempting to have occupational disease included in the state's workers' compensation laws (Green n.d., a:108). At the 1923 Hatters' Convention, the institution of New Jersey Department of Labor regulations for hat factories was reported. In addition, "It was further reported that mercury poisoning had wrought serious devastation among the Danbury and New York hatters" (107). Activism by the United Hatters grew stronger in the 1930s, beginning with the Connecticut locals under the leadership of Dennis Carroll. From 1935 to 1938, research studies on mercurialism among hat and hat fur workers in Connecticut were conducted by the USPHS. As a result of these studies, the USPHS recommended to the United Hatters' Union and to hat trade associations that mercury be prohibited in the carroting of fur felt (108). Finally, in 1942, with mercury deemed essential for the war effort, the War Production Board prohibited the issuance of mercury to the hatting industry (Felton et al. 1972).

Conclusion

The story of the hatters both fascinates and sobers us even today. There was at the time a surfeit of knowledge about the dangers of mercury; there were stated good intentions to protect the workers from it. The introduction of blowers, mandated by New Jersey law in 1904, led to improvements in dusty work conditions and alleviation of pulmonary disease for the hatters (NJDOL 1907:5–6; NJSLD 1908). Yet exposure to mercury persisted until 1940, when war emergency precluded mercury's use in the hatting trade. Economics drives American industry, including the hatting industry. Today, we have greater knowledge about toxic dangers in the workplace along with multiple federal and state bureaucracies and regulations to monitor them. The hatters' tale should caution us that even these may not be enough to protect workers, as long as corporate power and profit are paramount.

Notes

[1]The National Civic Federation, founded after the Pullman strike in 1894, had as one of its purposes to persuade management of the legitimacy of arbitration as a way of limiting labor strife. Management as well as labor union leaders and members served on its board. The federation sponsored meetings, conferences, and reports on social and political issues, as well as on industrial relations. By the 1930s, the more radical unions rejected the notion that labor and management could legitimately work together in one organization, and many labor union leaders and members withdrew from the federation, hastening its demise (Taft 1957:225–232). The federation had a special interest in labor legislation, especially workers' compensation (Brandeis 1935:575–576). Bates's study on mercury poisoning, which she did as a member of the Women's Welfare Department of the federation, reflects the organization's interest in workers' health.

[2]Green's official history of the union, *The Headwear Workers: A Century of Trade Unionism*, was published in 1944. The typescript of this manuscript, undated, in the Robert F. Wagner Labor Archives, Tamiment Institute, Elmer Holmes Bobst Library, New York University, is the source used in this chapter. The two sources vary, with the typescript offering a more comprehensive view of the industry itself, not only of its significant union achievements, which is the focus of the published version.

52

H. E. SHEEHAN AND R. P. WEDEEN

References

Aronow, R., Cubbage, C., Weiner, R., Johnson, B., Hesse, J., and Bedford, J. 1990. "Mercury Exposure from Interior Latex Paint—Michigan." *Morbidity and Mortality Weekly Report* 39:125–126.

Association of Life Insurance Medical Directors and the American Actuarial Society. 1913. *Effect of Occupation on Mortality.* Medicoacturial Mortality Investigation 3.

Bates, Mrs. L. W. 1912. *Mercury Poisoning in the Industries of New York City and Vicinity.* National Civic Federation, New York and New Jersey Section (Women's Welfare Department), and American Association for Labor Legislation.

Bensman, D. 1985. *The Practice of Solidarity: American Hat Finishers in the Nineteenth Century.* Urbana: University of Illinois Press.

Brandeis, E. 1935. "Labor Legislation." In *History of Labor in the United States, 1896–1932,* vol. 3. New York: Macmillan.

Chadwick, E. [1842] 1965. *Report on the Sanitary Condition of the Labouring Population of Gt. Britain.* Ed. M. W. Flynn. Edinburgh: University Press.

City of New York. Department of Health. 1915, December. *A Clinical and Sanitary Study of the Fur and Hatters' Fur Trade.* By L. I. Harris. Monograph Series, no. 12.

Corey and Stewart, Hatters. 1873. Advertisement. *The Successful Businessmen of Newark, N.J.* Syracuse, N.Y.: Van Arsdale.

The Directory of the Oranges. 1908. Price and Lee Co.

D'Itri, P. A., and D'Itri, F. M. 1977. *Mercury Contamination: A Human Tragedy.* New York: Wiley.

Felton, J. S.; Kahn, E.; Salick, B.; Van Natta, F. C.; and Whitehouse, M. W. 1972. "Heavy Metal Poisoning: Mercury and Lead." *Annals of Internal Medicine* 76, no. 5:779–792.

Foner, P. S. 1950. *The Fur and Leather Workers Union: A Story of Dramatic Struggles and Achievements.* Newark, N.J.: Nordan Press.

Freeman, J. A. 1860. "Mercurial Disease Among Hatters." *Transactions of the New Jersey State Medical Society:* 61–64.

"Garment Trades One-Eighth of Newark Industry." 1929. *Journal of Industry and Finance* (April): 75.

Glaberson, W. 1990. "Court Says Job Hazards May Be a Crime." *New York Times,* October 17, sec. B.

Goldwater, L. J. 1964. "Occupational Exposure to Mercury." The Harben Lectures. *Journal of the Royal Institute of Public Health* 27:279–285.

Green, C. H. n.d. Typescript for *The Headgear Workers.* a. "Adverse Business Conditions Have Their Effect (1916–1933)," b. "The Development of the Men's Hat Industry," 1–24; c. "The Men's Hat Industry in the 1870's and 1880's," 1–4; Box 64 (HRG), Robert F. Wagner Labor Archives, Tamiment Institute, Elmer Holmes Bobst Library, New York University.

———. 1944. *The Headwear Workers: A Century of Trade Unionism.* New York: United Hatters, Cap and Millinery Workers International Union.

Greenwald, R. A. 1990. "Work, Health and Community: Danbury, Connecticut's, Struggle with an Industrial Disease." *Labor's Heritage* 2, no. 3 (July): 4–21.

Hamilton, A. 1922. "Industrial Diseases of Fur Cutters and Hatters." *Journal of Industrial Hygiene* 4, no. 5:219–234.

Hat-Finishers Association of the City of Newark. 1853–70. Minutes Book. Box HRHF-3, Robert F. Wagner Labor Archives, Tamiment Institute, Elmer Holmes Bobst Library, New York University.

Hirsch, S. E. 1978. *Roots of the American Working Class: The Industrialization of Crafts in Newark, 1800–1860.* Philadelphia: University of Pennsylvania Press.

International Federation of Hat Makers. 1921. Ninth Congress, June 5–9. *Studies and Reports,* series A, no. 23, resolutions 9. Geneva: International Labour Office.

Kussmaul, A. 1861. *Untersuchungen über den constitutionellen Mercurialismus und sein Verhältniss zur constitutionellen Syphylis.* Wuetzberg: Der Staahel'schen Buch- und Kunsthandlung.

Neal, P. A., and Jones, R. R. 1937. "A Study of Chronic Mercurialism in the Hatters' Fur-Cutting Industry." *Public Health Bulletin* no. 234. U.S. Treasury Department, Public Health Service. Washington, D.C.: Government Printing Office.

———. 1938. "Chronic Mercurialism in the Hatters' Fur-Cutting Industry." *Journal of the American Medical Association* 110, no. 5:337–443.

Neal, P. A.; Edwards, T. L.; Reinhart, W. H.; Hough, J. W.; Dallavalle, J. M.; Goldman, F. H.; and Armstrong, D. W. 1941. "Mercurialism and Its Control in the Felt-Hat Industry." *Public Health Bulletin* no. 263. Federal Security Agency, Public Health Service. Washington, D.C.: Government Printing Office.

Newark German Hospital. From the Clara Maass Medical Center Archives, patient records. Belleville, N.J.

Newark (N.J.) Business Directories. 1893–94, 1903–4, 1913, and 1923.

New Jersey. Department of Labor. 1915. *Sanitary Standards for the Felt Hatting Industry.* L. T. Bryant, Commissioner.

New Jersey. Department of Labor. 1929. Industrial Disease Investigation Bureau. J. Roach and H. H. Kessler. *Industrial Bulletin* 3, no. 9 (September 8): 11–15.

New Jersey Review of Charities and Corrections 1904. 3, no. 5 (June): 100.

New Jersey State Legislative Documents. 1878. *Annual Report of the Board of Health (1878).* "Hatting as Affecting the Health of Operatives," By L. Dennis. Document no. 53, 67–85.

———. 1881. *Annual Report of the Board of Health (1880).* "Report of the Secretary of the Board." By E. M. Hunt Vol. 2, document no. 73, 5–64.

———. 1883. *Annual Report of the Board of Health (1882).* "Offensive Trades and Manufactories." By E. M. Hunt. Vol. 2, document no. 13. 5–34. 18–20 in "Report of the Secretary of the Board."

———. 1887. *Annual Report of the Board of Health (1886).* "Diseases of Hatters." By J. W. Stickler. Vol. 3, document no. 29, 157–200. 166–188 in "The Hygiene of Occupations," 157–200.

———. 1888. *Annual Report of the Board of Health (1887).* "Exposures and Diseases of Operatives: The Diseases of Potters." By David Warman. Vol. 3, document no. 27, 97–116.

———. 1890. *Annual Report of the Bureau of Statistics of Labor and Industries*

(1889). Vol. 2, document no. 13. Introduction, xiii–xvi; and "The Effect of Occupation on the Health and Duration of the Trade Life of Workmen," 3–43.

———. 1902. *Annual Report of the Bureau of Statistics of Labor and Industry (1901).* Vol. 1, document no. 8. "Diseases and Disease Tendencies of Occupations," 344–399.

———. 1907. *Annual Report of the State Sewage Commission (1906).* Vol. 2, document no. 26, 3–11.

———. 1908. *Annual Report of the Department of Labor (1907).* Vol. 1. Introduction, 5–6.

———. 1909. *Annual Report of the Board of Health (1908).* Vol. 3, document no. 16. "Excerpts from the Annual Report of Local Boards of Health," 455–470.

———. 1916. *Annual Report of the Department of Labor (1915).* Vol. 2, document no. 17, 3–80.

Ramazzini, B. [1713] 1964. *Diseases of Workers.* Translated from the Latin text *De Moribus Artificum* of 1713 by W. C. Wright. New York: Hafner.

Simon, J. 1887. *Public Health Reports,* vol. 2. Edited for the Sanitary Institute of Great Britain by E. Seaton. London: Offices of the Sanitary Institute, J. and A. Churchill.

Sonenscher, M. 1987. *The Hatters of Eighteenth-Century France.* Berkeley: University of California Press.

Stickler, J. W. 1886. "Hatters' Consumption." *New York Medical Journal* 43:598–602.

Taft, P. 1957. *The A.F. of L. in the Time of Gompers.* New York: Harper and Brothers.

Taylor, J. G. 1901. "Chronic Mercurial Poisoning, with Special Reference to the Dangers in Hatters' Furriers' Manufactories." *Guy's Hospital Reports* 40(3d series): 1271–1290.

Thackrah, C. T. [1832] 1985. *The Effects of Arts, Trades and Professions on Health and Longevity.* Reprint of second edition of 1832. Canton, Ohio: Science History Publications, Watson Publishing International.

Wedeen, R. P. 1989. "Were the Hatters of New Jersey 'Mad'?" *American Journal of Industrial Medicine* 16:225–233.

Weiss, H. B., and Weiss, G. M. 1961. *The Early Hatters of New Jersey.* Trenton: New Jersey Agricultural Society.

Wickes, S. 1892. *History of the Oranges in Essex County, N.J., from 1666–1806.* Newark, N.J.: Ward and Tichenor.

• CHAPTER 2 •

Dioxin at Diamond:
A Case Study in
Occupational/Environmental Exposure

ELLEN K. SILBERGELD, Ph.D.; MICHAEL GORDON, Esq.;
and LYNN D. KELLY

"Dioxin at Diamond" is an ongoing tale of toxic sprawl beyond the produc-
tion facility into the community, the Ironbound neighborhood of Newark,
New Jersey. This chemical calamity is recorded by Ellen K. Silbergeld, a
neuroscientist and spokesperson for the Environmental Defense Fund; Mi-
chael Gordon, a lawyer–politician; and Lynn D. Kelly, a paralegal assis-
tant. In early 1992, after a seven-week trial, the Ironbound community
settled for one million dollars from the Diamond Shamrock Company. The
company accepted no liability (Sullivan 1992). It did, however, accept the
contention of seventy-two former plant employees and their families, as
well as local residents, that "the company had recklessly endangered the
health of its workers and knowingly exposed residents and businesses near
its plant to the potentially harmful effects of dioxin" (Nieves 1991). Other
communities—Times Beach, Missouri, where dioxin was spread on road-
ways, necessitating the permanent evacuation of the residents in 1982 and
1983; and Seveso, Italy, where a plant emitted dioxin into the atmosphere
in the mid 1980s—share the Ironbound community's toxic exposure di-
lemma as do those exposed to dioxin in the form of Agent Orange during
the Vietnam War.

For two hundred years, factories and residential dwellings have coexisted
in the Ironbound district, so called for two popularly believed reasons—
one, that it is bordered by railroads, the other, that it is surrounded by iron
foundries. A second appellation, "Down-Neck," describes this neck of land
that follows a bend of the Passaic River as it flows east and then south

(Fidelity Union Trust Company 1953:2). Through the heart of the ethnically diverse Ironbound community runs Ferry Street, a thriving commercial center, dominated today by the Portuguese, who have settled there over the past thirty years. Begun in 1765, the Old Ferry Road was the first direct route between Newark and the Hudson River to the east, the gateway to New York City (3). This confluence of rivers, highways, and railroads formed a natural attraction for industry. "Foundries, planing mills, lumber yards and cement works lined the river bank" (9). Breweries and tanneries operated in the area, as did Sherwin–Williams Varnish Works (now Sherwin–Williams Paints) and Blanchard's Patent Leather Factory. Lister Agricultural Chemical Works, the original inhabitant of Diamond Shamrock's site on Lister Avenue, also overlooked the Passaic River. Along River Street (now Raymond Boulevard), the owners of these industries built their mansions, also facing the river (9). Workers lived in tenements interspersed among factories and commercial establishments. Hence, the stage for the disaster that struck the community in 1983 when dioxin was discovered was set from its early history as a bustling, congested industrial and residential center in which workers lived cheek by jowl with industry and its wastes.

During the 1960s, in support of the Vietnam War effort, the Diamond Shamrock Corporation manufactured Agent Orange, a chemical defoliant, for the United States government. Between 1951, when the chemical began to be made at the Newark site, and 1969, when production halted, dioxin, a byproduct, found its way into Ironbound backyards and playgrounds. Yet German manufacturers had warned the Diamond Alkali Company (predecessor of Diamond Shamrock) of the dangers of dioxin as early as 1957 and offered their help to manufacture the herbicide safely. In 1983, the Ironbound Community Corporation through its Ironbound Committee Against Toxic Wastes demanded an investigation by the New Jersey Department of Environmental Protection. For a while, local fears were intensified by media attention, but after a few years, both the community and state government shifted their attention to other environmental problems. Dioxin-contaminated soil remains stored in large shipping containers piled three deep behind barbed-wire fencing on the grounds of the defunct plant. Just a half mile away, a five-story toxic waste incinerator began operating in October 1990, accepting substances of questionable content from adjacent counties and exuding dioxin-containing combustion products into the air over Ironbound. In the future, Arnold Cohen of the Ironbound Community Corporation has pointed out, no one will be able to tell whether the Ironbound's dioxin came from the Diamond Shamrock plant or the incinerator (pers. comm. 1990). The Diamond Shamrock Corporation had also supplied chromate slag for landfill in Hudson County, New Jersey, as described in Chapter 7.

The dioxin problem in Newark poses what are becoming classic questions in cases of environmental contamination: Who can be held responsible for the contamination? Did the industry know of the toxin's effect at the time? What constitutes adequate cleanup of a contaminated industrial site? Are the standards for cleaning a residential site the same as or different from those of cleaning an industrial site? What redress do workers and community have for effects on their health, even if not clearly identifiable or evident at the time of the contamination or even years later?

In the 1970s, the New Jersey legislature enacted cleanup guidelines for contaminated sites, later adopted by the federal government in the Superfund Law. The procedures called for toxic site cleanup decisions to be made on a case-by-case basis. In 1991, New Jersey planned to address the issues raised above by drawing up a set of generic guidelines for the cleanup of two hundred toxic compounds, thereby enabling the establishment of standards for management of environmental problems (Strum 1991).

• • •

Dioxin, the toxic contaminant of Agent Orange, is an example of an occupational and an environmental health hazard. Frequently, the most intense exposure to toxic substances occurs within occupational settings where these materials are generated, used, and first released. The occupational setting may also release these same toxins into the general environment. While it is reasonable to expect that the clearest evidence of health effects associated with exposure to a toxic chemical may be found in exposed workers, the lack of evidence of adverse effects on workers cannot always be taken as an indication of the absence of risk for persons exposed—presumably to lower levels—in the general environment. The nonoccupational population includes persons of varying susceptibility—the very young and the aged, as well as those too infirm to work. Exposure may be continuous and occur at work as well as in the general environment away from work. Adverse effects not evident in the workforce may therefore be apparent in the general population if careful epidemiologic studies are performed over extended periods of time.

The alleged lack of clear health effects in workers has been cited as a reason for lack of concern regarding human health effects of the dioxins, particularly 2,3,7,8-tetrachlorodibenzo-p-dioxin (referred to here as TCDD) (Suskind and Herzberg 1984; Cook et al. 1986; Johnson 1990; Kimbrough 1990). To judge the safety of environmental exposure according to occupational studies that show no toxic effect, the workplace research must, at the very least, be scientifically sound. Negative studies must, therefore, demonstrate the following characteristics: (1) sufficient statistical power to exclude the possibility that lack of observed effect is erroneous; (2) accurate exposure assessment and no systematic bias; and (3) sufficient time for the expression of disease, particularly those of long latency, to occur. As noted by Monson (1986), problems with respect to any of these three criteria will result in a failure to find an association between the exposure and adverse health effects. Such studies are fundamentally flawed. Serious risk may be incurred by the general population from low-level environmental exposure despite negative findings in invalid studies.

The story of dioxin exposure at the Diamond Alkali (later Diamond Shamrock) facility in Newark, New Jersey, exemplifies many of the problems of using experience from occupational exposure for inferring more general human risks. For dioxin, the absence of occupational disease does not provide reliable evidence of the absence of environmental hazard. This chapter discusses the history of operations at Diamond Shamrock and then reviews the available medical data on the workforce at the facility. The second part of the chapter integrates this site-specific experience with larger issues related to the toxicology of dioxin and continuing controversies related to understanding its risks to human health. We use the term "dioxin" to refer to any halogenated dibenzo-p-dioxin and "TCDD" to refer only to 2,3,7,8-TCDD.

The heated debate about the human health effects from exposure to TCDD is an example of the difficulty of assuring the accuracy of studies of occupational cohorts. A large literature on occupational exposure to TCDD exists (Hardell and Sandstrom 1979; Hoar Zahm et al. 1986; Fingerhut et al. 1991), but we have selected Diamond because it exemplifies many of the social and methodological problems associated with understanding the history of occupational exposures and their associations with illness.

As of 1993, the story of Diamond Shamrock is incomplete. Considerable controversy continues to surround the history and present management of the facility, the consequences of past exposure for the workers, and the extent of contamination and its consequences for the nearby Ironbound community. Thus, this chapter is a commentary on a story in progress.

History of Diamond Shamrock

In 1951, Diamond Alkali purchased an existing agricultural chemical facility from Kolker Chemical Works, Inc., at 80 Lister Avenue in Newark (Figure 2.1 and 2.2). Over the next eighteen years, until the plant closed in 1969, Diamond manufactured a number of chemicals, including hexachlorobenzene and trichlorophenol, and the herbicides 2,4,5-trichlorophenoxyacetic acid (2,4,5-T) and 2,4-dichlorophenoxyacetic acid (2,4-D). A mixture of these herbicides, formulated by Diamond at this plant, was purchased by the Department of Defense as a defoliant for use in the Vietnam War. The defoliant was known as Agent Orange because of an orange stripe on the canister in which it was packaged. Production at this plant varied considerably between 1960 and 1970 (Table 2.1) (McBurney 1977), but by the end of the 1960s, the plant was one of the largest production facilities for these chemicals in the United States, with over sixteen million pounds of 2,4,5-trichlorophenol produced between 1952 and 1968 (Table 2.2).

The basic process used by Diamond Alkali to make 2,4,5-tricholorophenol (2,4,5-TCP), the precursor to 2,4,5-T, is important because it always yields the contaminant TCDD. The amount of TCDD generated depends upon the conditions and control of the process. In this process, 1,2,4,5-tetrachlorobenzene is reacted with sodium hydroxide to form the sodium salt 2,4,5-trichlorophenol. Sodium trichlorophenate is then reacted with sulfuric acid to yield 2,4,5-trichlorophenoxyacetic acid and, subsequently, either an ester or amine salt.

Dioxin, or TCDD, is a chemical byproduct of this reaction. The greater the temperature of the reaction, the greater the amount of dioxin formed. By the 1950s, industry chemists were aware that the temperature of the reaction vessel had to be kept below 155°C to reduce the formation of what were by then recognized as toxic byproducts (U.S. Environmental Protection Agency 1980; Schuck 1986).

Documents from the company's files indicate that Diamond was informed in 1957 by C. H. Boehringer Sohn, a German chemical

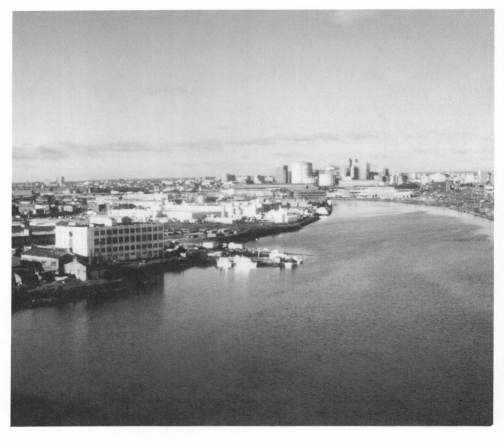

Figure 2.1. The Passaic River. The Ironbound district of Newark is in the foreground. The business district of Newark is in the distance. Photo by Lynn Butler. November 1990.

company, that dioxin was affecting the health of Boehringer's workers. Diamond was also told that dioxin was not formed in detectable amounts as long as the temperature in the trichlorophenol autoclave was not allowed to exceed 155°C and as long as the temperature of the dried trichlorophene caustic crude mixture was not allowed to exceed 120°C. Despite this knowledge, temperatures of the reaction at the Newark plant were reported to have fluctuated widely. After 1954, the reaction temperature ranges

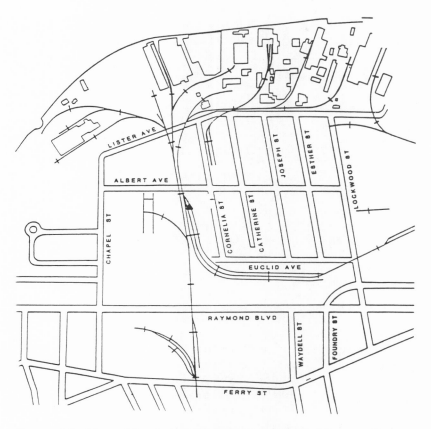

FIGURE 2.2   Map of Ironbound District, Newark, New Jersey. The Diamond Shamrock facility was located at 80 Lister Avenue. Source: New Jersey Department of Environmental Protection.

were often as high as 180°C (Burton 1960; Perkinsetal 1962). Despite Diamond's knowledge of dioxin's dangers to workers, dioxin was formed in every batch of trichlorophenol made at the Lister Avenue plant until it closed in 1969.

Fumes, ventilation, and drainage problems were frequently remarked upon by workers and the Newark plant manager. Air emissions were not controlled before 1963, at which time a caustic scrubber was installed to handle vent emissions. Waste management was relatively primitive. Wastewater discharges flowed into

TABLE 2.1.
Production, Exports, and Domestic Use (Including Agent Orange)
of 2,4-D and 2,4,5-T (Acid Basis) in the United States, 1960–70

	Production (lbs.)		Exports	Domestic use[a]	
Year	2,4-D	2,4,5-T	2,4,5-T	2,4-D	2,4,5-T
1960	36,185	6,337	8,796	31,131	5,859
1961	43,392	6,909	9,085	31,067	5,444
1962	42,997	8,369	10,192	35,903	8,102
1963	46,312	9,090	14,657	33,199	7,179
1964	53,714	11,434	13,037	43,986	8,912
1965	63,320	11,601	6,924	50,535	7,244
1966	68,182	15,489	5,419	63,903	17,080
1967	77,139	14,552	4,410	66,955	15,381
1968	79,263	17,530	3,391	68,404	15,804
1969	47,077	4,999	7,287	49,526	3,218
1970	43,576	———[b]	9,571	46,942	4,871

SOURCE: Kearney 1983.
[a]Includes military shipments abroad.
[b]Separate figure not available.

municipal sewers without pretreatment and spilled freely into the adjacent Passaic River. Several acid spills were reported in the 1950s, and their volume was estimated to be up to thirty thousand gallons per day in 1960 (Worthington 1983). Before 1954, no attempt was made to recover waste materials; after 1956, some recycling of organics was achieved. Solid wastes were hauled off-site to a nearby facility with no specific controls for hazardous waste; these are now known to have been heavily contaminated with dioxins. In 1967, these wastes totaled 8 tons; in 1969, they totaled 3.5 tons (Worthington 1983).

On February 20, 1960, a runaway reaction in the trichlorophenol autoclave caused it to explode, killing one worker, injuring a number of other employees, and destroying the building in which the autoclave was located. The explosion occurred when excessive pressure developed in the autoclave. The temperature recorder went off the scale at 200°C (Everett 1960). Apparently, this was not the first instance of a process accident involving blowing the rupture disk, a safety device on the autoclave, at Diamond's Newark plant, although it may have been the first explosion. Each of these inci-

TABLE 2.2
Production of Trichlorophenol at Diamond, 1952–68

1952	342,132 lbs.	1961[a]	1,206,222 lbs.
1953[a]	305,868	1962	1,301,754
1954	244,704	1963	1,472,813
1955	526,488	1964	1,343,877
1956	508,032	1965	685,427
1957	747,612	1966	678,674
1958	762,492	1967[a]	1,456,692
1959	912,840	1968	2,864,487
1960[b]	564,972		

SOURCE: Worthington 1983.
[a]Production capacity changes.
[b]Explosion, TCP works rebuilt February–March.

dents very likely released toxic substances, including TCDD, from the autoclave into the workplace. That the trichlorophenol process was liable to such incidents was well known: prior explosions had occurred at Monsanto's Nitro plant in West Virginia in 1949; at BASF's Ludwigshafen, Germany, plant in 1953; and at a Rhone–Poulenc facility in Grenoble, France, in 1956. The explosions and their consequences at BASF and Rhone–Poulenc were reported to the chemical industry by BASF and in the medical literature by Rhone–Poulenc (Hay 1982).

After the Newark explosion in 1960, the trichlorophenol works were shut down, only to reopen in 1961. The main process building was replaced with a new facility solely for the manufacture of trichlorophenol and derivative products, including 2,4-D, the other component of Agent Orange. The production facilities were expanded in 1967 to meet the demands of increasing defoliant usage by the Department of Defense in Vietnam (Kearney 1983). Diamond continued operations at dangerously high temperatures during this period, despite information from industry sources concerning the advisability of running the trichlorophenol reaction at lower temperatures to reduce formation of dioxins.

In 1969, manufacture of trichlorophenol and related herbicides ceased at Diamond Shamrock. At the same time, the United States reduced its heavy defoliation tactics in Vietnam in response to international scientific concerns about the ecological and health effects of these chemical agents (Hay 1982). Diamond Shamrock Company operations formally ceased at the facility, although manufacture of 2,4-D continued. In 1971, the original property was sold and leased to Chemicaland Corporation.

About ten years later, the second act of the story of dioxin at Diamond Shamrock began. In 1980, the U.S. Environmental Protection Agency published its first general statement on the sources and potential extent of environmental contamination with dioxins from trichlorophenol manufacture (USEPA 1980). In that document, the EPA mapped sites of trichlorophenol manufacture in the United States and raised the concern that these might be areas of significant off-site and on-site contamination by dioxins. The New Jersey Department of Environmental Protection (NJDEP) responded to this document as well as to the growing national controversy at Love Canal in New York (where dioxins and many other toxic chemicals had been dumped by Hooker Chemical Company). As noted by NJDEP, "Due to the large quantities of Agent Orange produced there over a short period of time," the Diamond Shamrock facility at Lister Avenue was the prime candidate in the state for on- and off-site contamination by dioxins (NJDEP 1984). In 1982, the state closed the Passaic River for fishing for eels and striped bass, with advisories issued for white perch and white catfish.

The Ironbound District

In 1983, the NJDEP and the EPA undertook a sampling and environmental monitoring program on the Diamond Shamrock site. The tests showed a zone of massive dioxin contamination at the plant site and in much of the surrounding neighborhood, the Ironbound District of Newark.

Although the Ironbound District contains a number of factories and industries, it is also a residential neighborhood, home to generations of immigrants that today include a large Portuguese population. Ironbound had a significant role in Newark's industrial growth, especially in the nineteenth century. A study of economic and social conditions in Ironbound was undertaken by a community organization, the Neighborhood House, shortly after 1900 (Roney 1912). Community workers were outraged by the impoverishment they found. Joseph Roney agreed with their findings, although he identified the roots of the problems as cultural rather than economic. Roney rejected the notion that the social conditions brought on by industrialization were the fundamental cause of the poor living conditions of the working-class Ironbound District. He feared the adverse publicity that social reformers gave to the condition of industrial workers would drive manufacturers away from Ironbound. Roney provides us with the community organizers' description of living conditions in Ironbound at the turn of the century, which still holds true today:

> The air is pregnant with dangerous acid fumes, smoke, and "unforgettable odors," of the manufacturers of the district, of the lowly looking tenements, of the dilapidated looking homes, of the saloons, the dance halls, the clubs and the pool rooms and the moving picture theaters. (15)

While acknowledging the pollution in the neighborhood, Roney finds it an acceptable price to pay for jobs. In support of the manufacturers, he noted:

> From the high chimneys of the manufacturing industries in the district come smoke and fumes that offend the olfactory organs, it is true. Must industrial establishments emit the sweet and fragrant odors of gardenias and forget-me-nots? The proprietors of these establishments have been experimenting at no little expense yearly to safeguard the health and the lives of the workmen they employ. To compare the present-day installation and methods of operating machinery with that of former years justifies this statement. The people of the district themselves rarely complain of the fumes, because they understand that these establishments furnish them a living. Only those whose faces, hands and clothing are not besmutted—through the chances of fortune or social survey work—with the soot and grime of a hard day's work can see nothing but death in the smoke and odors of the district. Smoke fumes and acids are inevitable accompaniments of these industries. They can, however, be reduced. (17)

Roney's presentation of this version of the American social compact—that national progress and individual economic advancement require the pollution of the environment and the sacrifice of workers' health and well-being—was voiced in the face of the first stirrings of what has grown into the occupational and environmental health movement. The story of dioxin at Diamond in the 1980s is a continuation of the struggle between reformers and the economic and political powers that contended in the pages of Roney's 1912 Newark document.

In Ironbound, NJDEP's environmental testing from 1983 onward showed that levels of dioxin on the site were as high as 51,000 parts per billion (ppb) (NJDEP 1984). Throughout the adjoining business and residential areas, levels of dioxin were in many places greater than 1,000 ppb. According to the federal Centers for Disease Control (CDC), dioxin concentrations in the soil of 1 ppb constitutes an "unacceptable risk to human health" (Kimbrough 1983).

Based on the NJDEP's finding, Governor Thomas Kean of New Jersey issued an executive order declaring a state of emergency. The Newark farmer's market, a major food distribution center one block from the Diamond Shamrock plant, was temporarily closed. In addition, orders were issued for some residents to evacuate their houses and all not to go outside during daylight hours while the cleanup operations were taking place. All train traffic in the area of the abandoned Diamond Shamrock site was stopped; further restrictions on access to the area and on fishing in the Passaic River were implemented.

At present, the Diamond Shamrock site is high on the national priority list for expedited cleanup under the federal Superfund Law. Most of the contaminated soil has reportedly been collected and contained on-site, in shipping containers stacked three deep, behind fences (Figure 2.3). Nothing further has happened. The dioxin-tainted soil is considered too toxic to be moved, and no waste facility has been found that will accept the material. One proposal is to permanently entomb the dioxin-tainted soil on-site, but this plan has not been approved.

Medical History of Diamond Shamrock

Health Effects   Investigations of occupational health at the Diamond facility go back to 1963, when the United States Public Health Service (USPHS) conducted the first of two special health surveys of the Newark workers. The first USPHS report was concluded in 1969. In 1977, the National Institute of Occupational Safety and Health (NIOSH) launched an official inquiry on the health status of workers at the facility—some ten years after peak

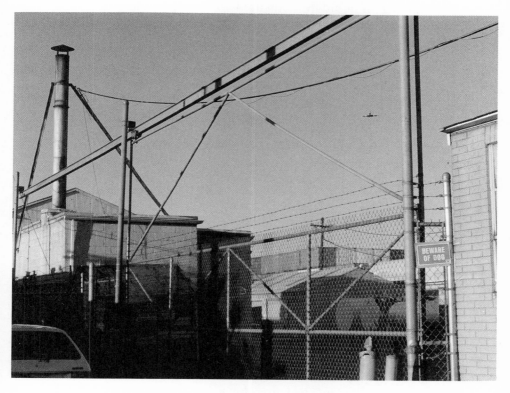

FIGURE 2.3. "Beware of Dog." Diamond Shamrock facility in the Iron-bound district of Newark, New Jersey. Stacked shipping containers storing dioxin-contaminated soil can be seen in background through gate. Photo by Richard P. Wedeen, November 1990.

production of 2,4,5-T. In the mid 1980s, part of the retired work-force was enrolled into the National Dioxin Registry under the direction of Marilyn Fingerhut at NIOSH. Thus, the occupational history of the workforce at Diamond has been unusually well documented in comparison with other industrial situations. Some of these studies have been published in the medical literature; others are still in progress. This official history is supplemented by materials revealed during litigation and investigations by state and federal officials of the site (Schuck 1986).

Corporate recognition of medical problems in the workers at Diamond Shamrock began in mid 1955, when (according to company files) Diamond experienced a "major outbreak of chloracne," a severely disfiguring acnelike condition related to relatively high levels of dioxin exposure (Silbergeld 1991b). Although the company's corporate medical director noted the potential for disease beyond the skin condition, Diamond ignored this finding, electing not to send any workers to outside medical experts at that time. Later, Diamond hired Jacob Bleiberg, a dermatologist, to treat the workers for their chloracne. Bleiberg noted the possibility of broad, adverse biologic effects in association with chloracne, and accurately diagnosed the source of the outbreak as overexposure to "chlorinated diphenyl ether," at the time a proposed molecular identity for the contaminant of 2,4,5-T production (Bleiberg et al. 1964). (A year later, doctors studying the workers at the Boehringer plant in Germany more specifically identified the causative agent as dioxin). The Boehringer group identified further adverse effects beyond chloracne, including conjunctivitis, loss of appetite, weakness in the legs, liver disorders, fatigue, and psychiatric disorders (Kimmig and Shulz 1957).

In 1963, more cases of chloracne were noted by Bleiberg and his new associate, Roger Brodkin. From 1961 on, the company had undertaken a particularly heavy production schedule to meet the increasing demand for Agent Orange (Kearney 1983; Worthington 1983). Bleiberg contacted Donald Birmingham, a dermatologist with the USPHS who had investigated a chloracne outbreak at Monsanto's Nitro plant ten years earlier. Birmingham and Marcus Key, also of the USPHS, visited the Newark plant in March 1963. They noted numerous signs of adverse effects beyond chloracne: red urine, altered skin pigmentation, and excessive hair growth. At this time, the first association between dioxin exposure and porphyria (a disorder of red-blood-cell metabolism in the liver) was made. Birmingham and Key recommended that all workers with severe chloracne, hyperpigmentation, and excessive hair growth be hospitalized for further medical evaluation (Birmingham and Key 1963:6). Once again Diamond ignored the recommendations and hospitalized only two workers rather than all those showing signs of systemic illness (Guidi 1963).

Based on the liver biopsies performed on those two workers and on urinalyses performed on others, Bleiberg and Brodkin pub-

lished an article in 1964 confirming the link between dioxin exposure and porphyria (Bleiberg et al. 1964; Silbergeld and Fowler
1989). In addition, Bleiberg and Brodkin's study noted other signs
and symptoms in the severely affected workers, including abnor-
mal skin pigmentation and hair growth, nerve damage, and conjunctivitis. Despite these findings, documents from Diamond's
files indicate that no other workers were hospitalized for further
study (Guidi 1963).

In 1965, Dow Chemical Company called Diamond and other
manufacturers of 2,4,5-T together to discuss the presence of dioxin
in their products, its toxicity, and methods to measure dioxin in the
manufactured product. Dow's goal was to disseminate its own information on techniques designed to reduce dioxin contamination and
to prevent worker exposure, as well as to propose an industrywide
standard for dioxin contamination of the final product. This strategy,
if it had been adopted, might have avoided much of the continuing
controversy. The toxic circle of recurrent disease, repeatedly ignored
warnings, and redundant documentation might have been prevented. In its survey of its own and competitors' products, Dow
found that Diamond was producing a product that contained quantities of dioxin at much greater levels than Dow was proposing for the
industry standard. During that same period, Diamond received
some reports of chloracne in customers using its chlorophenoxy-
acetic acid herbicide products, 2,4,5-T and 2,4-D. Diamond's response is unknown (Chandler 1962).

In 1969, the year trichlorophenol operations ceased at Diamond,
Alan Poland, a physician with the USPHS, was sent to the plant.
His findings on seventy-three workers showed a continuing prob-
lem of severe chloracne, liver injury, and neurological problems
(Poland et al. 1971).

Exposure   Understanding the exposure of the workforce at
Diamond in retrospect is complicated. No systematic monitoring or
industrial hygiene records are available. Moreover, with any study
where exposure occurs outside of a controlled environment, determining precise levels of exposure is difficult. Based on the information available on concentrations of dioxin in materials at the facility
during operations, however, it must be concluded that workers' exposure was high. One period of intense exposure probably took place
in connection with the 1960 explosion. Although no measurements

were taken within the facility at that time, in two comparable explosions concentrations of TCDD ranged from 10 to 25 ppm (Jirasek et al. 1974; Hay 1982). Exposure was likely to be particularly serious because of the lack of rudimentary worker protection at the plant. Not until after 1960 were adequate showering facilities and clothing changes made available to the workers. According to the workers, conditions at the plant were deplorable and safety precautions minimal (IHRAC and Brennan v. Diamond Shamrock 1989).

Some estimate of exposure can be made on the basis of analyses done of wastes, products, and environmental samples. Measurements made in 1965 at the Diamond plant revealed dioxin concentrations in unfiltered trichlorophenol solution between 25 to 40 ppm, and 73 ppm in recovered waste (Steward 1969). Some batches of 2,4,5-T acid analyzed that year had concentrations between 7 and 26 ppm TCDD. A 1968 report from the plant manager at Newark indicated that there were concentrations of dioxin of 75 ppm in the sump pit where the residues were stored (Kennedy 1968). The on-site analyses performed by the NJDEP and EPA after 1983 also indicate that considerable amounts of dioxin were generated and released within the facility during its years of operation (NJDEP 1984). Although it is difficult to construct accurate exposure profiles on this basis, there can be no doubt, based upon the reports of severe symptoms and the available analytic data, that the Diamond workforce was exposed to substantial amounts of TCDD.

This exposure information is difficult to interpret in terms of health effects. A systematic bias in exposure assessment may have entered into the studies at Diamond. The record fails to identify workers with exceptionally high exposure due to job history or work duties. As found by Fingerhut et al. (1991), the absence of detailed exposure profiles of Diamond Shamrock employees weakens the value of the clinical evidence. Another possible source of bias is loss of the most highly exposed members of the cohort to follow-up, a loss that may not be random. For example, the 1969 study by Poland was meant to be a follow-up to the study by Bleiberg and Brodkin. One worker had died in the interval, however. Since that worker's death was ignored, the completeness of Poland's study as a follow-up is limited and possibly skewed by the omission of a significant health effect of prior exposure (namely, death). Also, Poland never obtained treatment records from Bleiberg and Brodkin, even though many of the workers had been receiving treatment for their chloracne for years.

Future Health Studies at Diamond   Since 1969, no further studies have been conducted that might help evaluate the long-term consequences to Diamond's workforce of this exposure. A major report of increased cancer mortality in the National Dioxin Registry was published in 1991 (Fingerhut et al. 1991), but this study did not provide site-specific data on the Newark cohort. At this point, therefore, it is useful to consider what results could be expected from further study of this workforce. First, as noted at the beginning of this chapter, it is critical to ensure that accurate assessment of exposure is done in order to evaluate the relationship between exposure and outcome. From the information available, it seems likely that exposure assessment will remain imprecise. It may be improved with further biologic testing of residues in human tissue by NIOSH and others (Patterson et al. 1988), but the value of tissue testing diminishes with time. Second, it is important to exclude all systematic sources of bias from the study, such as nonparticipation. There are concerns that not all workers at Diamond were entered into the NIOSH registry. Third, it is important to determine that sufficient time has elapsed so that health effects with long latent periods, such as cancer, can be detected. Assuming that some workers' exposure to dioxin at Diamond commenced with operations in 1951, theoretically sufficient time—forty years—has elapsed so that a fairly definitive assessment of delayed adverse effects should be possible.

Of greatest importance in evaluating present or future epidemiologic studies at Diamond is the size of the cohort, that is, the number of workers in the group studied. From 1955 through 1969, 353 persons worked at Newark, with an apparent yearly average of about 75 (McBurney 1977). In 1969, at the time the USPHS did its first survey, 27 persons were employed in the trichlorophenol production area or in maintenance of that area. Of those 27, 10 had worked for more than fifteen years (most from 1951), while 11 had worked for five years or less (employment with Diamond, not all of that time necessarily in the trichlorophenol works). There are, therefore, only 14 workers with exposure histories such that by 1990 the time between onset of exposure and (potential) ascertainment of health status is greater than thirty years. This is a very small number of cases with which to discern any significant changes in incidence of disease or cause of death. Failure to identify adverse health effects may indicate only that the long-term exposure group is too small for useful interpretation.

A further complicating factor in this and many other cohort studies of trichlorophenol facilities is determination of an appropriate control group. The basic requirement for a control group is that the controls have no excess exposure to the toxin under study. This criterion cannot be met by fellow workers or individuals who reside in a contaminated community. Exposed controls make it impossible to discern toxic effects in the exposed group. Raymond Suskind and co-workers studying the Monsanto Nitro workforce have used other workers as controls, or even workers without recorded chloracne as controls for workers with chloracne, to investigate the long-term outcome of dioxin exposure (Suskind and Herzberg 1984). But chloracne is a sign of high-dose dioxin exposure; its absence cannot be construed to indicate lack of toxicologically significant exposure (Moses and Prioleau 1985; Silbergeld 1991b). The dangers inherent in this approach were revealed by another study of the Nitro workforce that showed a poor correlation between work history and chloracne as an indicator of exposure (Moses et al. 1984). Until more is known about the correlation between dose and chloracne, it is not wise to use this outcome as more than a crude index of exposure (Moses and Prioleau 1985). In contrast, Theiss et al. (1987), studying BASF workers, used the local population as controls and compared national death statistics with mortality patterns in the exposed group; in this study an excess of stomach cancer was reported in the exposed workers (Theiss et al. 1983; Rohleder 1989). Given the reports of general contamination of the site and the surrounding Ironbound neighborhood near Diamond, it is difficult to justify using any subset of the Diamond workforce or of the nearby population as controls. Since both groups were heavily exposed to dioxin, the failure to find increased numbers of cancers in the exposed group may reflect the high incidence of dioxin-induced cancer in inappropriate controls.

Dioxin at Diamond: The Larger Context

The risks of dioxin—in the workforce and in the general environment—remain hotly debated. The use of 2,4,5-T as a herbicide in the United States has been suspended by the EPA, and 2,4-D is under heightened scrutiny following several registry studies demonstrating increased risks of lymphoma in agricultural workers (Hoar Zahm et al. 1986; Silbergeld 1991a). Cleanup of former manufacturing facilities, such as Diamond, is now mandated under the federal Superfund Program, although the method of cleanup and eventual disposal of contaminated materials remains in dispute.

To a large extent, the uncontrolled chemical production that existed at Diamond for nearly twenty years has been phased out at major chemical companies in the United States. While these facilities are no longer major sources of dioxins, dioxins are still formed and released into the environment by such processes as paper pulp production, municipal solid waste incineration, and other chemical production processes (Silbergeld and Gasiewicz 1989). A municipal solid waste incinerator was built in the Ironbound District in 1991—despite community opposition—within a half mile of the 80 Lister Avenue site (Figure 2.4).

The ultimate effect of past and future releases of dioxin on local residents, although not yet known, is understandably of tremendous concern. It appears that, once again, because of their political powerlessness in the face of government and scientific expertise, Ironbound residents have lost their battle to control the quality of their environment. In a few years, it will be impossible to differentiate between dioxin from Diamond and dioxin from the solid waste incinerator in the Ironbound environment.

The history of dioxin contamination in Newark raises other troubling issues. The secrecy surrounding conditions at Diamond and other trichlorophenol facilities during the manufacture of material for the Department of Defense has made it difficult to determine the process of decision making and information gathering by companies and by the government, particularly during the 1960s (McCulloh 1984; Schuck 1986). More information on workplace conditions, levels of dioxin in the chemical building blocks, products and wastes, and exposure episodes, including medical records, may exist than has been made available to date. Whether these data will ever become part of the public record is unclear.

The events surrounding dioxin production at the Diamond plant exemplify the problems inherent in determining who knew what and when. Documentation gathered in the Agent Orange litigation (in which Diamond Shamrock was a defendant) and litigation involving workers at Diamond demonstrate that officials at Diamond,

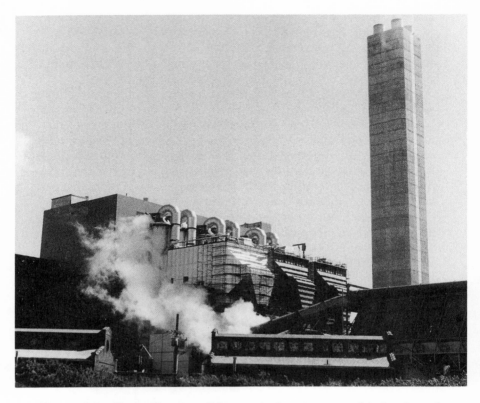

FIGURE 2.4.   Essex County solid waste incinerator opened in Ironbound district of Newark, 1990. Emissions include dioxin. Photo by Lynn Butler, November 1990.

along with those at other chemical companies, knew a substantial amount concerning the origin of persistent medical problems associated with trichlorophenol manufacture (Guidi 1963; Hay 1982). Within the industry, this knowledge arguably goes back to the 1950s. Persons involved in the internal investigations at Monsanto and BASF following their accidents in 1949 and 1953, respectively, showed considerable acumen in analyzing the sources and consequences of exposure to a potent toxic agent generated in trichlorophenol production. This knowledge was freely shared, first by BASF to Dow and then by Dow with the rest of the American industry in the mid 1960s. In March 1965, Kennedy and Cort from Diamond met with V. K. Rowe of Dow to discuss Dow's information on the etiology of chloracne. German chemists had identified the cause as 2,3,7,8-TCDD in 1957 (Kimmig and Schulz 1957). Diamond's files indicate that their own chemist had already suggested this identification in 1960 (Chandler 1965).

The occurrence of chloracne and other severe symptoms in workers in the synthetic organic chemical industry followed soon after the successful production of chlorinated napthalenes, benzenes, and phenols in the 1890s (Hay 1982; Silbergeld 1991b). The likelihood that these effects were due not to the identified precursor chemicals or products but rather to some contaminant or unintended byproduct was first raised by Thelwell Jones in 1941. This possibility was confirmed by further observations and studies of various products and waste fraction produced. Experimental research on the toxicity of these agents was begun in the 1930s. These studies demonstrated that they were systemic toxicants with a high degree of potency. Tetratogenicity has been clearly demonstrated in experimental animals (Couture-Haws et al. 1991). Oettel of BASF undertook some observational toxicology studies in the aftermath of the BASF explosion in 1953. He reported that rabbits placed in the vicinity of the exploded autoclave showed severe toxic reactions, including death. Ten years later, Philips Duphar scientists conducted a similar experiment by placing rats inside a building where a similar explosion had occurred. Many of the animals died, and others showed thymic atrophy and other signs of systemic intoxication (Hay 1982).

Tragically, while industry shared this information within its own circle, industry medical and toxicological staff withheld such knowledge from those most at risk, the workers. Although documents from Diamond's files show that the company knew in the late 1950s that dioxin exposure causes systemic damage and that reducing the temperature of the reaction would eliminate the creation of TCDD, some of the workers maintain that neither the company nor its doctors disclosed this information to the workers (IHRAC and Brennan v. Diamond Shamrock 1989; York 1955; Porter 1957; Holder 1959).

What we do know is that by the mid 1960s, at the latest, substantial information was available on the presence of dioxin in TCP manufacture and on the effect of this compound on workers. Industry has since argued that beyond chloracne, no serious health effects have been conclusively shown in humans exposed to TCDD.

Yet enough was known to convince certain firms to take rather extraordinary steps to reduce dioxin formation and to prevent human contact with dioxins. In some instances, companies, such as BASF, terminated TCP operations. BASF resumed these operations only after completely rebuilding its plant and altering the manufacturing process to eliminate the formation of dioxin. In other companies, such as Dow, procedures were instituted to control dioxin formation. Unfortunately, there was not a uniform response in the industry. Diamond never took these steps.

A second issue related to the larger picture of dioxins in industry is the fact that dioxins were never an intended product of chemical production. Did this make it easier or more difficult to deal with the problems they caused? In one sense, the fact that dioxins are unintended byproducts could have made resolution of the problem easier, since the commercial product was not in jeopardy. The first response to its presence in the product should have been to institute policies to reduce concentrations of dioxin in trichlorophenol and 2,4,5-T. In fact, Dow's stated policy was to keep contamination of trichlorophenol and 2,4,5-T below 1 ppm, since in this way the product could be made less toxic (Chandler 1965). In another sense, however, the fact that the dioxin problem was inadvertent complicated its resolution. The risks were transferred from the product to the waste stream. An acceptable product was produced without consideration of the continued problem of worker exposure from toxic effluents and the unresolved matter of eventual disposal. Diamond attempted recycling, even though BASF had already advised Diamond management that recycling of basic chemicals used to make Agent Orange aggravated the dioxin problem. Other measures that Diamond took, such as carbon cleanup, instituted after 1967, only transferred dioxin from trichlorophenol and 2,4,5-T to waste streams. While concentrations of dioxin in 2,4,5-T were probably reduced by this approach, thus perhaps reducing the exposure of the general population, it did not reduce exposure of the workforce or the community surrounding the Diamond facility or sites where its wastes were disposed. Similar environmental contamination for waste products occurred in Missouri and the Netherlands (Hay 1982; Kimbrough 1983). By the 1980s, industry and government attempted to catch up with the damage caused by unmanaged industrial waste disposal practices; dioxin contamination of industrial wastes represents the extreme of hazard and controversy in this painful game of catch-up.

The saga of Diamond clearly demonstrates the indivisibility of occupational and environmental health risks. The nature of the dioxin episodes at Diamond—both the occupational and the community exposure—exemplify many of the challenges to the study of health effects of toxic chemicals. As is frequently the case, the population available for study, the exposed workers, is very small—too small for useful statistical analyses (Phillips and Silbergeld 1985). Exposure undoubtedly varied among this small group, and retrospective assessment of that exposure is difficult, even with the biologic marker of lipid TCDD concentrations (Patterson et al. 1988). The legal and political controversies related to dioxin that have emerged since 1983 in Newark, and in other parts of the United States, do not make the task of the scientist easier (Finkel 1989). Understandably, people are reluctant to participate in studies conducted by agencies that they perceive have failed to protect them in the past, such as the USPHS, which came many times to visit Diamond Shamrock in Newark without effecting any substantial change in corporate behavior. Recent revelations challenging the integrity of many dioxin studies further erode the confidence of the affected population (Hardell and Eriksson 1991).

Corporate failure to address the problems of dioxin at Diamond and elsewhere has resulted in tragedy. Despite serial outbreaks of chloracne, repeated findings of systemic health effects, and specific knowledge of the chemical properties of dioxin, Diamond did not take the steps necessary to prevent further exposure, disease, and death. The full extent of unprevented disease and death remains to be determined. The greatest tragedy is that for the workers and community in the Ironbound, this final determination will not be aided by their experience, nor are they likely to benefit from the eventual consensus regarding the toxicity of dioxins to human health.

Update, 1993: Diamond's dioxin wastes in Newark Bay again made news when the EPA gave the Port Authority of New York and New Jersey permission to dredge its container-ship berths and have dioxin-contaminated sludge moved to the "Mud Dump" off Sandy Hook, lucrative East Coast fishing grounds. At stake were jobs of longshoremen and fishermen, a $20 billion-dollar waterfront industry, and a $100 million-dollar fishing industry (Johnson and Frank 1993; Strum 1993).

References

Birmingham, D. J., and Key, M. M. 1963, March 28. "Dermatoses Investigation." report to New Jersey State Department of Health. Occupational Health and Research Training Facility, Public Health Service, Cincinnati, Ohio.

Bleiberg, J.; Wallen, M.; Brodkin, R.; and Applebaum, I. 1964. "Industrially Acquired Porphyria." *Archives of Dermatology.* 84:793–797.

Burton, John (manager of Newark plant). 1960. Letter to Messrs. Conrad and Dole, CELA-GMBh, Ingelheim am Rhine, West Germanyy, 23 June.

Chandler, E. L. 1962. Diamond Alkali Company interoffice correspondence to R. A. Guidi regarding chloracne, July 9.

———. 1965. Report on Dow meeting on chloracne, Diamond Alkali Company interoffice correspondence to J. Cort, Jr., March 25.

Cohen, A. 1990. Personal communication.

Cook, R. R.; Bond, G.; Olson, R. A.; and Gonder, M. R. 1986. "Evaluation of the Mortality Experience of Workers Exposed to the Chlorinated Dioxins." *Chemosphere* 15:1969–1976.

Couture-Haws, L.; Harris, M. W.; Lockhart, A. C.; and Birnbaum, L. S. 1991. "Evaluation of the Persistence of Hydronephrosis Induced in Mice Following *in Utero* and/or Lactational Exposure to 2,3,7,8-Tetrachlorodibenzo-p-dioxin." *Toxicology and Applied Pharmacology* 107:402–412.

Everett, L. S. 1960. Report to Aetna Casualty and Surety Company, April 22.

Fidelity Union Trust Company. 1953. "Ironbound City." Newark, N.J.

Fingerhut, M. E.; Halprin, W. E.; Marlow, D. A.; Placetelli, L.; Honchar, P.; Sweeney, M., Greibe, A.; Dill, P.; Steenland, K.; and Suruda, A. J. 1991. "Cancer Mortality in Workers Exposed to 2,3,7,8-TCDD." *New England Journal of Medicine* 324:212–218.

Finkel, A. 1988. "Dioxin: Are We Safer Than Before?" *Risk Analysis* 8: 161–165.

Guidi, R. A. 1963. Diamond Alkali Company interoffice correspondence to R. W. McBurney, April 30.

Hardell, L., and Eriksson, M. 1991. "The Association Between Cancer Mortality and Dioxin Exposure: A Comment on the Hazard of Repetition of Epidemiological Misinterpretation." *American Journal of Industrial Medicine* 19:547–549.

Hardell, L., and Sandstrom, A. 1979. "Case Control Study: Soft Tissue Sarcomas and Exposure to Phenoxyacetic Acids or Chlorophenols." *British Journal of Cancer* 43:169–174.

Hay, A. 1982. *The Chemical Scythe.* New York: Plenum.

Hoar Zahm, S. K.; Blair, A.; Holmes, F. F.; Boysen, C. D.; Robel, R. J.; Hoover, R.; and Fraumeni, J. F. 1986. "Agricultural Herbicide Use and Risk of Lymphoma and Soft Tissue Sarcoma." *Journal of the American Medical Association* 256:1141–1147.

Holder, T. F. 1959. Diamond Alkali Company interoffice correspondence to J. Burton regarding Boehringer Company's experience with Chloracne, September 30.

IHRAC and Brennan v. Diamond Shamrock. 1989. Deposition testimony, Superior Court of New Jersey, Essex County.

Jirasek, L.; Kalensky, J.; Kubeck, K.; Pazderova, J.; and Lukas, E. 1974. "Acne Chlorina, Porphyria, Cutanea Tarda and Other Manifestations of General Intoxication During the Manufacture of Herbicides." *Ceskoslovenska Dermatologie* 49:276–283.

Johnson, E. 1990. "Association Between Soft Tissue Sarcomas, Malignant Lymphoma, and Phenoxy Herbicides/Chlorophenols: Evidence from Occupational Cohort Studies." *Fundamental and Applied Toxicology* 14: 219–234.

Johnson, T., and Frank, A. 1993. "EPA Edict Removes Barrier to Port Dredging." *Newark Star-Ledger,* March 31, 1 and 15.

Kearney, P. C. 1983. "Problems in Agriculture with TCDD." In *Accidental Exposure to Dioxins,* ed. F. Coulston and F. Pocchiari, 233–242. New York: Academic Press.

Kennedy, F. R. Diamond 1968. Letter to R. A. Guidi, Diamond Cleveland, February 26.

Kimbrough, R. D., ed. 1983. *Halogenated Biphenyls, Terphenyls, Naphthalenes, Dibenzodioxins, and Related Compounds.* Amsterdam: Elseview.

———. 1990. "How Toxic Is TCDD to Humans?" *Journal of Toxicology and Environmental Health* 30:261–271.

Kimmig, J., and Schulz, K. H. 1957. "Berufliche Akne (sog. Chlorakne) durch chlorierte aromatische zyklische Aether." *Dermatologica* 115: 540–546.

McBurney, R. W. 1977. Corporate Medical Director, Diamond Shamrock. Letter to John Finklea, M.D., Director, NIOSH, May 11.

McCulloh, J. 1984. *The Politics of Agent Orange.* Victoria, Australia: Heinemann Australia.

Monson, R. 1986. *Occupational Epidemiology.* Boca Raton, Fla: CRC Press.

Moses, M., and Prioleau, P. G. 1985. "Cutaneous Histologic Findings in Chemical Workers With and Without Chloracne with Past Exposure to 2,3,7,8-TCDD. *Journal of the American Academy of Dermatology* 12:497–506.

Moses, M.; Lilis, R.; Crow, K. D.; and Selikoff, I. 1984. "Health Status of Workers with Past Exposure to TCDD in the Manufacture of 2,4,5-T." *American Journal of Industrial Medicine* 5:161–182.

Nieves, E. 1991. "Dioxin and Former Maker Go on Trial." *New York Times,* December 3, sec. B.

New Jersey. Department of Environmental Protection. 1984. Dioxin investigation, Newark, N.J.

Patterson, D. G., Needham, L. L.; Pirkle, J. L.; Roberts, D.; Bagby, J.; Garrett, W.; Andrews J.; Folk, H.; Bernert, J.; Sampson, E.; and Houk, V. 1988. "Correlations Between Serum and Adipose Tissue Levels of TCDD in 50 Persons from Missouri." *Archives of Environmental Contamination and Toxicology* 17:139–143.

Perkins, Jewel H. Jr.; Borrar, Jack A.; and Guidi, Raymond. 1962. Patent application, U.S. service no. 196,507 invention, 21 May.

Phillips, A., and Silbergeld, E. K. 1985. "Health Effects Studies of Exposure from Hazardous Waste Sites: Where Are We Today?" *American Journal of Industrial Medicine* 8:1–7.

80   E. K. SILBERGELD, M. GORDON, L. D. KELLY

Poland, A. P.; Smith, D.; Metter, G.; and Possicle, P. 1971. "A Health Survey of Workers in a 2,4-D and 2,4,5-T Plant with Special Attention to Chloracne, Porphyria Cutanea Tarda, and Psychologic Parameters." *Archives of Environmental Health* 22:316–327.

Porter, D. J. 1957. Diamond Alkali Company interoffice correspondence to J. Burton regarding chloracne, September 18.

Rohleder, F. 1989. "A Reanalysis of an Occupational Cohort Exposed to 2,3,7,8-TCDD." Paper presented at the Seventh International Symposium on Chlorinated Dibenzodioxins and Related Compounds.

Roney, J. A. 1912. *Uplifting "Down-Neck,"* 2d ed. n.p.

Schuck, P. H. 1986. *Agent Orange on Trial.* Cambridge, Mass.: Belknap Press.

Silbergeld, E. K. 1991a. "Carcinogenicity of Dioxins." *Journal of the National Cancer Institute* 83:1198–1199.

———. 1991b. "Dioxin: Case Study of Chloracne." In *Dermatotoxicology,* 4th ed., ed. H. Maibach and F. Marzulli, 667–686. New York: Hemisphere.

Silbergeld, E. K., and Fowler, B. A., eds. 1989. "Mechanisms of Chemical Induced Porphyrinopathies." *Annals of the New York Academy of Sciences* 514.

Silbergeld, E. K., and Gasiewicz, T. A. 1989. "Dioxins and the Ah Receptor." *American Journal of Industrial Medicine* 16:455–474.

Steward, F. G. 1969. Diamond Newark. Letter to F. R. Kennedy, Diamond Cleveland, December 23.

Strum, C. 1991. "New Jersey Moves to Standardize the Cleanup of Toxic Waste." *New York Times,* December 8, sec. B.

———. 1993. "From Port to 17 Fathoms, Views on Dredging Differ." *New York Times,* January 30, sec. B.

Sullivan, J. 1992. "Company Settles Lawsuit over Exposure to Dioxin: Diamond Shamrock Will Pay $1 Million." *New York Times,* January 25, sec. B.

Suskind, R. R., and Herzberg, V. S. 1984. "Human Health Effects of 2,4,5-T and Its Toxic Contaminants." *Journal of the American Medical Association* 251:2372–2380.

Theiss, A.; Frentzel-Beyme, R.; and Link, P. 1983. "Mortality Study of Persons Exposed to Dioxin in a Trichlorophenol Process Accident." *American Journal of Industrial Medicine* 3:179–189.

Thelwell Jones, A. 1941. "The Etiology of Acne with Special Reference to Acne of Occupational Origin." *Journal of Industrial Hygiene and Toxicology* 23:290–312.

U.S. Environmental Protection Agency. 1980. *Dioxins.* EPA 600/2-80-197. Cincinnati, Ohio: EPA.

Worthington, J. B. 1983. Director, Environmental Affairs, Diamond Shamrock. Letter to Michael Catania, New Jersey Department of Environmental Protection, June 10.

York, J. M. 1955. Diamond Alkali interoffice correspondence to L. P. Scoville regarding chlorinated products at Newark, June 29.

• CHAPTER 3 •

Colorfast Cancer:
The Legacy of Corporate Malfeasance
in the U.S. Dye Industry

DAVID MICHAELS, Ph.D., M.P.H.

Bladder cancer arising from occupational exposure to "aniline dyes" (aromatic amines) at the Chambers Works in Deepwater, New Jersey, is one of two chemical catastrophes recorded in this book that originated at E. I. duPont de Nemours & Company located under the Deleware Memorial Bridge. Fatalities at the Chambers Works from tetraethyl lead are described in Chapter 6. Aromatic amines were also produced by the Allied Chemical Company, which plays a role in the dioxin (Chapter 2) and chromium (Chapter 7) episodes as well.

The epidemic of occupational bladder cancers that began in New Jersey has recurred in dye-manufacturing plants throughout the nation. The long latency between exposure and appearance of symptoms from bladder cancer, coupled with the relative infrequency of the tumor, enabled management to deny knowledge of causation and was used to justify indecision. Worker protection was deferred pending "conclusive proof." But the decision of when proof is sufficient to warrant preventive action is not a matter for science. Once the scientific data is in hand, what policies to formulate in view of the findings is fundamentally political. Prior to the creation of the U.S. Occupational Safety and Health Administration (OSHA), occupational exposure levels were set by corporate managers, often with advice from the American Conference of Government Industrial Hygienists (ACGIH), a nongovernment group of self-proclaimed experts, that came progressively under corporate control. Workplace safety was thus determined largely from inadequate studies and unpublished data held by the corporations. Not surprisingly, the corporate managers and scientists hired by Du Pont consistently found the evidence of causation of bladder cancers by aromatic amines to be inconclusive.

An earlier version of this chapter, "Waiting for the Body Count: Corporate Decision Making and Bladder Cancer in the U.S. Dye Industry," appeared in *Medical Anthropology Quarterly* 2:3 (NS) (Sept. 1988): 215–232.

*The asbestos tragedy has been repeated with aromatic amines. An impor-
tant difference is that in contrast to asbestosis and mesotheliomas, restitu-
tion for the work-induced bladder cancers could be obtained only through
workers' compensation. Toxic tort litigation was not feasible because no
"third-party" supplier could be identified who was not protected by workers' compensation laws. While requiring the company to pay medical bills,
workers' compensation laws preclude broader liability claims against the
primary employer on the part of the worker. Johns–Manville was forced
into bankruptcy not by its employees but by workers to whom it supplied
asbestos and who were employed by other corporations. Workers' compensation laws protect the company from liability from its own employees only.
Further protection for the company is provided by the statute of limitations, which requires that compensation claims be filed within two years of
injury. For the chronic diseases that appear decades after toxic exposure,
the statute of limitations makes it economic good sense for the company to
delay recognition of the problem.*

*The classic question, Who knew what, and when? is moot in compensa-
tion court. Financial settlements are meager, covering medical care only.
Neither the insurance carriers nor Du Pont had much impetus to establish
safe manufacturing procedures. Bladder cancers continue to appear among
Du Pont employees exposed decades ago, and the medical community continues to be surprised at the appearance of tumor clusters throughout the world
one hundred years after the carcinogenicity of these chemicals was first
described. Manufacturing of aromatic amines has been transferred to developing nations, with predictable scandals due in the twenty-first century.*

● ● ●

In February 1988, the Oil, Chemical and Atomic Workers Union,
representing workers at a Goodyear Tire and Rubber Company
plant in Buffalo, New York, requested that the National Institute for
Occupational Safety and Health (NIOSH) investigate what they believed to be an outbreak of bladder cancer among their members.
Since 1957, Goodyear had been using a chemical known as orthotoluidine, a suspected bladder carcinogen, in the production of
Wingstay, an antioxidant. Union officers, with the assistance of Ste-
ven Markowitz of the Mount Sinai School of Medicine, had counted
eight cases of bladder cancer between 1973 and 1988 among workers
exposed to orthotoluidine. They feared additional cases would be
discovered once a more comprehensive search was made.

Using data from the union, the company, and the New York State

Cancer Registry, NIOSH epidemiologists were able to determine that 13 Goodyear workers among the 1,749 workers employed at the plant developed bladder cancer during those years. Only 3.6 cases were expected to have occurred if no excess risk had been present. Six of the workers with cancer were among the 73 who had been employed for ten or more years in the department in which Wingstay was produced, mixing orthotoluidine with aniline and two other chemicals. The expected number of bladder cancer cases among the 73 was .22; NIOSH calculated that the exposure increased their risk of disease by more than 2700 percent (Ward et al. 1991).

Most of the orthotoluidine used at the Goodyear plant was purchased from two of the country's leading chemical companies: Du Pont[1] and Allied Chemical. It should have come as no surprise to these manufacturers that orthotoluidine was implicated as a human bladder carcinogen. The cancer outbreak at Goodyear's Buffalo plant occurred sixty years after the first cases were recognized at Du Pont and Allied's dye production factories, and almost forty years since the first appearance of cases in which orthotoluidine was implicated. Hundreds of workers at the Du Pont and Allied factories had already developed bladder cancer as a result of exposure to these chemicals.

For many years, orthotoluidine had been a mainstay of the dye industry, having been used to make magenta and several other important colors. The chemical is an aromatic amine, similar in structure to several other chemicals used in the dye and rubber industries and known to cause human bladder cancer. In failing to protect these workers from toxic exposure, Du Pont and Allied demonstrated that little had changed since the early decades of the century. When it came to the health of workers exposed to dangerous chemicals, manufacturers chose to ignore impressive quantities of scientific evidence. Only when workers, often in sizable numbers, started to develop cancer were the problems acknowledged and actions taken to decrease exposure.[2]

The Birth of the Synthetic Dye Industry and Discovery of Occupational Bladder Cancer

Since its inception, the synthetic dye industry has been dominated by the largest multinational chemical manufacturers. While the technology developed for dye production has resulted in important advances in chemical, munitions, and pharmaceutical manufacturing, the intermediate chemicals used in producing dyes have been responsible for a series of epidemics of bladder cancer in virtually every region of the world where the industry has located (Hueper 1969). The U.S. dye industry has been responsible for at least seven documented outbreaks of occupational bladder cancer, with at least 750 cases of the disease identified among dye workers since 1930.[3] New Jersey has been a particularly important center of the dye industry; the bladder cancer rate in Salem County, the site of the most important factory producing aromatic amines (and bladder cancer), is among the highest of any county in the country (Riggan et al. 1983).

Bladder cancer is an uncommon type of tumor, and for that reason the occurrence of more than one or two cases in any group of workers is cause for suspicion.[4] When outbreaks of the disease occurred at dye factories, the relative rarity of the cancer in the general population and the extreme magnitude of the increased risk associated with exposure to the dye intermediates generally made the occupational clustering of the cases so obvious that ultimately they could not be ignored. As a result, the manner in which the history of bladder cancer unfolded for each manufacturer, a process entailing the "discovery" of the epidemic, the communication of information about the risk of exposure, the overdue decision to institute initial control measures, and the eventual acknowledgment that the product could not be manufactured safely, is readily documented.[5]

The history of the synthetic dye industry can be traced to the 1856 discovery by William Henry Perkin, an eighteen-year-old British chemistry student, that coal tar could be transformed into a synthetic dye. Perkin had been attempting to prepare artificial quinine from coal tar, until then a useless byproduct of the distillation of coal to produce gas for lighting. Instead of quinine, he synthesized a delicate mauve solution, which he named mauvine (Borkin and Welsh 1943). Perkin's discovery was the first in a rapid series of scientific advances related to dyes that occurred throughout Europe in the second half of the nineteenth century. While not as colorfast as natural dyes, these artificial dyes were the beginning of an important new industry that provided textile dyers with bright and inexpensive colors.

Armed with the first patents, the English chemical industry

initially dominated the global dye market. The German industry, however, grew rapidly, with substantial public and private sector investment in the construction of research facilities and the education and employment of organic chemists. Seeing the opportunity for sustained industrial development, the German government built formidable university laboratories to train scientists and provide the basic research needed by the organic chemical industry. As a result, German scientists obtained hundreds of patents, which they then used successfully to dominate the world dye market for decades (Norton 1915; Scott 1962).

While the dye industry was notable for its size and financial return, its importance in economic history stems primarily from its relationship to the development of the synthetic organic chemical industry. The patents and production processes of the dye industry became the basis for the global expansion of organic chemical production, including pharmaceuticals (most notably sulfa drugs and aspirin), explosives, synthetic resins, petroleum additives, and numerous other materials (U.S. Tariff Commission 1946; Beer 1959).

The first bladder cancer cases among dye workers were seen by Rehn, a surgeon in Frankfurt-am-Main, a center of the German chemical industry. In 1895, Rehn reported that three of the forty-five workers employed in the production of the dye fuchsine developed bladder cancer. In addition, many more workers developed nonmalignant bladder disease. Grandhomme, the factory surgeon employed by Hoechst, one of the largest dye manufacturers, immediately disputed the report, claiming that while many workers had suffered severe irritation of the bladder, so few had cancer that it could not be work related. This debate continued for the next decade, as additional cases continued to appear. By 1906, Rehn had identified thirty-eight workers with bladder cancer, and other investigators reported more cases in subsequent years (Hueper 1969). Reports of an independent outbreak involving eighteen cases in Basel, Switzerland, and a total of one hundred cases in Germany presented at a conference of German factory physicians in 1913 finally confirmed for the scientific community the causal relationship between the dye intermediates and bladder cancer (International Labour Office 1921; Hueper 1969).

In the first outbreaks of occupational bladder cancer, it was difficult to differentiate between the carcinogenic effects of several of the most important substances used in dye production. Published reports consisted primarily of case series listing the exposures of each worker who was diagnosed as having bladder cancer. In 1921, the International Labour Office (ILO) issued a monograph entitled *Cancer of the Bladder Among Workers in Aniline Factories*. This work reviewed the exposure histories of all cases reported through 1920. Applying rigorous criteria for identifying the actual bladder carcinogens, the ILO asserted, correctly as it turned out, that the chemicals most likely to have caused these cases were benzidine and betanaphthylamine (BNA). The report concluded optimistically:

> Hygienic precautions, strictly applied, will assure at the end of a few years the diminution and even the disappearance of the disease. It is, therefore, absolutely necessary that in factories in which workers are exposed to the dangerous action of aromatic bases, the most rigorous application of hygienic precautions should be required. (ILO 1921:22)

The Spoils of War:
Du Pont and the Development of
the U.S. Dye Industry

The United States synthetic dye industry began on a small scale in the late 1800s and was soon dominated by the local output of European-owned plants. U.S. manufacturers were not able to compete successfully because German and Swiss dye producers controlled virtually all important patents in the field. The First World War radically changed this situation, when the U.S. government seized enemy-owned plants and patents and distributed them at low cost to U.S. chemical companies (U.S. Tariff Commission 1946). As a result, two New Jersey manufacturers, E. I. duPont de Nemours & Co. and American Cyanamid, along with Allied Chemical and Dye Corporation (later Allied Chemical, subsequently the Allied Corporation, and now Allied–Signal), became the three largest synthetic dye producers in the United States.

Du Pont chose the quiet town of Deepwater, New Jersey, for its first factory to be dedicated to the production of organic chemicals, a field in which Du Pont would become a global leader (Figure 3.1) (E. I. duPont de Nemours & Co. 1952; Hounshell and Smith 1988). The Chambers Works, as the factory complex was named, was located in Salem County, just across the Delaware

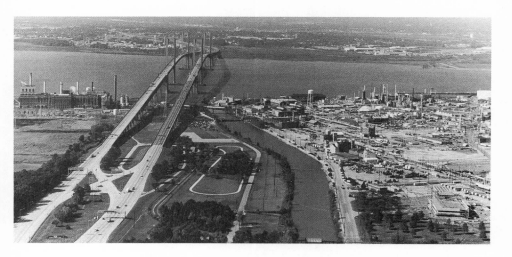

FIGURE 3.1.   I. E. duPont de Nemours & Company, Deepwater, New Jersey, in the shadow of the Delaware Memorial Bridge. Site of aniline dye and tetraethyl lead production. Photo by Lynn Butler, November 1990.

River from Wilmington, the center of the duPont industrial empire. Among the chemicals produced at the plant were BNA and benzidine, the two products that would soon be identified as powerful human carcinogens.

The Chambers Works, which opened during World War I, was soon the site of a major occupational disease outbreak, unrelated to dye production, accompanied by a national scandal. In the early 1920s, Du Pont and General Motors, which at the time was partly owned by Du Pont, agreed to manufacture and distribute leaded gasoline, a product designed to reduce automobile engine "knock." Du Pont chose the Chambers Works for its production facility. The neurological effects of organic lead exposure were so severe and widespread there that workers named the plant "the House of Butterflies," referring to the hallucinations of insects experienced by so many of the lead-poisoned workers. A *New York Times* reporter who investigated the situation reported that over three hundred workers were poisoned and eight killed by lead during the first two years of production (Rosner and Markowitz 1985).[6] The national notoriety Du Pont earned through the House of Butterflies scandal may have convinced the company that public disclosure of further outbreaks of occupational disease would most profitably be managed differently.

The first bladder cancer cases among workers at the Chambers Works were apparently recognized by Du Pont physicians in 1932, although the cancer may have started appearing some years earlier (Washburn 1936). For the next several years, these physicians documented both at national conferences and in the scientific literature the rapidly growing epidemic. In November 1933, twenty-seven cases were reported by G. H. Gehrmann, Du Pont's medical director, at a scientific symposium the proceedings of which were published in the *Journal of Urology* (Gehrmann 1934). Three years later, the medical superintendent at the Chambers Works, E. E. Evans, reported at a meeting of the New York branch of the American Urological Association that the number of cases of bladder cancer among workers at the plant was increasing rapidly (Evans 1936). By that date, the company knew of at least eighty-three cases, although other accounts suggest the actual number was higher (Washburn 1936).

After its initial flurry of publications, Du Pont decided to end its openness. For the next several decades, while the company's scientists continued to attend public meetings and participate in the scientific debate on occupational bladder cancer, they no longer presented data on the growing number of workers who developed the disease at the Chamber Works (Gehrmann et al. 1949). Internal reports by the medical department, however, noted that 140 cases were known to the company by 1946 (Hueper 1969).

During the decades in which the human cost of uncontrolled production of aromatic amines was withheld from the scientific literature, the number of bladder cancer cases continued to rise. A letter from Evans to Arthur Magelsdorff, of the Calco Chemical Company (predecessor of American Cyanamid) in Bound Brook, New Jersey, revealed the astounding carcinogenic strength of BNA. Evans declared that by 1947, less than two decades after the first cancer cases appeared, *every member of the original group engaged in the production of BNA had developed bladder cancer* (Evans 1947).

Du Pont eventually acknowledged publicly that, by 1981, it was aware of 316 workers at the Chambers Works who had developed bladder cancer (Mason et al. 1986). Since this registry was unlikely to include most workers who stopped working at Du Pont before developing the disease, the true number of victims is undoubtedly greater.

Du Pont Slowly Reduces BNA Exposure: A Chronology

The history of betanaphthylamine production at the Chambers Works, including the chronology of Du Pont's numerous changes in the production process over time, is provided in a 1958 memo by D. T. Smith, Protection Division supervisor at the Chambers Works. Smith wrote the memo to help the company determine the year and extent of exposure to BNA among workers who developed bladder cancer. Smith wrote:

> The manufacture of beta-naphthylamine was started in the Chambers Works in 1919. It was cast in open pans, broken with a pick, and transferred by hand into barrels, ground in an open mill, and shoveled by hand into operating equipment. There was no ventilation provided. Gross exposures occurred.
> In 1932, the occurrence of bladder tumors and their possible connection with beta-naphthylamine was first recognized. In the ensuing months a still, flaker and mill were installed in the low pressure autoclave building and positive ventilation was installed on all equipment handling this material. This equipment was put in operation in 1934, and the casting and grinding was discontinued. We consider that the period of general gross exposure was terminated April 1, 1934. (Smith 1958:1)

As the memo proceeds, it becomes clear that significant levels of exposure nevertheless continued throughout the 1930s and 1940s. Smith describes how Du Pont considered additional improvements in 1940 but moved slowly and eventually decided to delay any changes because of World War II. No further improvements in the BNA production process were implemented until 1948, when, Smith reports, exposure was finally eliminated in at least one of the production buildings. Total enclosure of the production process was completed in 1951, more than thirty-five years after BNA production began and twenty years after the epidemic was recognized. "After that date," Smith concludes, "possibility of exposure was greatly reduced" (2). The new building, which permitted safer production, was used for only four years; Du Pont terminated BNA production in 1955 (Smith 1958).

When Should Du Pont Have Known?

It is worthy of comment that the discovery of occupational bladder cancer among dye workers in this country was made by and initially publicized voluntarily by the industry. Rehn's reports met with such intense opposition in Germany that it was ten years before the causal relationship between dye manufacture and bladder tumors was recognized in that country (Hueper 1969). Even more unfortunate was the necessity to repeat Rehn's finding forty years later in the United States, without precautions having been instituted in the interim.

Could the Du Pont physicians have been unaware in the period 1916 to 1930 of occupational bladder cancer reports in central Europe? If they were, their ignorance is not attributable to a lack of published scientific information on the subject. The etiology, treatment, and prevention of that epidemic caused a major debate in the medical journals of Germany, Switzerland, and Austria, with at least fifteen articles appearing before World War I and many more in the years between the armistice and Du Pont's first reports. Germany and Switzerland made bladder cancer among dye workers a compensable occupational disease in 1925 (Hueper 1969).

It was not even necessary to read German to learn about the relationship between dyes and bladder cancer. A study conducted in 1925 by the National Research Council of Great Britain, which investigated cancer rates among members of different occupations and trades, found that chemical workers and textile dyers had elevated rates of bladder cancer, and the report suggested that benzidine and BNA were responsible (Young and Russell 1926). In addition, several other review articles and case reports of bladder cancer among dye workers were published in England during the 1920s (Bridge and Henry 1928; Wignall 1929).

Most important, the International Labour Office published its monograph on occupational bladder cancer in February 1921, ten years before the Du Pont epidemic was recognized. The explicit purpose of this report was to inform dye manufacturers in countries where the industry was young, such as the United States, of the dangers of dye production (International Labour Office 1921:2–3).

Furthermore, the Du Pont's obliviousness (and that of other American chemical companies) could not be attributed to lack of contact with the managements of the dye producers of central Europe and England. During the second and third decades of the century, Du Pont worked tirelessly with I. G. Farben, the huge German chemical cartel;[7] Imperial Chemical Industries (ICI), the British chemical giant that held monopolistic control of dye production and sales throughout the British Commonwealth; and the leading Swiss, French, and Italian chemical and dye producers, building collaborative business ventures and monopolistically dividing the world's chemical markets. Du Pont and Farben negotiated continuously from 1927 through 1929 to form a joint dye-producing venture, tentatively called the American Dyes Company. When the companies realized they would not be able to reach a successful agreement, they both accepted a state of "amicable cooperation" (Borkin and Welsh 1943; U.S. Tariff Commission 1946).[8]

Dr. Wilhelm Hueper:
Du Pont Makes an Enemy

Data provided by internal Du Pont sources show that the initial bladder cancer outbreak, reported in 1933, was not a surprise to the Du Pont management. The rapid onset of this epidemic was predicted by a physician, Wilhelm Hueper, who had been employed at the Cancer Research Laboratory of the University of Pennsylvania. Hueper eventually became one of the country's experts in chemical carcinogenesis and served as chief of the National Cancer Institute's Environmental Cancer Section from 1948 until 1964.[9] He originally met Irenee duPont in the early 1930s when he accompanied the laboratory's director, who at the time was also a duPont family physician, on house calls. Hueper told an interviewer that in 1932

> I had written to Mr. E. I. duPont, whom I knew personally at that time, that from my observations after visiting the dye works, I had come to the conclusion that their workers would have the same cancer hazards to the bladder as similar workers in European plants,

especially Germany, Switzerland and England and that an investigation would show that these men have an increased incidence of
bladder cancer. I didn't get any personal answers to this. My boss at
the cancer research laboratories at the University of Pennsylvania
told me several months later that they had come to the conclusion
that they had no cancer among their workers. "Well," I said, "that
may be, but they would get them." Then about four months later,
suddenly Gehrmann and the research director of the [Du Pont] research station came to us in Philadelphia and said, "We have some
now." I said, "How many?" And he said, "We now have 26." I said,
"You will have more. This is a going concern now." . . . At that time
I had already figured out that it would take about fifteen years. I told
them that men who are getting cancer now are those who your
company employed in 1917 when they created the dye work operation (Breslow 1979:1–2)

Hueper, who in 1934 published the first of his many articles on
occupational bladder cancer, was hired that same year by Du Pont
to join its newly formed Haskell Laboratory of Industrial Toxicology. Working for Du Pont, he was able to perfect the first animal
model for bladder carcinogenesis (Hueper et al. 1938). In his capacity as a Du Pont toxicologist, he requested permission to visit the
Chambers Works. The experience shocked him.

When the betanaphthylamine experiment had been well under way
for several months, I requested that I should be shown the incriminated operation in the Chambers Works, so that I could form an
enlightened judgment of the occupational hazard. Several associates
and I crossed the river a short time later to fulfill this task. The
manager and some of his associates brought us first to the building
housing this operation, which was located in a part of a much larger
building. It was separated from other operations in the building by a
large sliding-door allowing the ready spread of vapors, fumes and
dust from the betanaphthylamine operation into the adjacent workrooms. Being impressed during this visit by the surprising cleanliness of the naphthylamine operation, which at that occasion was not
actively working, I dropped back in the procession of visitors, until I
caught up with the foreman at its end. When I told him, "Your place
is surprisingly clean," he looked at me and commented, "Doctor,
you should have seen it last night; we worked all night to clean it up
for you." The purpose of my visit was thereby almost completely
destroyed. What I had been shown was a well-staged performance.
I, therefore, approached the manager with the request to see the
benzidine operation. After telling him what I just had been told, his
initial reluctance to grant my request vanished and we were led a
short distance up the road where the benzidine operation was
housed in a separate small building. With one look at the place, it

became immediately obvious how the workers became exposed. There was the white powdery benzidine on the road, the loading platform, the window sills, on the floor, etc. This revelation ended the visit. After coming back to Wilmington, I wrote a brief memorandum to Mr. Irenee duPont describing to him my experience and my disappointment with the attempted deception. There was no answer but I was never allowed again to visit the two operations. (Hueper n.d.:156–157)

Hueper's disagreements with Du Pont became acute, and he was told that he would not be able to publish all of his findings. He was dismissed in 1937. Du Pont refused him permission to publish or present data on his work on experimental induction of bladder cancer with aromatic amines, which was conducted while at Du Pont (Breslow 1979).

In 1942, Hueper nevertheless published his seminal text *Occupational Tumors and Allied Diseases*. It contained the most thorough review of world literature on occupational carcinogenesis to date. Never forgetting Du Pont's role in the bladder cancer epidemic at the Chambers Works, Hueper initially wanted the book's dedication to read, "To the victims of cancer who made things for better living through chemistry." This was a caustic allusion to Du Pont's well-known advertising slogan "Better things for better living from chemistry." In the end, probably fearful of the company's retribution, he dedicated the book, "To the memory of those of our fellow men who have died from occupational diseases contracted while making better things for an improved living for others" (Hueper n.d.; Agran 1977).

Benzidine:
Du Pont Protects a Valuable Asset

Virtually all the reports on occupational bladder cancer in the 1930s implicated both BNA and benzidine, since most workers who developed the disease worked in facilities where both chemicals were present. While Hueper's animal studies confirmed BNA's carcinogenicity in 1938, the coming of World War II interrupted the advancement of research in this area. According to Robert A. M. Case, the author of the most comprehensive study of the relationship between aromatic amine exposure and bladder cancer in humans, the British chemical industry and government were convinced that BNA and benzidine cause bladder cancer (Case 1983). As a result, a "gentleman's agreement" between the British government and the Association of British Chemical Manufacturers (ABCM) went into effect on January 1, 1939, providing the equivalent of workers' compensation payments to workers who developed occupational bladder cancer but not stopping the chemicals' use (Scott 1962; Case 1966). After the war ended, Case was appointed to a research fellowship created by the ABCM, and designed and conducted the first occupational cohort mortality study (Case et al. 1954).

Du Pont, however, took an alternative approach, much to the misfortune of its workforce. Hueper's animal studies made it impossible to deny that BNA was a carcinogen. Du Pont toxicologists had conducted a similar study on benzidine, involving only four dogs, and were not successful in causing bladder cancer. Du Pont considered a chemical innocent until proven guilty; in a 1948 international meeting, Gehrmann, its medical director, declared:

> We feel that it cannot be concluded that Benzidine is a cause of bladder tumours until conclusive proof that Benzidine workers who have developed tumours have never been exposed even in the slightest degree to Beta Naphthylamine (even an old Beta contaminated building constitutes exposure) and that the incidence of bladder tumours in workers exposed to Benzidine is greater than the incidence of idiopathic bladder tumours in such a group. (Gehrmann et al. 1949)

This enabled the company to justify continued production of benzidine, although Gehrmann himself, after a 1933 visit to Germany following the initial outbreak at Du Pont, recommended to the company that based on the evidence to date it should "take immediate steps to construct all operations so that there shall be absolutely no dust, no fumes nor any skin contacts [with benzidine]" (Case 1981).

What caused Gehrmann's change of heart? Research by Barry Castleman provides the answers.

> In the early months of 1949 the medical officer to the Imperial Chemical Industries Dyestuffs Division visited the DuPont Chambers Works dye plant. This man, the late Dr. Michael Williams, was accompanied by another British researcher, and they were shown around by the corporate medical director who had given the paper at

the London medical congress. After the plant tour, he drove Dr. Williams and his colleague to their next destination, quite a long drive. Dr. Williams, who often recounted the story, noticed that his companion in the back of the car had his eyes closed, and said to the DuPont doctor, "Look, you are company man, and Dr. So-and-So is asleep. Can you explain to me why, after the records and so on that you have shown to us today, you are so certain that benzidine is not causing any of the trouble?"

He got the reply, witnessed by the other Briton, who was in fact not asleep but thinking, "We here know very well that benzidine is causing bladder cancer, but it is company policy to incriminate only the one substance, Beta-naphthylamine." (Castleman 1979)

Case later confirmed the story, admitting that he was the "dozy Brit" in the back of the car. In the following year, 1950, studies supported by Allied Chemical provided the indisputable evidence that benzidine is a carcinogen. Corporate policy changed slowly. The 1954 edition of the textbook *Modern Occupational Medicine*, written and edited by Du Pont staff, stated that while BNA caused cancer, benzidine was only a "suspected cause of tumors" (Fleming et al. 1954). It was not until 1967—seventeen years after the Allied Chemical studies—that the production of benzidine was discontinued at the Chambers Works; Du Pont continued to use benzidine purchased from other manufacturers until 1972 (Mason et al. 1986). The following year, in response to a petition from the Oil, Chemical and Atomic Workers Union, the Occupational Safety and Health Administration (OSHA) issued an emergency temporary standard for benzidine, BNA, and twelve other carcinogens. Federal regulation made benzidine production no longer feasible in the United States; the last two manufacturers of the chemical ceased operations by 1976 (Walker and Gerber 1981). Benzidine-based dye manufacture, in which worker exposure to benzidine is virtually unavoidable, was also curtailed. Eight of the nine U.S. producers of these chemicals discontinued operations between 1974 and 1979; Fabricolor, of Paterson, New Jersey, was the only remaining producer (National Institute for Occupational Safety and Health [NIOSH] 1980). As a result, much production of benzidine-based dyes moved to developing countries, including Mexico, India, Egypt, and Poland, countries where labor and environmental regulation were weak or nonexistent (Samuels 1981). Importation into the United States of these dyes soared from 21,730 pounds in 1974 to 266,915 pounds in 1978 (Fishbein 1981).

Allied Chemical

The Allied Chemical and Dye Corporation began production of benzidine at its Buffalo, New York, plant in 1915, and product of BNA the following year (Johnson and Parnes 1979). Like Du Pont, Allied did nothing to protect its employees from these materials until 1935, when the first cases of workers with bladder cancer were discovered at the plant (Goldwater et al. 1965). During the next fifteen years, Allied continued to accumulate cases while sponsoring important toxicological experiments on benzidine carcinogenesis (Maguigan 1950; Spitz et al. 1950).

While the central European manufactuers had recognized benzidine as a human carcinogen decades earlier, there was evidently great debate within the U.S. dye-producing community regarding its carcinogenicity. In a 1950 article, W. H. Maguigan, a scientist employed by Allied's National Aniline Division in Buffalo, reviewed the state of knowledge on the subject to date and summarized Allied's ground-breaking laboratory experiments on benzidine carcinogenesis. Maguigan, referring to Du Pont's contention that benzidine was not a human carcinogen, wrote:

> More recently one group of investigators in this country have disputed the carcinogenicity of this material, pointing out that most of the benzidine cases were also exposed to beta-naphthylamine. Although I must admit that the evidence against benzidine is much less conclusive than that against beta-naphthylamine, I cannot agree with them. There are a few cases where exposure to benzidine is not complicated by exposure to beta-naphthylamne; there are more with a large exposure to benzidine and very slight or questionable exposure to beta-naphthylamine; and, as we shall see later, it has been possible to produce tumors in animals with benzidine. (Maguigan 1950:1360)

Allied funded the research that demonstrated in 1950 that benzidine was an animal carcinogen (Spitz et al. 1950). With publication of that finding, denying benzidine's hazardous nature was no longer possible. According to U.S. government investigators, however, the benzidine production process was not fully enclosed until 1957 (NIOSH 1972).

The elimination of exposure to benzidine came only after studies involving laboratory animals proved conclusively that the substance was a carcinogen (Ferber et al. 1976); perhaps no action was taken earlier because the numerous cases among workers at the plant and elsewhere were evidently not sufficiently convincing. Allied's lack of concern for the health of its workers is exemplified by its delay in implementing controls in BNA production. While there may have been a legitimate scientific debate about the carcinogenicity of benzidine, BNA had been shown to be both a human and an animal carcinogen decades before Allied's 1954 decision to eliminate the open distillation and flaking of the chemical (Ferber et al. 1976). Allied finally ceased production of BNA in 1955 but through 1962 continued to purchase it from other U.S. production facilities for use in dye production. In addition, until 1960 Allied produced a closely related chemical (alphanaphthylamine, or ANA) that was heavily contaminated with BNA (NIOSH 1972).

In contrast to Du Pont, Allied did not initially publish information about bladder cancer among its workers on its own initiative. In 1965, the New York State Health Department identified 96 workers at the plant who had developed bladder cancer, 46 of them dying from it (Goldwater, et al. 1965). Allied eventually made a public count of the number of the plant's bladder cancer victims in 1974; by that point, at least 151 workers were known to have developed the diseases, although, as with Du Pont, the actual number of cases was likely to have been substantially higher (Ferber et al. 1976). Allied continued producing benzidine until 1976 (Johnson and Parnes 1979).

Ignoring the Evidence from Home

The three largest Swiss chemical firms, Ciba, Geigy, and Sandoz (the first two eventually merging to form Ciba–Geigy), were among the first important dye manufacturers; as was the case in Germany, dye production formed the primary basis for the Swiss national chemical industry. From dyes, the firms expanded to pharmaceuticals, pesticides, and other chemicals, and these companies are now among the world's most important chemical manufacturers. Following the German model of I.G. Farben, in 1918 the Swiss dye manufacturers formed a cartel to control the production and marketing of dyes (U.S. Tariff Commission 1946; Erni 1979).

In the early 1920s, the Swiss I.G. established a manufacturing operation in the United States, the Cincinnati Chemical Works,

whose benzidine production facility opened in 1929. As early producers of dyes, the cartel's original manufacturing facilities in Switzerland had experienced numerous bladder cancer cases in the
pre–World War I era. The relationship of BNA and benzidine exposure to bladder cancer was so apparent at these factories that by
1925 the Swiss government recognized bladder cancer in workers
exposed to the materials as an occupational disease (Hueper 1969).
Ignoring the extensive epidemiologic evidence and the control measures in effect in factories at home, the Swiss managers designed
the benzidine production process in Cincinnati with no concern
about worker exposure. Laborers at the plant shoveled benzidine
by hand, with no protection provided. Furthermore, no provision
was made for medical screening or monitoring, or for keeping track
of past workers who left the plant's employ (Zavon et al. 1973;
Bingham, pers. comm. 1988).

Following the practices of Du Pont and Allied in this country,
the U.S. branch of the Swiss cartel treated the carcinogen as safe
until workers at its own factory actually developed the disease
and the problem could no longer be ignored. It is unlikely, however, that the Swiss I.G. was unaware of potential bladder cancer
problems in its overseas operations, since the first cases of benzidine-related bladder cancer appeared in 1938 at its British subsidiary, the Clayton Aniline Company, Ltd., of Manchester. T. S.
Scott (1952), Clayton's medical officer, reported that by 1951,
sixty-six workers, including twenty-three exposed only to benzidine, had developed bladder cancer.

When in 1956 the first recognized case of occupational bladder
cancer appeared at the Cincinnati Chemical Works, the company
management expressed surprise. A group of consultants from the
University of Cincinnati, brought in to start a bladder cancer screening program, later wrote:

> From the vantage point of 1972, it may appear strange that in 1958,
> eight years after Spitz et al. had used benzidine to induce bladder
> tumors in dogs and six years after Scott had reported 23 cases of
> bladder tumors in workers without contact with other known car-
> cinogens, there would be any question about the carcinogenicity of
> benzidine. Yet, it was obvious at the time that it was neither gener-
> ally known nor accepted that benzidine was a bladder tumorigen.
> Consultation with those engaged in the manufacture of the material
> in the United States indicated that, as of that time, they did not
> generally view benzidine as a tumorigen. Our statement that epide-

miological evidence strongly suggested that benzidine was a tumorigen came as a shock, and resulted in some troubled and anxious managements. (Zavon et al. 1973:1)

Since the personnel records at the plant were so poor, it was difficult to identify exposed workers other than those employed at the time the first case was discovered. Of the twenty-five workers in this group, however, thirteen had developed the disease by 1972 (Zavon et al. 1973).

The Upjohn Company

The history of benzidine production in the North Haven, Connecticut, factory originally operated by the Carwin Company and then purchased by the Upjohn Company is illuminating because its production of dye intermediates *began* more than a decade after the highly publicized Du Pont epidemic. In this case, there is clear documentation that the manufacturer knew from the onset of production of the carcinogenic nature of benzidine; took only limited precautions; and after realizing that the precautions were insufficient, later actually denied having known the substance was a human carcinogen.

Carwin began benzidine operations at its North Haven plant in 1946 (Johnson and Parnes 1979). The following year, clearly worried about the cancer risk at the plant, the company contracted with several scientists associated with the Institute of Occupational Medicine and Hygiene at the Yale School of Medicine. With the collaboration of the U.S. Public Health Service (USPHS), this group conducted a series of studies on the routes of benzidine exposure and biologic metabolism of the substance among those exposed. Benzidine air levels were regularly monitored, and individual exposure levels determined. As a result, the group was able to develop a rapid technique to measure benzidine metabolites in urine (Meigs et al. 1951; Murray 1973). The level of activity focused on benzidine must have been substantial, since the research team produced at least five scientific papers describing different facets of its work at the plant (Rye et al. 1970). It seems likely that as a result of these studies exposure to benzidine was reduced. In retrospect, however, the limited value of these new procedures seems clear. By the mid 1950s, Allied had already acknowledged that there was no safe level of exposure to this carcinogen and had installed an enclosed system for benzidine production (Ferber et al. 1976).

Upjohn purchased the benzidine plant from Carwin in October 1962. Ignoring the extensive and well-publicized scientific work related to benzidine that had been going on at the North Haven plant for over a decade, corporate officials date Upjohn's knowledge of the carcinogenicity of benzidine to 1964 and claim that the discovery was somewhat fortuitous. According to a sworn statement by William M. Murray, manager of the plant's Process Development and Control Department:

> In late October 1964, the Upjohn Company was informed by another manufacturer that they had evidence of human carcinogenesis through industrial experience limited solely to benzidine. Following the receipt of this information, a thorough and exhaustive re-examination was conducted of existing toxicological data. After engineering considerations we determined that it was not economically feasible to obtain the known levels of exposure warranted by a known human carcinogen and thus The Upjohn Company decided to terminate manufacture of Benzidine. (Murray 1973:4–5)

While Murray was aware of the Yale studies done at the plant throughout the 1950s, he suggested that Upjohn had no prior knowledge of reports of benzidine-related bladder tumors in exposed workers at other facilities. This seems unlikely since on the first page of the first article the Yale investigators published on exposure at the North Haven plant, they cited five studies containing evidence that "workers who have been involved in manufacturing benzidine for periods of 10 years or more have an unusually high incidence of bladder cancer" (Meigs et al. 1951:533).

A second "official" account of Upjohn's discovery of benzidine's carcinogenicity can be found in a 1970 article defending the safety of several related aromatic amines. In "Facts and Myths Concerning Diamine Curing Agents," (1970) authors W. A. Rye and P. F. Woolrich, respectively director and chief of Industrial Health Services for Upjohn, and R. P. Zanes, director of Health Services for the North Haven plant and a member of the Yale faculty, recount the history of Upjohn's knowledge about benzidine. They assert, contrary to extensive scientific evidence, that it was only in 1964 that it became clear that benzidine by itself was a carcinogen.

Prior to 1964, investigation of the experience and practices of other American, English, and European plants in which tumors had occurred pointed to concurrent exposure to beta-naphthylamine. As workmen in this plant and one other producer were not exposed to beta-naphthylamine, and *neither had experienced bladder tumors,* it had been concluded that the carcinogenicity of benzidine alone, if carefully handled, was not yet proved. Animal experimentation added little since tumor induction was not comparable to the human experience. (Rye et al. 1970:212; emphasis added)

It is worth noting that Upjohn was here taking the same position as did the other dye manufacturers, thirty (or, if we count the European experience, sixty) years earlier. Yet the absence of identified bladder cancer cases at North Haven did not prove benzidine was not a carcinogen, no matter what the manufacturer hoped. Evidently, it was only the warning of a medical officer of Imperial Chemical Industry's Dyestuffs Division, coming on the day before Christmas 1964, that convinced Upjohn to treat benzidine as a carcinogen (212).

A 1972 inspection of the North Haven plant by the NIOSH found evidence that working conditions had been quite dangerous: "Open centrifuges and filter presses had been used in the manufacture of benzidine, and past exposures to workers in these operations appeared obvious after viewing first hand some of the old equipment" (Johnson and Parnes 1979:280). While the NIOSH scientists located six cases of bladder cancer among past workers at the plant, there is no evidence of whether these cases were known to Upjohn.

The human cost of these years of exposure is only now being measured. A cohort mortality study, published in 1986 by one of the Yale scientists originally asked by Carwin to help reduce exposure, determined that the rate of bladder cancer among the workers with the highest exposure levels was more than ten times that of the Connecticut population (Meigs et al. 1986:7).

Denouement at Du Pont:
Orthotoluidine "Discovered" to Cause
Bladder Cancer

With the promulgation of an OSHA standard in the early 1970s, the last remaining U.S. producers of BNA and benzidine ceased operation (and the importation of dye products manufactured overseas skyrocketed) (Samuels 1981). But the gap between scientific knowledge and regulatory action remained. Tens of thousands of U.S. workers remained exposed to numerous other chemicals that were carcinogenic in animal studies but were never regulated as carcinogens by OSHA, although U.S. and international agencies recommended they be treated as such.

Orthotoluidine, implicated in the bladder cancer outbreak at Goodyear's Buffalo plant, was one of these chemicals. It had been widely used in the dye industry for many decades, especially in the production of magenta, one of the early important commercially manufactured dyes. Subsequently it was adopted by the rubber industry as an antioxidant, used to improve resistance to oxidation and the effects of aging and exposure to the sun. Orthotoluidine was incriminated in earlier bladder cancer outbreaks, although most workers in these cases were also exposed to other powerful carcinogens. The first reports of bladder cancer among workers exposed only to orthotoluidine were published in the early 1950s; there were five cases at one factory where magenta was produced and where no other suspect carcinogens were present (Scott 1952; Case et al. 1954). Over the next three decades, several reports and studies were published in the world literature implicating orthotoluidine in outbreaks of bladder cancer (Borneff 1965; Khlebnikova et al. 1976; Rubino et al. 1982).

The animal evidence on orthotoluidine's carcinogenicity developed in a similar progression. The results of early animal studies (Morigami and Nisimura 1940; Satani et al. 1941; Strombeck 1946; Ekman and Strombeck 1947) suggested that this chemical might be carcinogenic, although utility of animal models in this period was limited. By the early 1970s, however, several studies demonstrated increased incidence of tumors in laboratory animals exposed to orthotoluidine (Homburger et al. 1972; Russfield et al. 1973), prompting the National Cancer Institute (NCI) to conduct its own bioassay of the chemical's carcinogenicity. The results of this study, published in 1979, showed definitively that ortho-toluidine is also an animal carcinogen (NCI 1979), prompting the International Agency for Research on Cancer to conclude that "ortho-toluidine should be regarded, for practical purposes, as if it presented a carcinogenic risk to humans" (IARC 1982:170).

NIOSH estimates that in the early 1980s, almost thirty thousand workers were still exposed to orthotoluidine (Ward et al. 1991).

Unfortunately, neither Du Pont and Allied's unfortunate history of having presided over the development of hundreds of bladder cancer cases among workers exposed to similar chemicals nor the mounting evidence of orthotoluidine's carcinogenicity prompted either of these companies to warn other companies purchasing this product that it had the potential to cause cancer.

The human cancer cost attributed to orthotoluidine was not limited to the workers at Goodyear's Buffalo plant. In 1990, a thirty-four-year-old worker who had been employed in the orthotoluidine production area at Du Pont's Chambers Works was diagnosed with bladder cancer.

Allied stopped producing orthotoluidine in the late 1970s; Du Pont has continued, in the face of considerable evidence that there is no safe level of exposure to this substance. Only after NIOSH's publication of the Goodyear study did Du Pont begin to collect data to determine if there was an increased incidence of bladder cancer among its workers exposed to orthotoluidine. Almost one hundred years after Rehn's first report and sixty years after the first bladder cases were discovered at the Chambers Works, the lessons of the bladder cancer epidemic have yet to learned.

Conclusion

The German dye industry discovered in 1895 that two of its most important (and profitable) chemicals were bladder carcinogens. With the publication and dissemination of the 1921 International Labour Office report, the uncontrolled exposure of dye workers to these carcinogens should have been eliminated. Instead, each U.S. manufacturer went through its own discovery process, ignoring well-publicized warnings and allowing uncontrolled exposure to occur until the human cost became so obvious that it was no longer acceptable. Du Pont, with a high public profile and a production facility that had received extensive public scrutiny connected with an organic lead disaster a few years earlier, was successfully able to manage public discussion of the situation. While Du Pont scientists openly presented data on the outbreak at a series of scientific meetings, its managers were slow to institute changes in the production process and attempted to muzzle their own toxicologist. In contrast,

Allied made little effort to protect its workers during this period and avoided public discussion of the number of cases at its plant until decades after the epidemic began. The Swiss I.G. repeated Du Pont's behavior twenty-five years later, allowing uncontrolled exposure until the epidemic began, while Upjohn, making little attempt to identify bladder cancer cases and ignoring the well-developed scientific literature, became concerned only after a strong warning from a physician employed by another dye manufacturer.

What thoughts went through the minds of these managers while production was occurring? It is plausible that the corporate managers of Du Pont and Allied were actually unaware of the scientific literature on bladder carcinogenesis when they began production, although once the first cases appeared at their own facilities, this ignorance could not have continued. A lack of information could not have characterized the managers at Ciba–Geigy, Sandoz, and Upjohn, since they were aware of the scientific literature on occupational bladder cancer. The tragic experiences of earlier manufacturers did nothing to encourage these newer ones to install the environmental controls necessary to protect exposed workers from bladder carcinogens. As a result, hundreds of workers died.

This review of the scientific and industrial record on aromatic amine dye products is most profitably considered as part of an emerging literature on the history of occupational health (Rosner and Markowitz 1987). There are striking parallels between the history of dye production and that of the industrial production of asbestos products (Castleman 1984; Brodeur 1985; Kotelchuck 1987), beryllium (Zwerling 1987), and tetraethyl lead (Rosner and Markowitz 1985; Graebner 1987). Workers employed in the manufacture of these products were exposed to extremely toxic materials, while corporate managers and scientists ignored scientific evidence (much of it gathered by the industry itself) about the hazardous nature of the exposure. Furthermore, in each of these cases, corporate scientists played an important role in justifying management production policies and attempted to limit the epidemiologic information released to the scientific community and the public.

The dissemination of scientific information about bladder cancer outbreaks at other plants had little impact on the decision-making process of corporate managers as it related to decisions to protect the health of workers in their employ. This chronology underscores the limitation of voluntary compliance with workplace health regulation. Acknowledging that it could not be manufactured safely, Switzerland banned BNA production in 1938, and Great Britain followed in 1952. In the absence of regulation in the United States, Du Pont did not stop producing this carcinogen until 1955; Allied continued to manufacture BNA-containing chemicals through 1960 and to purchase it for two additional years. Smaller companies maintained production, often with virtually no protection for their workers, until federal intervention finally began a decade later (Johnson and Parnes 1979; Stern et al. 1985). This same tragic sequence was repeated for benzidine, although with a slower chronology, attributable to Du Pont's refusal to recognize the chemical's carcinogenicity. The sequence was then repeated once again, decades later, with orthotoluidine, a chemical for which substantial evidence of its carcinogenicity existed. As a result, over a dozen workers developed bladder cancer, with many more inevitably to follow.

In each case, manufacturers ignored the mounting evidence and assumed the chemical was innocent until proven guilty, as demonstrated by the appearance of cancer among workers. Given the documented recalcitrance of some of the country's largest and most profitable chemical manufacturers in protecting their workers from exposure to known human carcinogens, it seems extremely unlikely that employers will voluntarily protect workers from less obvious hazards. Decades after BNA and benzidine were shown to be human carcinogens, manufacturers chose not to protect workers until bladder cancer cases began to appear and an epidemic was inevitable. The presence of a national workplace safety and health regulatory apparatus did little to prevent the bladder cancer outbreak at Goodyear that occurred following exposure to orthotoluidine.

The U.S. chemical industry has not considered itself responsible for acquiring, interpreting, and applying information contained in the extensive scientific literature about the relationship of aromatic amine exposure to bladder cancer. The findings of this case study demonstrate the weakness of current federal regulation of workplace exposure, as well as the need for much stronger government and worker-controlled workplace safety and health regulatory mechanisms.

Notes

[1]This large chemical manufacturer was founded and is still controlled by the duPont family and is known as E. I. duPont de Nemours & Company, or, in its shortened form, Du Pont. For this reason, the spelling "duPont" is used here only for individual members of the family or for the family itself; "Du Pont" is used for the name of the enterprise.

[2]The objective in this chapter is to investigate the development and communication of knowledge about bladder cancer within the U.S. chemical industry by focusing on four companies: Allied Chemical, the Swiss-owned Cincinnati Chemical Works, Du Pont, and Upjohn. More data about the production of dyes, and of bladder cancer, exist for Du Pont than for any other producer, in part because Du Pont has traditionally been in the forefront of the design and provision of corporate occupational health services. It has long encouraged its physicians to publish in academic journals, and Du Pont occupational health specialists are responsible for one of the most important early U.S. texts in the field (Fleming et al. 1954). For these reasons, many other manufacturers have looked to Du Pont for leadership in the area of occupational health, and for these same reasons data from Du Pont play a significant part in this article.

In focusing on Allied, Cincinnati Chemical, Du Pont, and Upjohn, I do not seek to indict these four manufacturers in particular. There is substantial evidence that other important U.S. dye producers (Lieben 1963; Kleinfeld 1967; Johnson and Parnes 1979; Markowitz and Lyons 1979), as well as dye producers in Germany, Great Britain, France, Italy, and Japan (Temkin 1963; Hueper 1969), treated the bladder cancer epidemics for which they were responsible in ways very similar to those profiled here. I have selected this group of corporations for study because their policies and actions are documented in published studies, in testimony submitted to hearings and trials, and in internal memoranda that have become available as a result of legal suits.

[3]This figure was calculated by adding the results of several recent studies to the compilation of cases performed by Hueper in 1969. As an estimate, it is likely to be an extremely conservative one since it includes only cases identified in published epidemiologic studies and case reports.

[4]Occupational bladder cancer generally appears fifteen or more years after first exposure to the carcinogen. while it is sometimes fatal, most people who develop bladder cancer currently are cured. The five-year survival rate, the statistic epidemiologists use to approximate the cure rate, is now about 78 percent among whites and 56 percent among blacks. This has been improving consistently in recent decades; in the early 1960s, only 53 percent of whites and 24 percent of blacks who developed the disease survived five years after diagnosis (American Cancer Society 1990).

[5]There is little discussion in this chapter of the activities of either the workers at these companies or, where they existed, their unions. The history of workers' struggles to obtain safer workplaces is generally more difficult to examine than corporate policies because written documentation of worker efforts, when it exists, is often not easily obtained. A study of

workers' reactions to the bladder cancer epidemics would serve as a very useful complement to this case study.

[6]The history of the development and uncontrolled use of leaded gasoline, resulting in a particularly severe and global public health problem, has been doucmented by David Rosner and Gerald Markowitz (1985). Their fascinating study raises many of the same questions about the relationship of scientific knowledge, public health, and corporate decision making that are addressed in this chapter.

[7]In the aftermath of World War I, the six German chemical manufacturers, including three that are still of paramount importance in the global economy (Hoechst, BASF, and Bayer), formed a cartel, named I.G. Farben, in an attempt to dominate the world chemical industry. Dyes and dye-related chemicals were their most important products; *Interessen Gemeinschaft Farbenindustrie* translated is the "Community of Interest of the Color Industry."

Farben's chemical production played a vital role in the Nazi war effort. Farben produced synthetic rubber and petroleum, without which Hitler's tanks could not have stormed through Europe. Using production techniques perfected in manufacturing dyes, Farben's factories also produced pharmaceuticals and munitions, as well as Zyklon B, the poison gas used in extermination camp gas chambers throughout the Reich. Farben built its own synthetic rubber and oil factory at Auschwitz (known as I.G. Auschwitz). An estimated twenty-five thousand prisoners were worked to death there, sometimes dying at a rate greater than 1 percent per day (Borkin 1978).

[8]These agreements were not only in the area of dye production and sales. Beginning in November 1919, with the ink on the recently signed armistice barely dry, Du Pont began negotiations with the companies that constituted the Farben cartel for the organization of a "world company" for the synthetic manufacture of ammonia. By 1926, Du Pont, Farben, and ICI had also successfully divided up the international gunpowder market (Borkin and Welsh 1943).

Multinational cartel agreements remained in effect into World War II, with U.S. and British chemical manufacturers secretly continuing their collaborations with important Nazi companies. In May 1942, a federal grand jury indicted the five leading U.S. dye manufacturers, Du Pont, Allied Chemical, American Cyanamid, GAF (owned by I.G. Farben), and Cincinnati Chemical Works, for restraint of trade. They were accused of price fixing, setting quotas for foreign markets, preventing other companies from entering the field, and a host of other charges. Several foreign manufacturers, including ICI and Mitsui Enterprises of Japan, were also named as parties in the case. The trial, however, was delayed to avoid interference with the U.S. defendants' war production activities. The case was settled in 1946, when all defendants entered pleas of nolo contendere and were fined a total of $111,000 (U.S. Tariff Commission 1946).

[9]Dr. Wilhelm C. Hueper, at one time one of the leading U.S. scientists in the field of occupational and environmental carcinogenesis, devoted much of his life to the investigation and prevention of occupational bladder

cancer. His books, which contain the most important and complete chronologies of this tragic history (Hueper 1942, 1969), along with his unpublished autobiography, served as a primary source of information and inspiration for this chapter. Throughout his life, Hueper continually refused to separate his scientific work from his dedication to public health and social justice. For a summary of Hueper's career, see Samuel Epstein's (1975) presentation speech when Hueper was awarded the Society of Occupation and Environmental Health's First Annual Award.

References

Agran, L. 1977. *The Cancer Connection*. Boston: Houghton Mifflin.

American Cancer Society. 1990. *Cancer Facts and Figures*. New York. American Cancer Society.

Beer, J. J. 1959. *The Emergence of the German Dye Industry.* Urbana: University of Illinois Press.

Bingham, E. 1988. Personal communication, April 26.

Borkin, J. 1978. *The Crime and Punishment of I.G. Farben*. New York: Free Press.

Borkin, J., and Welsh, C. H. 1943. *Germany's Master Plan: The Story of Industrial Offensive*. New York: Duell, Sloan and Pearce.

Borneff, J. 1965. "Carcinoma of the Bladder Found in Workers Employed in Tar Distilleries." *Zentralblatt für Arbeitsmedizin und Arbeitsschutz* 15:288–292.

Breslow, L. 1979. *A History of Cancer Control in the United States 1946–1971*. Appendix 9. Department of Health, Education, and Welfare pub. no. (NIH) 79-1519.

Bridge, J. C., and Henry, S. A. 1928. "Industrial Cancers." *Proceedings of the International Cancer Conference*. London: Wright Bristol.

Brodeur, P. 1985. *Outrageous Misconduct: The Asbestos Industry on Trial*. New York: Pantehon Books.

Case, R.A.M. 1966. "Tumors of the Urinary Tract as an Occupational Disease in Several Industries." *Annals of the Royal College of Surgeons of England* 39:213–235.

———. 1981. Letter in *Corporate Criminal Liability*. Hearings before the Subcommittee on Crime of the Committee on the Judiciary, U.S. House of Representatives 71:101–103.

———. 1983. *The Misbegotten Camel*. Unpublished manuscript.

Case, R.A.M.; Hosker, M. E.; McDonald, D. B.; and Pearson, J. T. 1954. "Tumours of the Urinary Bladder in Workmen Engaged in the Manufacture and Use of Certain Dyestuff Intermediates in the British Chemical Industry." *British Journal of Industrial Medicine* 11:75–96.

Castleman, B. T. 1979. "Du Pont's Record in Business Ethics: Another View." *Washington Post*, July 15, sec. E.

———. 1984. *Asbestos: Medical and Legal Aspects*. New York: Harcourt Brace Jovanovich.

E. I. duPont de Nemours and Co. 1952. *Du Pont: The Autobiography of an American Enterprise.* New York: Scribner's.

Ekman, B., and Strombeck, J. P. 1947. "Demonstration of Tumorigenic Decomposition Products of 2,3-Azotoluene." *Acta Physiologica Scandinavica* 14:43–50.

Epstein, S. S. 1975. "Presentation of the First Annual Award of the Society for Occupational and Environmental Health to Dr. Wilhelm C. Hueper." *Annals of the New York Academy of Sciences* 271:457–459.

Erni, P. 1979. *The Basel Marriage: History of the Ciba–Geigy Merger.* Zurich: Ciba–Giegy.

Evans, E. E. 1936. "Causative Agents and Protective Measures in the Anilin Tumor of the Bladder." *Journal of Urology* 38:212–215.

———. 1947. Letter to Dr. Arthur Mangelsdorff, June 18.

Ferber, K. H., Hill, W. J.; and Cobb, D. A. 1976. "An Assessment of the Effect of Improved Working Conditions on Bladder Tumor Incidence in a Benzidine Manufacturing Facility." *American Industrial Hygiene Association Journal* 37:61–68.

Fishbein, L. 1981. "Aromatic Amines of Major Industrial Importance: Use and Occurence." In *Environmental Carcinogens: Selected Methods of Analysis.* Vol. 4, *Some Aromatic Amines and Azo Dyes in the General and Industrial Environment,* ed. H. Egan, 3–113. Publication no. 40. Lyon, France: International Agency for Research on Cancer.

Fleming, A. J.; D'Alonzo, C. A.; and Zapp, J. A. 1954. *Modern Occupational Medicine.* Philadelphia: Lea and Febiger.

Gehrmann, G. H. 1934. "The Carcinogenic Agent: Chemistry and Industrial Aspects." *Journal of Urology* 31:126–137.

Gehrmann, G. H.; Foulger, J. H.; and Fleming, A. J. 1949. "Occupational Carcinoma of the Bladder." Ninth International Congress on Industrial Medicine, 472–475. London: Bristol Wright.

Goldwater, L. J.; Rosso, L. A.; and Kleinfeld, M. 1965. "Bladder Tumors in a Coal Tar Dye Plant." *Archives of Environmental Health* 11:814–817.

Graebner, W. 1987. "Hegemony Through Science: Information Engineering and Lead Toxicology, 1925–1965." In *Dying for Work: Workers' Safety and Health in Twentieth-Century America,* ed. D. Rosner and G. Markowitz, 140–159. Bloomington: Indiana University Press.

Homburger, F.; Friedell, G. H.; Weisburger, E. K.; and Weisburger, J. H. 1972. "Carcinogenicity of Simple Aromatic Amine Derivatives in Mice and Rats." *Toxicology and Applied Pharmacology* 22, no. 2:280.

Hounshell, D. A., and Smith, J. K. 1988. *Science and Corporate Strategy: Du Pont R & D, 1902–1980.* Cambridge: Cambridge University Press.

Hueper, W. C. n.d. Unpublished manuscript. Washington, D.C.: National Library of Medicine.

———. 1942. *Occupational Tumors and Allied Diseases.* Springfield, Ill.: Thomas.

———. 1969. *Occupational and Environmental Cancers of the Urinary System.* New Haven, Conn.: Yale University Press.

Hueper, W. C.; Wiley, F. H.; and Wolfe, H. D. 1938. "Experimental Production of Bladder Tumors in Dogs by Administration of Beta-Naphthylamine." *Journal of Industrial Hygiene and Toxicology* 20:46–84.

International Agency for Research on Cancer. 1982. *IARC Monographs on the Evaluation of the Carcinogenic Risk of Chemicals to Humans.* Vol. 27, *Some Aromatic Amines, Anthraquinones and Nitroso Compounds, and Inorganic Fluorides Used in Drinking-water and Dental Preparations.* Lyon, France: International Agency for Research on Cancer.

International Labour Office. 1921. *Cancer of the Bladder Among Workers in Aniline Factories.* Studies and Reports Series F, no. 1. Geneva.

Johnson, W. M., and Parnes, W. D. 1979. "Beta-Naphthylamine and Benzidine: Identification of Groups at High Risk of Bladder Cancer." *Annals of the New York Academy of Sciences* 329:277–284.

Khlebnikova, M. I.; Gladkova, Y.; Kurenko, L. T.; Pshenitsyn, A. V.; and Shalin, B. M. 1976. *Problems of Labor Hygiene and the State of Health of Workers in the Production of o-Toluidine.* Gorky, U.S.S.R.: Institute of Labor Hygiene and Occupational Diseases.

Kleinfeld, M. 1967. "Cancer of the Urinary Bladder in a Dye Plant." In *Bladder Cancer: A Symposium,* ed. W. B. Deichmann and K. F. Lampe, 136–143. Birmingham, Ala.: Aesculapius.

Kotelchuck, D. 1987. "Asbestos: 'The Funeral Dress of Kings'—and Others." In *Dying for Work: Workers' Safety and Health in Twentieth-Century America,* ed. D. Rosner and G. Markowitz, 192–197. Bloomington: Indiana University Press.

Lieben, J. 1963. "An Epidemiological Study of Occupational Bladder Cancer." *Acta Unio International Contra Cancrum* 19:749–750.

Maguigan, W. H. 1950. "Occupational Bladder Tumors." *Acta Unio International Contra Cancrum* 6 (suppl):1359–1364.

Markowitz, S., and Lyons, C. 1979. "Bladder Cancer at Bound Brook: Malignant Neglect." New York. Montefiore Medical Center Report.

Mason, T. J.; Prorok, P. C.; Neeld, W. E.; and Vogler, W. J. 1986. "Screening for Bladder Cancer at the Du Pont Chambers Works: Initial Findings." *Journal of Occupational Medicine* 28:1011–1016.

Meigs, J. W.; Brown, R. M.; and Sciarini, L. J. 1951. "A Study of Exposure to Benzidine and Substituted Benzidines in a Chemical Plant." *Archives of Industrial Hygiene and Occupational Medicine* 4:533–540.

Meigs, J. W.; Marrett, L. D.; Ulrich, F. U.; and Flannery, J. T. 1986. "Bladder Tumor Incidence Among Workers Exposed to Benzidine." *Journal of the National Cancer Institute* 76:1–8.

Morigami, S. and Nisimura, I. 1940. "Experimental Studies on Aniline Bladder Tumors." *Japanese Journal of Cancer Research (GANN)* 34:146–147.

Murray, W. M. 1973. Affidavit concerning 3,3'-dichlorobenzidine. Submitted to the U.S. Department of Labor, Occupational Safety and Health Administration, May 15.

National Cancer Institute. 1979. *Bioassay of o-Toluidine Hydrochloride for Possible Carcinogenicity.* Department of Health, Education, and Welfare pub. no. (NIH) 79–1709.

National Institute for Occupational Safety and Health. 1972. Field survey of Allied Chemical Corporation, Specialty Chemical Division, 340 Elk Street, Buffalo, N.Y., October 16.

———. 1980. *Special Occupational Hazard Review for Benzidine-Based Dyes.*

DHEW (NIOSH) publication no. 80-109. Washington, D.C.: Government Printing Office.

Norton, T. H. 1915. *Dyestuffs for American Textile and Other Industries.* U.S. Department of Commerce, Special Agent Series no. 96. Washington, D.C.: Government Printing Office.

Public Health Reports. 1965. "Pennsylvania Prohibits Beta-Naphthylamine Use." *Public Health Reports* 80:126.

Riggan, W. B.; Van Brugger, J.; Acquarella, J. F.; Beaubier, J.; and Mason, T. J. 1983. *U.S. Cancer Mortality Rates and Trends, 1950–1979* vol. 2. EPA 600/1-83-0156. Washington, D.C.: Government Printing Office.

Rosner, D., and Markowitz, G. 1985. "A 'Gift of God'?: The Public Health Controversey over Leaded Gasoline in the 1920s." *American Journal of Public Health* 75:344–351.

———. 1987. *Dying for Work: Workers' Safety and Health in Twentieth-Century America.* Bloomington: Indiana University Press.

Rubino, G. F.; Scansetti, G.; Piolatto, G.; and Pira, E. 1982. "The Carcinogenic Effect of Aromatic Amines: An Epidemiological Study on the Role of o-Toluidine and 4,4'-Methylene bis (2-Methylaniline) in Inducing Bladder Cancer in Man." *Environmental Research* 27:241–254.

Russfield, A. B.; Homburger, F.; Weisburger, E. K.; and Weisburger, J. H. 1973. "Further Studies on Carcinogenicity of Environmental Chemicals Including Simple Aromatic Amines." *Toxicology and Applied Pharmacology* 25:446.

Rye, W. A.; Woolrich, P. F.; and Zanes, R. P. 1970. "Facts and Myths Concerning Aromatic Diamine Curing Agents." *Journal of Occupational Medicine* 12:211–215.

Samuels, S. W. 1981. "The International Context of Carcinogen Regulation: Benzidine." *Banbury Report* 9:497–512.

Satani, Y.; Tanimura, T.; Nishimura, I.; and Isekawa, Y. 1941. "Clinical and Experimental Examination of Bladder Papillomas." *Japanese Journal of Cancer Research (GANN)* 35:275–276.

Scott, T. S. 1952. "The Incidence of Bladder Tumours in a Dyestuffs Factory." *British Journal of Industrial Medicine* 9:127–132.

———. 1962. *Carcinogenic and Chronic Toxic Hazards of Aromatic Amines.* Amsterdam: Elsevier.

Smith, D. T. 1958. "History of Beta Naphthylamine Manufacture: Chambers Works." Du Pont confidential memo, September 22.

Spitz, S.; Maguigan, W. H.; and Dobriner, K. 1950. "The Carcinogenic Action of Benzidine." *Cancer* 3:789–804.

Stern, F. B.; Murthy, L. I.; Beaumont, J. J.; Schulte, P. A.; and Halperin, W. E. 1985. "Notification and Risk Assessment for Bladder Cancer of a Cohort Exposed to Aromatic Amines: III. Mortality Among Workers Exposed to Aromatic Amines in the Last Beta-Naphthylamine Manufacturing Facility in the United States." *Journal of Occupational Medicine* 27:495–500.

Strombeck, J. P. 1946. "Azotoluene Bladder Tumors in Rats." *Journal of Pathology and Bacteriology* 58:275–278.

Temkin, I. S. 1963. *Industrial Bladder Carcinogenesis.* New York: Pergamon Press.

U.S. Tariff Commission. 1946. *Dyes: War Changes in Industry Series.* Report no. 19. Washington, D.C.: Government Printing Office.

Walker, B., and Gerber, A. 1981. "Occupational Exposure to Aromatic Amines: Benzidine and Benzidine-Based Dyes." *National Cancer Institute Monographs* 58:11–13.

Ward, E.; Carpenter, A.; Markowitz, S.; Roberts, D.; and Halperin, W. 1991. "Excess Number of Bladder Cancers in Workers Exposed to Ortho-Toluidine and Aniline." *Journal of the National Cancer Institute* 83, no. 7:501–506.

Washburn, V. D. 1936. "Abstract of Discussion." *Journal of the American Medical Association* 107:1438–1439.

Wignall, T. H. 1929. "Incidence of the Bladder in Workers in Certain Chemicals." *British Medical Journal* 2:291–293.

Young, M., and Russell, W. T. 1926. *An Investigation into the Statistics of Cancer in Different Trades and Professions.* London: Medical Research Council.

Zavon M.; Hoegg, U.; and Bingham, B. 1973. "Benzidine Exposure as a Cause of Bladder Tumors." *Archives of Environmental Health* 27:1–7.

Zwerling, C. 1987. "Salem Sarcoid: The Origins of Beryllium Disease." In *Dying for Work: Workers' Safety and Health in Twentieth-Century America,* ed. D. Rosner and G. Markowitz, 103–118. Bloomington: Indiana University Press.

• CHAPTER 4 •

Scrotal Cancer in Wax Pressmen

JOHN J. THORPE, M.D., and JOHN G. LIONE, M.D.

The development of scrotal cancers in petroleum workers preparing candle wax is a remarkable story recounted by two occupational health physicians who spent their careers with the Exxon Corporation. Drs. John J. Thorpe and John G. Lione describe the events that followed the discovery of a cluster of scrotal cancer cases in Standard Oil of New Jersey's Bayonne refinery in the midtwentieth century. The cancers occurred after ten years of exposure in 12 percent of the wax pressmen, almost all of whom were foreign born. The episode is reminiscent of the first recognition of occupational cancer in chimney sweeps almost two hundred years earlier and many subsequent miniepidemics of scrotal cancers among workers exposed to industrial oils. In this case report, the etiology was determined by the corporate medical staff. Standard Oil identified the source and attempted to modify the candle wax/lubricating oil production process until the development of a new manufacturing technology in 1951 obviated the need for wax pressmen. Debate on whether prevention of scrotal cancers required more hygienic working conditions or cleaner wax pressmen came to an end. The toxic circle was broken, at least in Bayonne.

Bayonne, a peninsular town extending into Newark Bay and the Kill van Kull, is part of the New York City–New Jersey harbor. A farming and fishing community in earlier times and a seaside resort for New Yorkers in the nineteenth century, the town was transformed into an industrial center in the early twentieth century. The "hook" section of the town juts into the bay and the Kill van Kull; here the oil companies settled—Standard Oil Company of New Jersey, the Gulf Oil Company, and the Tidewater Oil Company—attracted by the port and overland transport connections to New York and west (Thomas 1925). As in other East Coast cities, the turn of the century marked the migration of eastern and western Europeans to Bayonne. Polish immigrants formed a large component of the Standard Oil workforce. In July 1915, while Standard Oil was busily supplying oil to the

European countries engaged in World War I, a series of strikes for higher wages and better working conditions was led by Polish and Italian workers. At the time, no agreements regulated company–employee relations. Foremen decided hiring and firing policies, promotions, discipline, and work conditions as they saw fit, a system that often seemed arbitrary, capricious, and sometimes coercive to the workers (Dorsey 1976). A series of bloody confrontations ensued, ending in the fall of 1916. As a result, Standard Oil established an annuity and benefit plan, including death, accident, and sickness benefits. Personnel and training departments were created to handle wage and discipline policies and to provide oversight of working conditions (Dorsey 1976). These immigrant workers of an earlier period thus helped set the stage for an effective corporate response to the cluster of cases of scrotal cancer in wax pressmen half a century later.

• • •

UNDER ordinary circumstances, the receipt of a medical disability report from a petroleum refinery employee's private physician does not occasion much comment by the medical department staff. One day in 1947, however, at one of the original Standard Oil Company refineries in Bayonne, New Jersey, the staff member who reviewed one particular report remarked to a colleague that the diagnosis "cancer of the scrotum" was the second one he had seen within the last two months. The observation was relayed to the senior plant physician, who was aware that this condition was rarely seen in the general population, and its occurrence in an employee population of about twenty-five hundred required more than routine investigation. His concern increased markedly when a review of the medical files of both employees with this diagnosis indicated that not only did they both work in the wax production area of the plant but also that both were wax pressmen.

Thus begins a story that recalls the history of one of the first cancers attributed to occupational exposure and its reappearance in several settings during the Industrial Revolution. The story also illustrates how a number of social factors affected what appeared superficially to be a straightforward clinical problem. This chapter summarizes the clinical, epidemiologic, industrial hygiene, and experimental studies that these two index cases generated. A historical review of scrotal cancer follows, as well as a social portrait of Bayonne. The development of medical care systems in the private, company, state, and federal sectors is also presented, with an explanation of the role these entities could have played in earlier recognition and prevention of this problem. Finally, some explanations of why the connection between exposure, social context, and the specific disease process was not recognized earlier are offered.

Returning to the story of the index cases: the preliminary information was rather quickly passed up through the two higher echelons of the company medical organization. Within a short time, the refinery medical staff of two physicians, nurses, and secretarial personnel was receiving assistance from new staff at the company's headquarters, namely, a toxicologist, two industrial hygienists, and an assistant medical director. Local and higher-management personnel were concerned and supportive. Operating and technical people were made available to help gather job classification and employment history information requested by the medical personnel. Six steps were taken in examining the work environment of the wax pressmen and in attempting to resolve the problems identified in the review. These were as follows:

1. A review of the entire wax-manufacturing operation. The method for obtaining wax from an oil substrate was developed about 1850 by James Young in Britain and was first applied to shale oil (Benton 1956). With the discovery of practical commercial production of petroleum by well-drilling in the United States in 1857, a less expensive substrate for wax production became available. By 1867, the first recorded commercial paraffin wax production from petroleum began in Corry, Pennsylvania. The technique used at that time involved hanging large canvas bags filled with an oil of high wax content in commercial ice boxes. As the oil oozed out of the bags, chilled, solidified wax remained behind, where it could be harvested (Zwicker 1988).

After several years of experimentation with solvent extraction of the oil fraction by means of solvents such as gasoline in conjunction with chilling, a method was developed in the 1880s that became standard well into the next century. Not long after, this new "wax-pressing" method was installed at the Standard Oil Company Bayonne refinery (Hidy 1955). The new method involved initial fractional distillation of a paraffinic crude oil to remove the most volatile portions, and then separation of the middle oily fraction from the heavy bottoms containing tar, pitch, and so on. The oily fraction, containing the wax, was then cooled by refrigeration in what were known as Carbondale or Vogt chillers, which caused the wax to come out of solution in a fine suspension. This material in turn was pumped into Moore presses under high pressure so that the oil oozed out into small spaces between alternating steel and canvas discs. As the temperature was lowered further, the wax was deposited on the canvas discs. The pressure was held at a high level for many hours until much of the oil was removed. At that point, the pressure was reduced to normal so that the discs could be separated manually by the pressmen, using steel scrapers to knock the wax off the canvas into a trough below. There a screw conveyor moved the wax to another area for further processing. During the process just described, the wax contained between 20 and 40 percent oil, some of which invariably contaminated the iron bars located on either side of the press. Removing the wax and shifting the steel discs was heavy work, and for the pressmen to avoid contacting the bar at groin level was practically impossible (Figure 4.1). As a result, work clothing quickly became oil soaked, as did the skin of the lower abdomen and genitalia. Although the men made some effort to protect the area by tying gunnysacks over their clothing, investigation revealed that the clothing still became oil soaked. Furthermore, many of the pressmen cleaned their clothes infrequently and did not bathe on a regular basis.

Subsequent steps in handling the slack wax, which, as noted, still contained 20 to 40 percent oil, reduced the oil content to about 0.5 percent. The last step in the process was the production of large cakes of wax, warm liquid wax, and flake wax for sale to intermediate manufacturers of consumer products. During these later steps in wax manufacture, employee contact with the product was minimal, except for the large wax cakes, which were hand carried to bags or boxes for final packaging (Hendricks et al. 1959; Lione and Denholm 1959).

2. A review of the medical records of all employees who had worked one day or more at the refinery beginning January 1, 1937. The review was carried forward through December 31, 1956. This effort yielded a total of eleven cases of squamous cell carcinoma of the scrotum over the twenty-year period. All occurred within a group of eighty-two men who had worked as wax pressmen (Hendricks et al. 1959). Detailed clinical studies made on ten of these employees (see Table 4.1) were summarized as follows: the age of onset varied from forty-seven to sixty-two years; the average being fifty-six years. The period of potential exposure to unrefined wax varied from fourteen to thirty-seven years. The average potential exposure was approximately twenty-three years. No case of carcinoma of the scrotum occurred in wax pressmen with fewer than ten years of exposure to crude wax. Recurrences were not infrequent, as shown by the development of eight additional lesions in four of the patients. Metastases occurred in three members of the group. Of the ten reported cases, nine occurred in persons of foreign birth, but practically all wax pressmen were of foreign birth. There was surprisingly little labor turnover on the presses; hence, men working forty years as pressmen were by no means a rarity. Generally, personal hygiene was poor in the entire group (Lione and Denholm 1959).

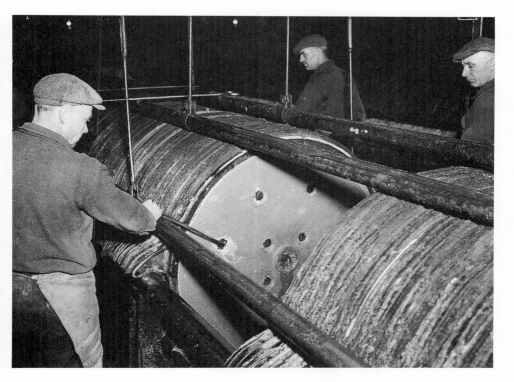

FIGURE 4.1. A team of four wax pressmen is separating the steel discs and canvas filters to which the slack wax clings. The wax is being knocked off the canvas to fall into a screw conveyor below. Note the steel bar of the press frame, which became coated with oil during the pressing phase of the operation. From time to time the pressmen leaned over this at groin level and their trousers became soaked with oil. The pressman on this side of the frame wears a burlap gunnysack in an effort to protect himself from the oil. From Hendricks et al. 1959. Reprinted with permission of the Helen Dwight Reid Educational Foundation. Published by Heldref Publications, 1319 18th Street, N.W., Washington, D.C. 20036-1802. Copyright 1959.

As shown in Table 4.2, the age-adjusted cancer incidence for the entire refinery population was the same as that for the general population. The incidence for the wax department population, exclusive of the wax pressmen group, was slightly higher than the general population but not significantly so. The handlers of finished wax had no cancers of the skin in areas that had actual contact with the wax.

TABLE 4.1

Data from Ten Cases of Cancer of the Scrotum

Case no.	Age at original diagnosis, yr.	Yrs. potential exposure	Birthplace	Status	Remarks
1	53	14	Ireland	Died, age 55	Died of cancer of scrotum
2	56	28	Poland	Living, age 67	3 lesions "cured"
3	62	22	Poland	Died, age 65	Extensive surgery, died of cancer of scrotum
4	58	31	Italy	Living, age 67	3 lesions "cured"
5	53	32	Lithuania	Living, age 62	3 lesions "cured"
6	58	20	Poland	Living, age 67	3 lesions "cured"
7	58	20	U.S.A.	Living, age 66	1 lesion "cured"
8	56	18	Poland	Living, age 70	1 lesion "cured"
9	59	37	Poland	Died, age 65	Died 6 years later of coronary thrombosis
10	47	15	Poland	Died, age 51	Died 2 years later of cancer of stomach

SOURCE: Hendricks et al. 1959. Reprinted with permission of the Helen Dwight Reid Educational Foundation. Published by Heldref Publications, 1319 18th Street, N.W., Washington, D.C. 20036-1802. Copyright 1959.

TABLE 4.2
Incidence of Cancer Among Workers Engaged in Wax Manufacturing

Group	Average annual rate/100,000
General white male population	338.0[a]
Refinery workers as a whole	338.0
Wax department workers so engaged 10 years or more	563
Pressmen so engaged 10 years or more	1,383
Wax department workers engaged in wax manufacturing 10 years or more (exclusive of pressmen so engaged 10 years or more)	402

SOURCE: Hendricks et al. 1959. Reprinted with permission of the Helen Dwight Reid Educational Foundation. Published by Heldref Publications, 1319 18th Street, N.W., Washington, D.C. 20036-1802. Copyright 1959. [a]Donn, H. F., and Cutler, S. J. 1955. "*Morbidity from Cancer in the United States,*" pt. 1. Public Health Monograph no. 29. Public Health Series no. 418, p. 12.

Some additional steps were taken, not long after the original cases came to light.

3. Communication to employees. Once the industrial hygiene review had indicated what the probable route of exposure was and what could be done to remedy it, the situation was reviewed with the pressmen and the refinery union.

4. Introduction of personal protective measures. Pressmen were provided with protective rubber aprons, double-layered long underwear (which was laundered by the company each day), separate lockers for street clothes and work clothes, and a changing room equipped with showers. An intensive campaign was carried out to persuade the men to take showers after work "on company time."

5. Introduction of frequent skin examinations. Pressmen were seen in the medical department at intervals of three months, at which time a complete skin examination was done. If any suspicious skin lesions were noted, the employee was referred to a consulting specialist for an opinion and, where indicated, a biopsy, at company expense. Several of the cancers that developed after the signal scrotal malignancies were detected by these special examinations. Some of these cancers developed within a very short period of time and were promptly removed. In a few instances, several new lesions developed in other areas. In addition to paying special attention to the wax pressmen, the medical staff emphasized the importance of

complete examination of the skin during regularly scheduled periodic examinations of other refinery employees (Lione and Denholm 1959).

6. Expansion of toxicologic studies. In 1945, the company had contracted with the Sloan–Kettering Institute for Cancer Research to carry out studies on high-boiling aromatic oils derived from catalytic cracking. Soon after the scrotal cancer problem surfaced, samples of slack wax were added to the list of materials under test. The samples proved to have a low order of carcinogenicity in mice. When extracts of the oil from the slack wax were tested, however, they showed much greater potency (Smith et al. 1951). On the other hand, subsequent studies of purified wax (less than 0.5 percent residual oil) at Sloan–Kettering and by other investigators confirmed the fact that the purified wax was noncarcinogenic (Shubik et al. 1962).

Technological Changes in Wax Manufacture

Although not specifically related to the scrotal cancer problem under discussion, a new method for extracting wax from the middle cut of paraffinic crude had been under development for some time. This new process, introduced into the refinery in 1951, eliminated the wax presses and the jobs of wax pressmen. The new technology involved solvent extraction of the oil by methyl ethyl ketone and was carried out in a closed system, making worker contact with the oil unnecessary. This process eliminated the more stringent elements of the personal protective program described above (that is, rubber aprons and gloves), but the importance of personal hygiene continued to be stressed and the skin examination program was continued (Hendricks et al. 1959).

Historical Review of Scrotal Cancer

Kipling and colleagues believe that the first pathological description of scrotal malignancy should be credited to Treyling, who in 1740 described the condition in a Bavarian cavalryman (Kipling et al. 1970). Although Treyling raised the question whether chronic irritation from the saddle played a major causative role, most medical historians have felt that the first definitive description of the occupational nature of the lesion was published by Sir Percival

Pott, a distinguished English surgeon. In 1775, in "Chirurgical Observations," Pott noted that he had seen the lesion fairly often in chimney sweeps (Waldron 1983:390). He related it to the appalling life histories of many of the sweeps he had treated. Most of them began working as sweeps when they were young children, as they were small enough to crawl up and down the narrow, angular chimneys built in London after the Great Fire of 1666. Their clothes, of poor quality, were rarely cleaned; the sweeps frequently slept in them. They had no decent bathing facilities, and as a result, the soot to which they were exposed was ground into their skin. Pott believed that the long-term lodgment of soot in the rugae of the scrotum produced enough irritation to result in the malignant lesion. A number of surgeons who began to report cases after Pott's initial report appeared to accept his observation but puzzled over the fact that most of the patients were in their thirties or forties before the lesions appeared. They also could not explain why most sweeps did not develop the cancer or, if they did, why the lesion might not appear for a decade or two after they moved on to some more fortunate occupation. Another fact, not studied until the late nineteenth century, was why this ailment was not seen in chimney sweeps on the Continent. Henry Butlin, a surgeon at St. Bartholomew's Hospital in London, studied this question from 1889 through 1891 (Butlin 1892). In Holland, Belgium, Germany, and Switzerland, the chimney sweeps wore outer work clothing and hoods or woolen caps, which they removed after work; they then scrubbed their entire bodies thoroughly with soap and hot water. Cancer of the scrotum was very rarely seen at all in the hospitals and not more often in sweeps than in other people. In northern France and Paris, where Butlin considered the clothing and the personal hygiene of the "lower classes" inferior to that of the rest of northern Europe, but still better than that of England, he felt that the brown coal or wood used there was not as "nocuous" as the hard coal used in the other areas. Various theories about the mechanism of irritation and the existence of a specific cancer-inducing agent in soot were debated in the late nineteenth and early twentieth centuries. In 1922, R. D. Passey settled the matter by inducing skin tumors in mice with repeated application of ether extracts of soot (Passey 1922).

In light of our interest in the social factors that relate to the occurrence of occupational cancer, we must go back to the early days after Pott's publication of his observations on the life of a chimney sweep. By the beginning of the nineteenth century, the reformers of the Industrial Revolution added the sweeps' cause to the list of changes they desired. In 1803, a society was formed to substitute in place of boys a mechanical method for cleaning chimneys. This proposed reform made little headway until a committee of the House of Commons introduced it in an act in 1817. The proposal was passed by the House of Commons but vetoed by the House of Lords in response to heavy lobbying by fire insurers and master chimney sweeps. Success came to the reformers in 1840 when a bill banning the use of boys passed and took effect in 1842. The custom of using young sweeps continued in other parts of the country, however, for at least twenty years. Even then, the incidence of cancer of the scrotum remained higher in sweeps than in any other occupational group in Britain until the 1940s (Waldron 1983).

The challenge of chimney soot had scarely been recognized and attempts at control made when another agent appeared on the scrotal cancer scene. In 1873, von Volkmann, speaking at the Third Surgical Congress in Berlin, described three cases of scrotal cancer in workmen engaged in brown-coal tar and paraffin manufacture (von Volkmann 1875). The cancers were described as identical in clinical course and anatomical structure to the chimney sweeps' cancer in Britain. The growing use of coal-derived tar, pitch, and paraffin worldwide led to a growing number of scrotal cancer case reports over the next fifty years. By 1907, "scrotal epitheliomata occurring in chimney sweeps and epitheliomatous cancer or ulceration of the skin occurring in the handling or use of pitch, tar and tarry compounds" was added to the Third Schedule of the Workmen's Compensation Act in Britain (Waldron 1983). These clinical case reports led to increased efforts to identify the active carcinogenic agents by a number of laboratory research scientists using animal models. Hanau in Germany is credited with the first attempts in 1889, using the rat as the test animal (Hanau 1889). His efforts were unsuccessful, as were those of a number of other scientists, until 1914 when Yamagiwa and Ichikawa succeeded in producing papillomas on rabbit ears by the repeated application of coal tar (Yamagiwa and Ichikawa 1918). In the 1920s and 1930s, Kennaway narrowed the probable causes down to high-boiling tar fractions and then showed that synthetic pure 1,2,5,6-dibenzanthracene could produce skin tumors in mice (Kennaway 1925). His work was subsequently extended by Cook and co-workers, who isolated benzo(a)pyrene from pitch and showed it to be highly carcinogenic in mice (Cook et al. 1932).

Two additional materials used in the latter half of the nineteenth century must be considered in relation to scrotal cancer. The first, oil derived from shale, made a relatively brief and geographically localized appearance in 1850 in Scotland. It was a source for naphtha (used as a solvent), lubricating oil, and solid paraffin. The method of extracting and separating the latter two compounds required a refrigerating and pressing technique that, as noted previously, was later applied to petroleum. James Bell described cases of scrotal cancer in shale oil workers in 1876 (Bell 1876–77). A total of thirty-one cases were ascribed to this material in the period 1900 to 1921 (Scott 1922). Other cases of scrotal cancer were reported in the textile industry, initially related to exposure to shale oil but later to lubricating oil derived from petroleum. The lesions were called "mule spinner's cancer" because they developed from contact of the groin of a mule spinner leaning against an oil-soaked "faller bar" to repair broken threads in the yarn being spun (Leitch 1924). The "mule" is the spindle on which the yarn is wound.

Although because of competition from petroleum-derived oil the use of shale oil diminished markedly by 1872, some was still made in Scotland until 1962, supported by government subsidy (Waldron 1983). Thus, while a relatively small number of cases of scrotal cancer were attributed to shale oil, a growing number of cases reported in the latter part of the nineteenth century and first quarter of the twentieth century were causally ascribed to "mineral oil," the name given to lubricants derived from petroleum. By 1914, the British Workmen's Compensation Act schedule included cancers associated with exposure to "bitumen, mineral oil or paraffin or any compounds or products or residue of any of these substances." During the 1920s, the number of scrotal cancer cases in the textile industry approached epidemic proportions, causing the Home Office to appoint a committee to study the problem. In 1926, only a year after it was appointed, the committee identified spindle oil as the culprit and recommended protective measures and periodic medical examinations every four months (Henry 1946). In addition, animal research was carried out over the next twenty years and demonstrated that various oils had different carcinogenic potencies (Twort and Twort 1930). By 1945, lighter oils were thought to be less harmful, but this was not universally true. By 1954, however, inert white oils could be manufactured consistently, and their use in textile manufacture was mandated by law (Waldron 1983).

The story of spindle oils was repeated at a later date with cutting oils, which were essential for technological progress in the metal-working industry. Although not directly related to the story of the wax pressmen, it is of interest that a 1987 study of Swedish metal workers exposed to cutting fluids for at least five years during the period 1958 to 1983 yielded seven cases of scrotal cancer in 250 "turners," where no cases would be expected. All worked with straight cutting oils. On the other hand, no cases of scrotal cancer occurred in 559 "grinders," who used emulsified mineral oils (Jarvholm and Lavenius 1987).

Wax Pressmen
and Their Community Environment

The city of Bayonne, New Jersey, the site of the refinery where the story of the wax pressmen unfolded, is located on a peninsula between Upper New York Bay and Newark Bay, in northeastern New Jersey. Temporary settlements by Dutch traders with the Indians of the area date back to 1614. By 1654, permanent grants of land were given by the Dutch government to more permanent settlers; the city considers this the date of its official founding. Over the next two hundred years Bayonne was a pleasant village with a maximum population of about five hundred whose main livelihood came from farming or fishing. The majority were of Dutch or English ancestry, with the addition of a few Irish and German families who arrived in the early part of the nineteenth century. In the second quarter of the nineteenth century, large estates were built on the waterfront properties and a small hotel did a thriving weekend and vacation business. For a time, the town was known as the "Newport of New York."

With the extension of the Central Railroad of New Jersey from the mainland of New Jersey across the inner bay to Bayonne, the area became economically attractive for industrial expansion. By the last quarter of the nineteenth century, several oil refineries had been built and extensive dock facilities constructed, and many new manufacturing companies were in business. All of these enterprises needed people to make them function. By 1880, the population reached 9,372, and by 1904, it was 41,000 and still growing. The increase in population came primarily from immigration from Europe. Unpropertied people left their homelands because the agrarian economies could not support them. The Industrial Revolution in those countries reduced them to the level of slavery and many political systems removed their freedom and their cultural heritage. America was the "land of opportunity," a dream reinforced by letters from relatives who had crossed the Atlantic earlier, by steamship advertising, and by the glowing promises of labor recruiters. The first major influx came from Ireland in the 1840s and 1850s as a result of the potato famine and, from the late 1860s into the 1880s, in response to job scarcity and political oppression. Germans came after the suppression of the 1848 revolution and again about the time of the Franco–Prussian War. In the 1890s, an influx of immigrants from the Austro–Hungarian empire, Russia, Poland, and the Baltic States began, and shortly afterward from Italy and other Mediterranean countries (Sinclair 1940; Robinson 1961). Many of these newcomers had come from rural communities or overcrowded cities where educational opportunities were limited. Those who had trade skills or professions found opportunities to exercise them. The majority, however, qualified only for unskilled jobs at low pay.

By the second decade of the twentieth century, the Standard Oil workforce in Bayonne was predominantly of central and eastern European origin. In October 1915, 30 percent of these employees could not read, write, or speak English (Gibb and Knowlton 1956). Housing was in short supply, with many buildings overcrowded. The infrastructure of the community could not keep pace with the demands of an increasing population. The first city water supply, constructed in 1881, was unfit to drink and was used only for manufacturing purposes. The first garbage collection began about 1890. Living conditions in Bayonne were described as follows:

> The houses were crowded with hard-working people who were glad to have homes so near their jobs. Modern bathrooms were mostly unknown. Behind the rows of houses stood rows of small structures characteristic of "backyard plumbing." Only a few houses had . . . city water piped to faucets and sinks. The houses on the side streets . . . relied on several central street-side faucets and a few wells. From these the housewife and the older children had to carry

in pails and buckets every drop of water used in cooking, washing and bathing. (Robinson 1961:no page no.)

The writer describes the problems of heating these dwellings with one large coal-fired stove. Small wonder that workers in the nearby factories, refineries, and presumably wax presses did not bathe or change their work clothes frequently!

Although significant improvements in water supply and sewage disposal occurred as time went on, these changes may have taken place in newer parts of the city sooner than in the older sections. Records show that the old part of the city described above was razed after World War I to make room for industrial expansion. Although a private sector Bayonne Housing Corporation, financed by a number of major industries including Standard Oil Company, completed one hundred units of model garden apartments by 1925, what happened to the refinery workers in the meantime is not clear (Thomas 1925). We do not know how many of these workers were able to secure apartments in the new housing. And there is no documentation of what changes occurred in their personal hygiene when, and if, they relocated to better housing.

Hygienic conditions in the refineries into the first part of the twentieth century were not significantly different from the home environment described above.

Little attention was paid to sanitation, little thought to personal comfort or health protection. Crudely constructed latrines were few and far between. Drinking water was carried to the men by water boys equipped with galvanized tin pails and long-handled tin dippers, which were promiscuously used by thirsty workers. . . . Soap and water were seldom used as the water faucets were scarce. This indeed was a heyday for bacteria. (Goodrich 1939:14)

Medical Resources in Bayonne

In the latter part of the nineteenth century and the first half of the twentieth century, Bayonne was served by physicians in general practice, a number of whom performed surgery when the first hospital and dispensary with forty beds opened its doors in 1890. As time passed, the profession followed a pattern similar to that of cities with populations between 50,000 and 100,000. Specialization appeared, at first based on individual physicians limiting their practices to specific areas in which they had a particular interest. Initially, special training was obtained by apprenticeship with an older, experienced practitioner and later by special didactic training at metropolitan teaching centers. After the establishment of specialty organizations (for example, the American College of Surgeons and the American Board of Internal Medicine), residency training for a number of years at approved teaching hospitals became the standard in medical education. While the local hospitals provided primary and secondary care, highly specialized care was usually obtained at medical centers, teaching hospitals, or specialty hospitals in nearby locations in the New York metropolitan area.

While this sketch presents a simplified overview of medical practice in a small city like Bayonne, it serves to emphasize the focus on curative medicine. Injuries, burns, suffocations, and electrical shock would generally be regarded as occupational in origin, provided they occurred on the job. Medical disorders, like silicosis and asbestosis, would not be so categorized until the early 1940s. Skin diseases, including skin cancer, were treated; however, their etiology was not ascribed to job exposure unless immediate cause and effect was clearly evident. Preventive medicine meant immunization against smallpox, quarantine of infectious disease patients, and early diagnosis and treatment of tuberculosis, not the identification of certain kinds of cancer with job exposure.

In the refinery itself, no organized medical care was provided prior to 1905. In principle, employees were expected to arrange for their own care and to pay for it whether the health problem had any relationship to their work or not. In practice, in the case of obvious, serious work-related injuries, local management authority paid for medical care and wage loss on a case-by-case basis (Hidy and Hidy 1955:595). If no help was offered, the employee had the right to sue under tort law, but few had the knowledge or the money to do this. After the state Workmen's Compensation Law came into existence in 1911, the company was obliged to pay for care and also wage loss in instances of work-related disability.

In 1905, the first refinery-supported first aid program began. Management assigned this task as an additional responsibility to a clerk in the boiler shop. The clerk had no previous, or subsequent, medical training and was expected to use "his good judgement and common sense" (Goodrich 1939). A healing salve, hydrogen peroxide, cotton, and bandages constituted his therapeutic equipment. When he considered the problem a "serious" one, he sent the employee to the local hospital. In what appeared to be minor problems, the employee was on his own. He could decide, if he wished, to consult his own physician or not. By 1907, the first-aider had acquired a wooden box containing additional items such as scissors; tinctures of ginger, arnica, and iodine; and carbolic acid and iodoform. He could take this kit to provide treatment at the scene of the emergency. By 1913, a full-time physician and clerk were employed; they worked in a large room in the labor department building. In 1914, a Ford ambulance was purchased and, in 1916, a new three-room medical building was built. Two aid men were employed to provide coverage for two shifts, from 4:00 P.M. to 8:00 A.M. (Goodrich 1939) In theory, the medical staff was to provide care only for occupational injuries. In practice, the staff undoubtedly took care of nonoccupational problems that occurred at work. It is unlikely that in the early days much of the time of the medical department personnel was devoted to preventive aspects of employee health.

These responsibilities changed, however, in 1918, when the Standard Oil Company of New Jersey headquarters in New York acquired a medical director. Appointment of a medical director was related to the implementation of a new, companywide employee benefit program. This significant social agenda was undertaken to address the underlying causes of the serious strikes at the Bayonne refinery in 1915 and 1916. The program included disability allowances, retirement pensions, centralized employment and placement, training, a stock purchase plan, and death benefits (Gibb and Knowlton 1956). While the creation of a central medical department, with coordinating responsibility for field units—refineries, pipelines, ships—was tied in with administration of the disability program, the first medical director, Willard J. Denno, had a strong background in preventive medicine and public health. His principal consultant, W. Gilman Thompson, a professor of medicine at Cornell Medical College, organized the first occupational health clinic in the United States in 1910. Thompson, the author of "Occupational Diseases," was also a consultant in industrial hygiene to the United States Public Health Service (USPHS) ("Medical Service Staff" 1918). Thompson was an internist with a broad-based knowledge of, and interest in, preventive medicine and brought credibility as well as expertise to the new medical program. These individuals played a role in the development of a medical policy that called for preplacement physical examinations and periodic examination programs, immunizations, and health education programs for employees ("Medical Service" 1918).

Over the next two decades, despite the pressures of economic depressions, the medical department increased its personnel to meet the demands of the new program. Initially, the emphasis was on the control of infectious diseases, particularly tuberculosis. A special program developed for victims of this disease included payment for hospitalization in company-sponsored beds in a nationally known sanitorium in Liberty, New York. Programs were also developed for the control of potential exposure to toxic materials such as lead, benzene, and silica. It is ironic to note that cancer began to be recognized as a potential health hazard subsequent to the Tworts' report on the induction of cancer by the repeated application of cracked mineral oil to the skin of mice in 1935 (Twort and Twort 1935). Catalytic cracking was believed to be able to produce cancer-causing compounds, whereas the old process of wax pressing was overlooked. This report stimulated a special survey on skin cancer carried out that very year on employees potentially exposed to petroleum products in refineries. When no unusual number of cases were discovered, the special examinations were incorporated into the regular periodic program (Wade et al. 1951). With the onset of World War II, a number of medical department employees entered the armed forces, and no replacements were obtainable. The refinery medical departments carried out the basic parts of the program with emphasis on keeping as many employees on the job as possible. No special clinical investigative programs could be initiated during this critical period.

At Standard Oil headquarters and among company researchers, however, there was concern about the potential health impact of high-boiling, catalytically cracked aromatic compounds. Catalytic cracking was a new technology introduced in the early 1940s; it had the potential for accelerating the development of the petrochemical side of the industry. The probability that the production of potentially carcinogenic compounds would grow undoubtedly resulted in the start of animal testing of these compounds at Sloan–Kettering Institute for Medical Research, referred to previously. It may have played a role in the decision to add a toxicologist and an industrial hygienist to the headquarters' medical department staff in the immediate postwar period.

The Role of Government Agencies in Health

The role of government during the early years of the growth of the refinery, at the top of its growth curve, and at the time when the scrotal cancer problem became evident is not clear. Initially, the growth of all types of industry in the late nineteenth century proceeded without much local government regulation. Industry provided jobs and a secure tax base. In exchange, the city provided basic sanitary services and the fire and police protection available to all taxpayers. There is no evidence that local authorities intruded on day-to-day operations of industries like the refinery.

The state government assumed more responsibility for overseeing certain aspects of industrial operations. Details of the evolution of the state Department of Labor from the Bureau of Statistics of Labor and Industry and, later, a Factory Inspectorate are covered in other sections of this volume. Initial reports of the New Jersey Factory Inspector on the employment of children in industry are reminiscent of Dickens's novels of the early Industrial Revolution era (New Jersey 1883). Standard Oil's Bayonne refinery appears on the list of industries inspected during the years 1891 through 1903. Apart from occasional notations about a few unguarded machine belts, the general working conditions were described as good (New Jersey 1884–1904). A review of the state worksite inspections indicates that the wax-pressing operation drew no adverse comment.

New Jersey was the fourth state to enact compensation laws, in 1911, but in 1914, it was the first state in which such laws withstood the test of constitutionality (New Jersey 1956–57). Initially, the administration of the new laws was carried out by the Employers' Liability Commission, which in the course of a few years evolved into a bureau, and then a Division of Workmen's Compensation in the Department of Labor. In the beginning, the major focus of Workmen's Compensation was on gross physical trauma to limbs, eyes, and brain, secondary to mechanical accidents, fires, and explosions. As time went on, loss of function or disability due to falling, lifting, bending, and so on, was included. With the recognition that disability could be related to disease caused by exposure to certain materials, these diseases were added by name to the accepted causes for occupational disability—for example, silicosis and asbestosis. Finally, in 1949, as the number of disease entities that could be ascribed to occupational exposure continued to grow, the legisla-

ture amended the law to "make compensable all occupational diseases contracted as a result of exposure hazards in employment but
only when exposure stated has occurred during employment; ex-
punges from present act enumeration of specific diseases which are
compensable" (New Jersey 1949:18). Under this broadened coverage of the Workmen's Compensation Law, individuals suffering
from cancer of the scrotum had their medical bills paid and received
disability benefits.

Of particular interest to this story is the start in July 1941 of an
industrial hygiene program within the New Jersey Department of
Health, with a staff of two physicians, a nurse, an engineer, a
chemist, a technician, and a clerk. The growth of industries during
World War II, at first supplying the anti-Axis forces in Europe and
later helping the American defense effort, accounts for the development of this specialized program. In the first twelve months of its
existence, this unit carried out 246 inventories of 168 large and small
plants and began an industrial employee chest X-ray survey program (New Jersey 1942). In 1943, this activity acquired the status of
Bureau of Industrial Hygiene Service (New Jersey 1944). In 1944,
the bureau began to operate an industrial hygiene laboratory, and
by 1945 it had surveyed by questionnaire the status of health services in all plants with over one hundred employees. Of the 1,452
plants queried, 1,317 (90.7 percent) cooperated in the survey (New
Jersey 1945). By 1944, the organization was known as the Bureau of
Industrial Health, which in turn became the Division of Adult and
Industrial Health in 1946. By 1947, a new, separate Division of
Cancer Control came into being (New Jersey 1947). Over the next
few years the Department of Health underwent repeated reorganization with many name changes as well as shifts in organizational
reporting levels. What effect all this reshuffling had on efficiency is
unknown, but it certainly obscured the history of the health department's development when reviewed forty years later! The problem
of tracing the history of the multiple departments' work is exemplified by the fate of a cancer survey in industry undertaken in 1952
with the support of a USPHS grant. The annual report for 1952
describes the study as being in its final stages of the analysis of 663
cancer deaths in 415 industrial plants in the state. Three succeeding
annual reports do not mention the study, nor are there any traces of
it in the Records Retention Division of the Health Department or
the State Archives Department. One may surmise that the study

results were either negative or inconclusive (New Jersey 1952). No reports of a scrotal cancer problem appear in the annual reports from 1948 through 1956.

At the federal government level, industrial health concerns during the first half of the twentieth century centered on the collection of statistical data. Vital statistics on the general population by age, sex, and cause of death according to accepted diagnostic categories provided a base upon which to evaluate statistics collected on occupational populations. Federal data also included reporting of occupational and nonoccupational injury and illness data in various types of occupations. A study entitled "Cancer Mortality in the U.S.: Trends 1900–1935" concerned itself with the experience of the general population (Gover 1939). Only one other federal study, by the USPHS, entitled "Disabling Morbidity and Mortality from Cancer Among Male Employees of an Oil Refining Company with Reference to Age, Site, and Duration, 1933–38, Inclusive," was published (Gafafer and Sitgreaves 1940). In this report, seventy cases of cancer were recorded in a population with 60,000 exposure years over a 5-year period. Forty-six of these died. Almost 70 percent of the deaths were related to the digestive system. No cancers of the genitourinary system were noted; in particular, no scrotal cancers (Gafafer and Sitgreaves 1940).

During World War II, the federal government's concern about occupational exposure to potentially toxic materials led to the development of industrial hygiene as a major discipline in the occupational health team. Occupational cancer, however, was not an important topic for concern until after World War II.

Conclusion

This review of a relatively small group of workers with an uncommon neoplasm, cancer of the scrotum, in a single, large oil refinery during the mid 1940s and 1950s illustrates the complexity of recognizing illness caused by occupationally related cancer. From the time cancer of the scrotum was first associated with occupation, over two hundred years ago in Britain, it was apparent that the social aspects of its occurrence were as important as the pure exposure factor. British chimney sweeps and their helpers faced dirty and dangerous working conditions; their housing and sanitary conditions were equally bad. The latent period for the development of scrotal cancer was long, and the termination of their exposure provided no guarantee that they would not develop the disease many years later. After seventy-five years of struggle, laws were enacted to minimize exposure; over time, the number of cases appeared to decrease. The occurrence of more than the expected number of cases in sweeps, however, continued for another hundred years. The fact that scrotal cancer did not occur more often than "background" in chimney sweeps on the Continent, where workers used their clothing in a protective manner and supplemented this with rigorous personal cleanliness, indicates the role of individual habits in disease prevention. Basic patterns of personal hygiene were among the only effective measures in the absence of legislation regulating workplace conditions.

The occurrence of scrotal cancers in Scottish shale extraction operators and, later, in workers involved with oil from brown coal or petroleum from which wax was then removed reinforced the link between poor personal hygiene and the disease. The story was repeated with mule spinners' cancer (scrotal cancer) and contact with lubricants in the British textile industry. Later, a similar relationship appeared with certain cutting oils used in metal working. The Swedish experience of the 1950s and 1960s suggests that this particular hazard was not understood universally. In the first quarter of the twentieth century, the discovery, through animal experiments, that the active carcinogens were aromatic hydrocarbons demonstrated the common thread linking all the cited incidents. While intellectually satisfying, this finding did not diminish the contributing role of social factors in exacerbating workers' exposure to these agents.

With the benefit of hindsight and the landmark reviews of Henry (1946) and Waldron (1983) as well as a significant body of research since the 1940s, one may wonder why the scrotal cancer story in Europe was repeated in Bayonne. Several possible explanations are offered here.

The pace of industrial development in the late nineteenth and twentieth centuries emphasized worker productivity, not safety or comfort. Concerns about work conditions changed in the Standard Oil Company at New Jersey companies after 1918, with the introduction of the progressive employee benefit program (Gibb and Knowlton 1956). Off-the-job lifestyle patterns, such as good personal hygiene, were not immediate concerns of the newly formed workplace medical department. The rapid influx of immigrants, many of them from poor agricultural or city slum environments, created competition for the dirty, heavy-labor jobs. The primary concern of the worker was housing, food, and clothing for himself and his family. Heat and water for bathing were, in many cases, luxuries not necessities; work clothing was worn for days, perhaps weeks, without washing. Language, cultural, and educational differences were barriers to health education.

After 1918, the refinery's medical service, begun in 1905, added a strong preventive emphasis to the good-quality, curative treatment already in place. Over time, prevention expanded from a narrow focus on infectious disease to include concern about the long-term effects of exposure to toxic substances such as lead and benzene. By the 1930s, concern about the relationship between job exposure and cancer was growing. Awareness of the Tworts's work on the carcinogenicity of certain aromatic hydrocarbons produced by cracking (Twort and Twort 1935) led to special skin examinations of workers in all the refineries beginning in 1935. In like vein, concern about the potential of high-boiling aromatic hydrocarbons derived from catalytic cracking led to the Sloan–Kettering animal studies beginning in 1945 (Smith et al. 1951). With this degree of interest, there must have been knowledge of the work of the Manchester group (including Kennaway, Cook, and Twort), initiated in response to the mule spinners' cancer epidemic. One can only theorize that the relationship of scrotal cancer to paraffin/wax manufacture was overlooked. Chimney sweeps' cancer focused on soot; mule spinners' cancer was related to the end users' exposure to lubricating oil. This theory is supported by the fact that the publications detailing the relationship of wax manufacture to scrotal cancer were available relatively early in the unfolding of the story. Butlin's paper of 1892 referred to a handful of cases of scrotal cancer described by von Volkmann (1875) and Bell in the 1870s (1876–77) in production workers who were extracting naphtha, paraffin, and tar from brown coal and shale. A few similar cases were described by Leitch, A. (1922) and Scott, A. (1922). After this time, the primary focus was on mule spinners' cancer. While the wax extraction process in Bayonne yielded lubricating oil as a companion product, the latter is the one that would have been more likely to have drawn attention as a potential hazard for scrotal cancer than would the wax extraction side of the process. The record does not indicate, however, whether it did or not during the period of interest in our story.

Local, state, and federal labor and health agencies had public health problems to address—infectious diseases, water supply, sewage disposal—and, in the workplace, gross mechanical hazards, and industrial dust and fume exposure to consider. In 1941, the New Jersey Health Department embarked on an industrial health program with federal money and in 1946 established a cancer control program that was initially concerned with occupational cancer. From the official records surveyed, however, there is no indication that anyone was concerned about exposure to slack wax or was aware of the historical background of scrotal cancer.

Would a health professional (plant physician, industrial hygienist, or member of the state health and labor departments) on the Bayonne scene in the 1920s or 1930s have been familiar with the publications of Butlin, Leitch, or Scott? Would he or she have observed the wax pressmens' trousers soaked with oil in the groin area and made the connection with the mule spinners' similar exposure?

We do not know the answer to these questions. We do know that there is no record that a plant physician ever made such an observation or logical connection. We also know that the first industrial hygienist did not arrive at the refinery until 1946 or 1947, on the eve of the recognition of the signal cases.

One final speculation is whether the attitudes of management and the union toward productivity, medical cost containment, and the potential hazard of job exposure bore any relationship to an earlier investigation of the work environment. Prior to the diagnosis of the original cases, local management probably would have resisted changes with regard to the provision of work clothes, showers, and other protective measures, since these would have reduced productivity. Management probably would not have been concerned about medical cost containment, because this concept had not evolved at that time. The existing medical benefit policy/ Workmen's Compensation plan coverage would have been considered adequate. In that era, the union was primarily interested in wages, benefits, and safety. By safety it meant, for the most part, mechanical hazards. Concern about long-term outcomes (for example, cancer, chronic respiratory disease, etc.) would come later, with the rise in public anxiety about the chronic health effects of potentially toxic exposure. Both management and union would probably not have been moved to action by the "potential" of scrotal cancer. After the diagnosis of the two initial cases, however, both parties appear to have acted responsibly.

References

Bell, J. 1876–77. "Paraffin Epithelioma of the Scrotum." *Edinburgh Medical Journal* 22:135–137.

Benton, W. 1956. *Encyclopedia Britannica* 17:253-B, S. V. "paraffin."

Butlin, H. T. 1892. "Cancer of the Scrotum in Chimney Sweeps and Others." *British Medical Journal* 2:66–71.

Cook, J. W.; Heiger, I.; Kennaway, E. L.; and Mayneord, W. V. 1932. "The Production of Cancer by Pure Hydrocarbons." *Proceedings of the Royal Society of London* 111:455–484.

Dorsey, G. 1976. "The Bayonne Refinery Strikes of 1915–1916." *Polish American Studies* 33, no. 2 (Autumn): 19–30.

Gafafer, W. M., and Sitgreaves, R. 1940. "Disabling Morbidity and Mortality from Cancer Among the Male Employees of an Oil Refining Company with Reference to Age, Site and Duration, 1933–1938, Inclusive." *Public Health Reports* 55, no. 34: 1517–1522.

Gibb, G. W., and Knowlton, E. H. 1956. *The Resurgent Years: 1911–1927.* New York: Harper and Brothers.

Goodrich, S. L. 1939. "Thirty-three Years of Medical Service in Bayonne Refinery." *Medical Bulletin* 4:14–19.

Gover, M. 1939. "Cancer Mortality in the U.S.: Trends 1900–1935." *Public Health Bulletin* 248.

Hanau, A. 1889. "Erfolgreiche experimentelle Übertragung von Carcinom." *Fortsher. Med.* 7:321–330.

Hendricks, N. V.; Berry, C. M.; Lione, J. G.; and Thorpe, J. J. 1959. "Cancer of the Scrotum in Wax Pressmen: I. Epidemiology." *A.M.A. Archives of Industrial Health* 19:524–529.

Henry, S. A. 1946. *Cancer of the Scrotum in Relation to Occupation.* London, New York, Toronto: Humphrey Milford, Oxford University Press.

Hidy, R. W., and Hidy, M. E. 1955. *Pioneering in Big Business 1882–1911.* New York: Harper and Brothers.

Jarvholm, B., and Lavenius, B. 1987. "Mortality and Cancer Morbidity in Workers Exposed to Cutting Fluids." *Archives of Environmental Health* 42:361–366.

Kennaway, E. L. 1925. "Experiments on Cancer-Producing Substances." *British Medical Journal* 2:1–4.

Kipling, M. D.; Usherwood, R.; Varley, R. 1970. "A Monstrous Growth: An Historical Note on Carcinoma of the Scrotum." *British Journal of Industrial Medicine* 27:382–384.

Leitch, A. 1922. "Paraffin Cancer and Its Experimental Production." *British Medical Journal* 3:1104–1106.

———. 1924. "Mule Spinners' Cancer and Mineral Oils." *British Medical Journal* 3:941–943.

Lione, J. G., and Denholm, J. S. 1959. "Cancer of the Scrotum in Wax Pressman: II. Clinical Observations." *A.M.A. Archives of Industrial Health* 19:530–539.

———. "Medical Service." 1918. *Lamp* 1:15.

"Medical Service Staff." 1918. *Lamp* 1:22.

New Jersey. 1883. *First Annual Report of the Inspector of Labor of Children.* Trenton, N.J.: John L. Murphy.

———. 1884–1904. *Second Through the Twenty-second Reports of the Inspector of Factories and Workshops.* Trenton, N.J.: John L. Murphy.

———. 1942. *Annual Report of the Commissioner of Health* 65:7, 91–95.

———. 1949. *Annual Report of the Commissioner of Health* 72:18.

———. 1944. *Annual Report of the Health Department* 67:9, 71–74.

———. 1945. *Annual Report of the Health Department* 68:14–83.

———. 1947. *Annual Report of the Health Department* 70:11, 125–127.

———. 1952. *Annual Report of the Health Department* 75:18, 210–211.

———. 1956–57. *Department of Labor and Industry Annual Reports.*

Passey, R. D. 1922. "Experimental Soot Cancer." *British Medical Journal* 2:1112–1113.

Robinson, W. F. 1961. *Bayonne Centennial Historical Review.* Bayonne, N.J.: Progress Printing.

Scott, A. 1922. "On the Occupational Cancer of the Paraffin and Oil Workers of the Scottish Shale Oil Industry." *British Medical Journal* 2:1108–1109.

Shubik, P.; Saffiotti, V.; Lijinsky, W.; Pietra, G.; Rappaport, H.; Toth, B.; Raha, C. R.; Tomatis, L.; Feldman, R.; and Ramaki, H. 1962. "Studies on the Toxicity of Petroleum Waxes." *Toxicology and Applied Pharmacology* 4 (suppl.): 1–62.

Sinclair, G. M. 1940. *Bayonne Old and New.* New York: Maranatha.

Smith, W. E.; Sunderland, D. A.; and Sugiura, K. 1951. "Experimental Analysis of the Carcinogenic Activity of Certain Petroleum Products." *A.M.A. Archives of Industrial Hygiene and Occupational Medicine* 4:299–314.

Thomas, A. J. 1925. *Industrial Housing: The Bayonne Housing Corporation, Bayonne, N.J.* New York: Currier and Harford.

Twort, C. C., and Twort, J. M. 1930. "The Relative Potency of Carcinogenic Tars and Oils." *Journal of Hygiene* 29:373–379.

———. 1935. "Induction of Cancer by Cracked Mineral Oils." *Lancet* 2:1226–1228.

von Volkmann, R. 1875. *Beiträge sur Chirurgie.* Leipzig: Breitkopf und Hartel.

Wade, L. J.; Hansen, H.; Nevins, T. J.; Lione, J. G.; Berry, C. M. 1951. "Cancer Control Program for High-Boiling Catalytically Cracked Oils." *Medical Bulletin* 11:416–429.

Waldron, H. A. 1983. "A Brief History of Scrotal Cancer." *British Journal of Industrial Medicine* 40:390–401.

West, K. A. 1985. *New Jersey Spotlight on Government: League of Women Voters of New Jersey Education Fund.* 5th ed. New Brunswick, N.J.: Rutgers University Press.

Yamagiwa, K., and Ichikawa, K. 1918. "Experimental Study of the Pathogenesis of Carcinoma." *Journal of Canadian Research* 3:1–29.

Zwicker, D. H. 1988. "The Wonders of Wax." *Lamp* 70, no. 4:8–11.

• CHAPTER 5 •

The New Jersey Radium Dial Workers: Seventy-five Years Later

WILLIAM D. SHARPE, M.D.

William D. Sharpe is in a unique position to recount the facts surrounding the New Jersey radium dial workers. A distinguished medical historian and former editor of the Bulletin of the New York Academy of Medicine, *Dr. Sharpe was also a fellow pathologist and collaborator with Dr. Harrison S. Martland, chief medical examiner of Essex County, who first recognized the cause of death in the young radium dial painters (Sharpe 1971). Dr. Martland measured the radioactivity in the bodies of the dial painters and, in 1925, published the information connecting their bone disease and aplastic anemias with radium. The young painters had been directed to Dr. Martland by the concerned women of the New Jersey Consumers League, founded in 1899. This organization had among its objectives the improvement of working conditions for women and children, including the reduction of occupational disease (Handen 1990). From Dr. Martland, Dr. Sharpe inherited pathological specimens, medical records, and a voluminous correspondence relating to the dial painters.*

Nowhere is industry's "ignorance" defense more plausible than in the radium dial episode. Sabin A. von Sochocky, founder of the United States Radium Corporation (Figure 5.1), died from the same radiation exposure that killed twenty-two female employees (Bale 1987). As a nuclear physicist, Sochocky knew of the dangers of radium. The fact that he subjected himself to the risk was a compelling demonstration of self-delusion. Such a blatant disregard for safety seemed unworthy of so learned an entrepreneur. A chemist who worked for the company also died of radium poisoning, again indicating no intent on the part of the company to subject the dial painters to special risk. In the eyes of some, the total disregard of the danger of radiation relieved the company of responsibility for injury to the dial

This piece appears in its original, unedited form because the essay was subpoenaed in draft form and entered as evidence in a 1992 federal court case (*Street et al.* vs. *Chevron U.S.A. Inc.*). Thus, the essay, as it stands, is part of the public and historical record. These circumstances underline how important the radium dial workers remain over half a century later.

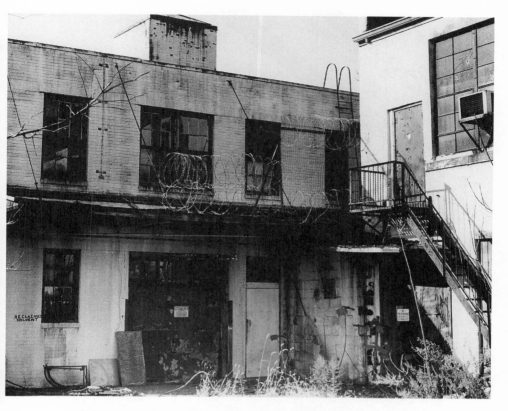

FIGURE 5.1. Abandoned radium dial factory, United States Radium Corporation, Orange, New Jersey. Photo by Lynn Butler, November 1990.

painters. Others suggested that the young women knowingly accepted the risk because of good salaries and, therefore, were responsible for their own fate. Because they died slowly, some observers suspected a hoax designed to extract money from the U.S. Radium Corporation. The company's president steadfastly denied a causal relationship between radium and disease and enlisted experts from Columbia University's College of Physicians and Surgeons, and Harvard's School of Public Health to research the matter with the stipulation they not publish their findings (Clark 1987). The experts, in conjunction with the statute of limitations, workers' compensation laws, and lawyers, effectively prevented payment of any but token amounts to the twenty-two women who died.

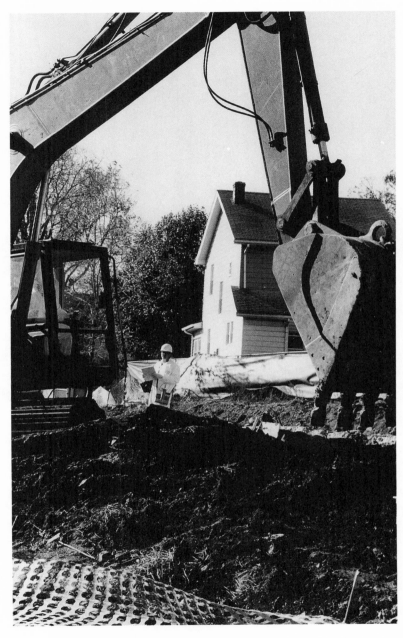

FIGURE 5.2.　Removing radium-contaminated landfill from residential site in Montclair, New Jersey. Photo by Lynn Butler, November 1990.

In the 1920s, radium was considered a boon to health, not a detriment. From 1925 until 1931 (when prohibited by the Federal Trade Commission), the Bailey Radium Laboratories of East Orange, New Jersey, sold 400,000 bottles of a patent medicine called "Radiothor" at one dollar apiece (Macklis 1990). This alleged tonic and sexual rejuvenator contained one microcurie of radium 228 and one microcurie of radium 226 in each bottle. It was guaranteed to contain no "drugs." Although no longer a tonic, radium is still used to treat cancer. Radiation therapy was given for a radium-induced osteogenic sarcoma in at least one of the dial painters (Sharpe 1971).

The legacy of the radium dial industry lives on in New Jersey. Radium-laden soil from the United States Radium Company in Orange was transported to suburban Montclair to be used as landfill. Since 1984, five thousand barrels of contaminated soil have been stored in Montclair awaiting decent burial; but no burial grounds have yet been found. In 1990, the U.S. Environmental Protection Agency demolished several homes it acquired in Montclair because the homes had been constructed on radium-contaminated landfill (Figure 5.2).

References

Bale, T. 1987. "A Brush with Justice: The New Jersey Radium Dial Painters in the Courts." *Health/PAC Bulletin* 17:18–21.

Clark, C. 1987. "Physicians, Reformers, and Occupational Disease: The Discovery of Radium Poisoning." *Women and Health* 12:147–167.

Handen, E. 1990. "Juliet Clannon Cushing, 1845–1934." In *Past and Promise: Lives of New Jersey Women*, Editor-in-Chief Joan N. Burstyn. ed. the Women's Project of New Jersey, 119–120. Metuchen, N.J., and London: Scarecrow Press.

Macklis, R. M. 1990. "Radiothorium and the Era of Mild Radium Therapy." *Journal of the American Medical Association* 264:614–618.

● ● ●

[I]t still remains true that for most of our knowledge concerning new compounds in industry we must depend on human experiments, the workman himself is the guinea pig.

Alice Hamilton, 1943[1]

About 1910, radium-containing luminous paint was used on the dials of expensive Swiss and German watches.[2] Toward 1913, a cheaper but commercially acceptable paint was developed by Dr. Sabin A. von Sochocky, part-owner of the United States Radium Corporation plant in Orange, New Jersey, until his death on November 14, 1928, of radium intoxication. Aub et al.[3] state that until about 1925, practically all of the self-luminous compound in the United States was mixed by von Sochocky himself who, from 1917 to 1923, was exposed to approximately 10.2 *curies* of ^{228}Ra(MsTh$_1$) and 8.2 *curies* of ^{226}Ra. This ratio averaged 10.2/8.2, but the paint was usually aged to permit ^{228}Th(RdTh) to grow in from ^{228}Ra(MsTh$_1$), and the predicted ratio of 1:1 was confirmed by Petrow's assays forty-odd years later.[4]

Radioluminous dials were widely used during World War I in submarines, aircraft, and for watches. After the war, radioluminous paint was used for a variety of novelty items as well as for watch and clock dials, but after about 1925, the U.S. Radium Corp. stopped painting dials and thereafter confined itself to the manufacture of the paint. Table 5.1 shows the quantities of radium used, 1917–1927. Hundreds of people painted instrument dials during World War II, and clocks with radium dials were manufactured at least until the early 1970s, but much more safely.

TABLE 5.1

Use of ^{226}Ra and ^{228}Ra(MsTh$_1$) in Self-Luminous Compounds by the United States Radium Corporation, 1917–1927[a]

	1917–1923	1926	1927
mg. ^{226}Ra used	6953	1452	2421
mg. ^{228}Ra(MsTh$_1$) used	6012	390	471
^{226}Ra content of ^{228}Ra(MsTh$_1$) in mCi, if 20% ^{226}Ra	1200	78	94
MsTh$_1$ content of ^{228}Ra(MsTh$_1$) in mCi, if aged 3 years	7500	490	590
Ratio of mCi MsTh$_1$ to mCi ^{226}Ra after 3 years of aging	0.92	0.32	0.23

SOURCE: J. C. Aub, R. D. Evans, L. H. Hempelmann, and H. S. Martland, 1952. The Late Effects of Internally-Deposited Radioactive Materials in Man. *Medicine 31:* 221–329, at p. 304. Copyright © by Williams and Wilkins, 1952. Reprinted with permission.

The Paint

The exact composition of the radioluminous paint was apparently never reduced to writing. Later analyses indicate that about 1920, a typical paint consisted of 0.4 to 0.7 μCi of "luminizer," ^{226}Ra and/or ^{228}Ra(MsTh$_1$), the latter matured to permit ingrowth of ^{228}Th(RdTh) unless demand for the paint was so great that it had to be used without aging, for each 100 grams of dry heat-crystallized zinc sulfide with hundredths or thousandths of a percent by weight of cadmium, copper and manganese to produce bright fluorescence when alpha particles bombarded the zinc sulfide phosphor.

Until about 1918, only ^{226}Ra sulfate or bromide was used as the luminizer, but after 1918, ^{228}Ra(MsTh$_1$), a less expensive but shorter-lived byproduct of the local gas mantle manufacturing industry, was added in variable amounts depending on the probable useful life of the watch dials. This dry paint was ground in small mortars (about twice the size of a thimble) with distilled water, gelatin and gum arabic, diluted to the consistency of heavy cream, and issued in 10 ml. lots. The texture was described as "gritty." Water-based paint required brush application; that used outside New Jersey was usually oil-based and was applied using pen nibs. Like most water colorists, the painters (chiefly teenaged girls and young women) pointed their brushes using their lips, despite contrary instruction and the addition of a bitter substance (probably quinine) by von Sochocky early during the 1920s to discourage this. By licking the brushes, each painter swallowed considerable paint—perhaps as much as 12 to 125 μCi of radioactive material weekly. Workers were also exposed to aerosols of radioactive dust, and to penetrating gamma radiation from inevitably contaminated workplace surfaces.

Radium

^{226}Ra is an alkaline earth that decays by alpha and beta emission, with some gamma rays, through a series of daughters that includes ^{222}Rn (radon), an inert noble gas, itself radioactive and decaying through a number of daughters to stable lead. Table 5.2 diagrams the disintegration patterns of ^{226}Ra and of ^{228}Ra(MsTh$_1$). Although human bodies normally contain traces of radium from air, food and water, it is required in no metabolic process. Quantities of ^{226}Ra and

TABLE 5.2
^{226}Ra and ^{228}Ra(MsTh$_1$) Disintegration

Th	Ac	Ra	Fr	Rn	At	Po	Bi	Pb	Tl	Symbol	Classical Name	Physical Half-Life	Mode of Decay
		226								^{226}Ra	Radium	1622 years	α, γ
				222						^{222}Rn	Radon	3.825 days	α, γ
						218				^{218}Po	Radium-A	3.05 min.	$\alpha, \beta-$
								214		^{214}Pb	Radium-B	26.8 min.	$\beta-, \gamma$
							214			^{214}Bi	Radium-C	19.7 min.	$\alpha, \beta-, \gamma$
						214				^{214}Po	Radium-C'	164 microsec.	α
								210		^{210}Pb	Radium-D	19.4 years	$\beta-, \gamma$
							210			^{210}Bi	Radium-E	5.00 days	$\alpha, \beta-$
						210				^{210}Po	Radium-F	138.40 days	α, γ
								206		^{206}Pb	Radium-G	Stable	
		228								^{228}Ra	Mesothorium$_1$	5.75 years	$\beta-$
	228									^{228}Ac	Mesothorium$_2$	6.13 hours	$\beta-, \gamma$
228										^{228}Th	Radiothorium	1.91 years	α, γ
		224								^{224}Ra	Thorium-X	3.62 days	α, γ
				220						^{220}Rn	Thoron	55.6 sec.	α, γ
						216				^{216}Po	Thorium-A	0.16 sec.	α
								212		^{212}Pb	Thorium-B	10.64 hours	$\beta-, \gamma$ 35% 65%
							212			^{212}Bi	Thorium-C	60.5 min.	α $\beta-, \gamma$
						212				^{212}Po	Thorium-C'	0.304 microsec.	α
									208	^{208}Tl	Thorium-C"	3.1 min.	$\beta-$ γ
								208		^{208}Pb	Thorium-D	Stable	

SOURCE: W. D. Sharpe. 1983. Radium (Ra). In H. Zumkley, ed., *Spurenelemente: Grundlagen, Ätiologie, Diagnose, Therapie*, pp. 174–180, at p. 174. Stuttgart and New York: Georg Thieme Verlag. Reprinted with permission.

^{228}Ra(MsTh$_1$) involved in clinical situations are so small that they are *chemically* negligible, and merge with the body's calcium pool. Danger comes from accumulated damage caused by radioactive decay products over years and decades. Alpha particle radiation from internally deposited sources is always nonhomogeneous, sometimes extremely so, but tissue damage is focal because cells outside reach of alpha particle tracks are not directly radiated.[5]

Most (90% or so) ^{226}Ra ingested is quickly eliminated in feces, urine and bile, acting in that respect like lead, but a variable part of that ingested and all of that injected enters the blood stream. Some is stored in bone mineral, where ^{226}Ra enters into the hydroxyapatite crystals, randomly substituting for calcium. Inhaled particulates enter the pulmonary lymphatic drainage and are taken up by the reticuloendothelial system. Radium harms both by its direct alpha and beta bombardment of bone and marrow, and by the circulation of its decay products, particularly ^{222}Rn. ^{222}Rn, although inert, is soluble in body fluids and fat, and approximately half of that formed in subjects with longstanding ^{226}Ra burdens is exhaled from the lungs after circulating dissolved in blood. ^{222}Rn from decay of ^{226}Ra also accumulates in the airspaces of the accessory sinuses of the skull and contributes to the danger of carcinoma of these sinuses. ^{222}Rn, although forming no compounds by itself, emits alpha particles during its decay, and so far as cell damage goes, the decay products of ^{222}Rn are probably more dangerous than the ^{226}Ra itself.

The half-life of ^{226}Ra is so long relative to the human lifespan that physical decay does not lead to significant loss of radioactivity. The tissue dose of ^{226}Ra is high immediately following a single exposure and during continuing exposure, but once acquisition of ^{226}Ra ceases, total body ^{226}Ra content declines within about a year to a relatively stable level. A year following a single intravenous dose of ^{226}Ra, between 0.2 percent and 2.3 percent of the administered dose is retained.

When concentrations in blood are high, actively forming bone (particularly growing epiphyses and forming haversian systems) picks up large quantities of activity. These areas of high activity ("hotspots") are buried by subsequent bone deposition and remodeling. Long-term exchange of alkaline earth ions between blood and the bone mass produces a diffuse radioactive component that continues even without active bone deposition and resorption. Long-lived radioactive elements deposited in bone resist efforts to accelerate their normally slow excretion.[6] Twenty years after administration, with very considerable individual variation, patients excrete only about 0.008 percent of the ^{226}Ra in their bodies each day. More than 95 percent of this is excreted in the feces, and less than 5 percent in urine. The stable distributions of ^{226}Ra in the human skeleton is extremely variable, but an individual pattern persists for years.[7] No correlation exists between regions of bone with focally high levels of ^{226}Ra and the sites at which bone malignancies actually developed. The distribution of ^{226}Ra in bone is decidedly not homogeneous, and individual "hotspots" may have 10 or 100 times the radioactivity of surrounding bone.

^{228}Ra(MsTh$_1$) is soluble in body fluids, deposits on bone surfaces (periosteum and endosteum), and is diffusely deposited in bone mineral through resorption and remodeling.[8] A large fraction is excreted before long-term storage occurs and one year after injection, only about 2.5 percent of the quantity injected is retained. ^{226}Ra and ^{228}Ra(MsTh$_1$) have very similar behavior, but ^{228}Ra(MsTh$_1$) in equilibrium with its disintegration products is, in an acute dose, extremely toxic and in this respect resembles plutonium and polonium rather than radium. However, its half-life (5.75 years) is short enough that significant decrease in radioactivity does occur through physical decay, although the half-life (55.6 seconds) of ^{220}Rn (thoron) is so short that little is exhaled through the lungs and therefore remains in the body. (For practical purposes, thoron decays completely in about 5 minutes.) Another decay product, ^{228}Th(RdTh), seeks the organic matrix of bone rather than its crystalline lattice, but ^{228}Th(RdTh) has the chemical properties of thorium, not radium.

Because ^{228}Ra(MsTh$_1$) has a comparatively short half-life, subsequent measurements of its activity contain large errors whereas ^{226}Ra is fairly accurately measured even decades later. Some of the workers may, in addition, have ingested ^{228}Th(RdTh), radiothorium, an element so insoluble that absorption was probably minimal. ^{228}Ra(MsTh$_1$) in equilibrium with its ^{228}Th(RdTh) emits 5 alpha particles to ^{226}Ra's 4, but has particles of greater velocity and penetration than ^{226}Ra, hence it is biologically more active and destructive than ^{226}Ra. In man, the main difference in dose effects is that most of the ^{226}Ra daughters decay outside the body, ^{222}Rn (radon) being exhaled through the lungs, while practically all of the ^{228}Ra(MsTh$_1$) daughters decay fairly close to the anatomic sites where deposited. Maletskos et al.[9] fed normal elderly men and women volunteers mock radium paint containing ^{224}RaSO$_4$, ^{234}Th(SO$_4$)$_2$, BaSO$_4$ carrier and ZnS phosphor, and found intestinal absorption of about 20 percent for ^{224}Ra but only about 0.02 percent for ^{234}Th, concluding that the ^{228}Ra(MsTh$_1$) in the real dial paint was unlikely to have contributed a significant radiation dose ($\leq$5 percent that of the ^{226}Ra) to the dial painters' bones. Be that as it may, ^{228}Th(RdTh) measured in dial painters most likely grew in from their ^{228}Ra(MsTh$_1$), even though some ^{228}Th(RdTh) may have been incorporated in the paint.

The Workers

The New Jersey Radium Research Project identified, using at least two independent sources, by name, 978 individuals who had worked in the radium industry in the state at any time during its existence.[10] Some worked only a few days, at no time do more than about 300 seem to have been at work simultaneously, and median duration of employment approximated one year. Women were just beginning to enter the labor market in large numbers around the time of World War I, and most of the dial painters came from blue-collar backgrounds—teenaged girls who had finished seventh or eighth grade, and who would work until they married. Jobs were scarce for untrained and uneducated young women, and dial-painting studios were attractive: pay was good, piecework meant that diligent workers were rewarded, work was light, and working conditions seemed pleasant enough. Workers agreed: "It wasn't like the usual factory job at all." Some regarded themselves as artists.[11]

But in October, 1922, an Orange physician reported "phosphorus necrosis" of the jaw in a dial painter who had worked two-and-a-half years but had left the radium plant in good health two-and-a-half years before her diagnosis. Local and state health departments had investigated the radium plants but found no phosphorus in use and therefore no violation of state law. On January 30, 1923, and again on April 6, 1923, Dr. Martin Szamatolski, a state health department chemist, ascribed (although without proof) jaw necrosis to radium, not phosphorus or zinc.[12] Dentists encountered many refractory cases of mandibular and maxillary osteomyelitis, and were sometimes reluctant to work on or to pull dial painters' teeth from fear of precipitating or aggravating "jaw rot." In 1924, a physician–

dentist, Theodor Blum, first mentioned "radium jaw" as a one-sentence footnote.[13]

Deaths began in the fall of 1922, and between 1922 and 1924, seven dial painters died.[14] Nothing suggested foul play and autopsies were not done. Death certificates included such diagnoses as ulcerative stomatitis, syphilis, gingivitis, primary anemia, sepsis, Vincent's angina, jaw necrosis due to phosphorus intoxication, and occupational poisoning (character unknown). Osteonecrosis and aregenerative anemia had not yet been described, and local physicians faced a new and hitherto unknown disease.[15]

These deaths had not at first been attributed to any occupational hazard, but by the time that the sixth victim, Miss H. K., died on December 9, 1924, radium was seriously suspected. Her story got very substantial publicity, not only because of five previous deaths within walking distance of the factory in Orange, but because of the number of other workers who suffered bone pain, fractures of the shafts of long bones, necrosis of the jaws, hip, thigh, and other painful disabilities.

By 1924, the U.S. Radium Corp. was also concerned about the possibility of an industrial intoxication, and Arthur Roeder, the president, invited W. B. Castle, Katherine R. Drinker and C. K. Drinker, of the Harvard School of Public Health, to visit the plant on April 16–18, 1924. Phosphorus had been excluded as a possible toxic agent, and Castle and the Drinkers regarded the zinc phosphor as nontoxic. Radioactivity had been documented in some of the living workers, and these investigators suggested that the skin, lungs and gastrointestinal tract were probable portals of entry. They could prove no relationship between radium and the workers' illnesses, but thought it prudent to assume one. Their paper was published in August, 1925,[16] after the company had been less than forthcoming in its report of their findings to the New Jersey State Department of Labor.[17] They acknowledged the "complete co-operation" of the company's executives and employees, and commented on the "excellent hygienic conditions of the work" in the factory, concluding, "It thus appears as if the only constituent of the luminous material which can do harm must be the radium." Dental X-ray films placed throughout the factory fogged, and examination of 22 workers demonstrated that none had normal hematologic values: total leukocyte counts were reduced, polymorphonuclear leukocytes were deceased and lymphocytes increased. They concluded also, "The amounts of radium in this paint are extremely minute, so slight as to cause no one in this plant or in other plants employed in similar work to consider the possibility of a radium hazard." Mouth-pointing of brushes was said to have been stopped late in 1923, six months before their visit.

On June 7, 1925, thirty-six-year-old Dr. E.D.L., chief chemist since 1912 of the U.S. Radium Corp., died in East Orange, and his physician reported his death to the Essex County Medical Examiner, Dr. Harrison S. Martland. Autopsy demonstrated a regenerative anemia, and postmortem assays yielded 14 μCi of radioactive material in his body, 5 percent of it ^{226}Ra and the balance ^{228}Ra(MsTh$_1$). On June 12, 1925, Dr. Philip Conlon asked Dr. Martland to see a dial painter in St. Mary's Hospital, Orange, who was also profoundly anemic. When Mrs. S.T.M., the tenth known victim, died on June 18, 1925, Martland was able to prove that their deaths were caused by radioactive material. Martland reported these cases to the New York Pathological Society on October 8, 1925.[18] In May 1925, Martland examined two dial painters with jaw necrosis and severe anemia; both later died and Martland, as county medical examiner, performed autopsies. Thus, by October 1925, Martland had defined radium intoxication as a new disease. On the basis of two autopsies and clinical data from five still-living workers, he proved how radium entered the body, its form when ingested, its storage in the reticuloendothelial system, its recovery from and demonstration in exhaled air and in the body's tissues, its characteristic anemia, and its hopeless prognosis.[19] Deaths continued at the rate of a few a year, and on November 14, 1928, Dr. Sabin von Sochocky died of aplastic anemia, a victim of the paint he originated.

In September 1927, Martland did an autopsy on a thirty-five-year-old woman who had quit dial painting in good health in 1919. She was anemic, had an osteogenic sarcoma, and her body contained about 50 μCi of radioactive material, most of it ^{228}Ra(MsTh$_1$). Martland regarded the sarcoma as secondary to previous radiation osteitis, and by 1931, reported five osteogenic sarcomas among eighteen dead radium workers. Other radium workers complained of severe bone pains and arthralgia, and some had spontaneous fractures through the shafts of long bones. Workers continued to develop osteonecrosis and malignant tumors, and to die. The first deaths seem to have been from infectious complications of a peculiar anemia; the second were from complications of osteonecrosis, especially osteogenic sarcoma.[20]

Reaction

The National Consumers' League, founded in 1899, busied itself with extending basic legal protection to factory workers, especially women and adolescent girls. Its label on garments, for example, was supposed to improve factory working conditions because "the conscientious consumer . . . did not want to buy goods manufactured in substandard factories or finished in tenements."[21] Mrs. Florence Kelley was general secretary, with an office in the Protestant Charities Building at 22nd Street and what is now Park Avenue South, New York—just short of an hour from Orange by train and subway.

The Consumers' League of the Oranges was concerned about objectionable fumes from one of the radium plants: a radium chemist reported that "acid fumes ate clothes right off the line" and an aspiring singer's voice had been ruined by the same fumes. In 1924, Leonora Young, Orange's health officer, struck by the number of deaths among young women who had worked at the radium plant, shared her concern with the League's state secretary, Katherine G. T. Wiley, who interviewed some workers and the families of some workers who had died. Miss Wiley referred a number of these workers to Dr. Martland, Essex County Medical Examiner, and the deaths to the attention of the State Board of Health and of the State Department of Labor as possible industrial deaths. The Board of Health had no jurisdiction over occupational diseases, and the Department of Labor could not identify the radium workers' illness and deaths as falling within any of the then defined occupational diseases. The closest they came, considering maxillary and mandibular osteonecrosis, was phosphorus poisoning, but the radium factory used no phosphorus and this was excluded.

Miss Wiley, although the dangers of radium were unknown in 1924, contacted Mrs. Kelley, and they later persuaded Dr. Frederick L. Hoffman, a Newark insurance company statistician, to review some of their data. The *New York Times*, on May 30, 1925, under the headline, "New Radium Disease Found," reported Hoffman's paper read before the Section on Preventive and Industrial Medicine and Public Health at the American Medical Association meeting at Atlantic City on May 29, 1925. He described the symptoms and deaths among women who had painted watch dials and urged that expert studies begin at once to avoid further deaths.[22]

Mrs. Kelley also contacted Dr. Alice Hamilton, probably after radium osteonecrosis was reported among Connecticut dial painters who used paint manufactured by the U.S. Radium Corp. A meeting was held in Manhattan in 1928, including Dr. Hamilton, Dr. Martland, and Dr. Charles Norris, Chief Medical Examiner of the City of New York, and it was determined to ask the Surgeon General of the United States to call a conference to consider the problem. Mrs. Kelley recruited Walter Lippmann, who supported this in a *New York World* editorial on July 16, 1928. Further support came from the important Committee on Public Health of the New York Academy of Medicine (in which Martland was very active) and from the New York City Commissioner of Health. At the National Consumers' League annual dinner in November, 1928, with Mrs. Franklin D. Roosevelt as toastmaster, Dr. Norris demonstrated roentgenograms of bones from both living, dead and exhumed dial painters. Prodigious public interest in the dial painters continued, indeed, Ben Hecht even had a Broadway play—*Hazel Flagg*—based on a dial painter's experience.[23]

On December 20, 1928, a conference was held in Washington by specialists in occupational hygiene and public health, including representatives of the Bureau of Standards, National Research Council, Public Health Service, and Bureau of Labor Statistics, under the auspices of Surgeon General Hugh Cumming. Representatives of industry blamed careless workers for licking their brushes; occupational physicians blamed radioactive dusts, radon and external gamma radiation. Radioactivity had also been found in workers, including many men, exposed only to radioactive dust and to gamma radiation from contaminated work surfaces, who had not licked brushes.[24]

Another meeting was held in Washington on February 25, 1929, devoted entirely to discussion of techniques for the measurement of body burdens of radium. In addition to Martland, those present included essentially everyone then actively working in the field: William Duane (Harvard), Herman Schlundt (University of Missouri), S. C. Lind (University of Minnesota), Alice Hamilton (Harvard), Gioacchino Failla (Memorial Hospital, New York), C. F. Burnam (Johns Hopkins) and O. H. Gish and L. F. Curtis of the Federal Bureau of Standards. Mrs. Kelley was pleased with this response, and on March 28, 1929, wrote Martland:

> It is our idea that that Bureau [Federal Bureau of Standards] is better qualified than any other agency for preventing such horrors as the

Bayonne deaths from the manufacture of gasoline, and the radium
cases, and that agitation with Congress for provision would keep the
horrors of industry before the public mind and at least tend to make
manufacturers more cautious.[25]

Elaborate protective procedures were eventually defined,[26] and
although World War II required many times the quantity of industrial radium than did World War I, things were vastly safer.[27] Employees who retained more than 0.1 μCi of ^{226}Ra were dismissed or
rotated to other jobs, and this 0.1 μCi became the "occupational
standard"—presumed "safe" for industrial workers, but not for the
general public.[28]

Litigation

Unfavorable publicity continued for the radium company. Families
of victims—ailing, disabled and dead—blamed radium exposure
for their problems. In 1927, five women joined, having been given
"a year to live," and filed a lawsuit against the company. The U.S.
Radium Corp. denied the complaint on two grounds: that the company was not negligent, and that the statute of limitations outlawed the suit. After some postponements, Federal Judge William
Clark, for humanitarian reasons, voluntarily urged the parties to
compromise so that the victims could obtain some relief while they
were still alive. Vice Chancellor Backes, in Essex County Chancery
Court, ruled that the statute of limitations would not halt the action
for damage.

The *New York Times,* in a front page story on June 5, 1928, described
the settlement with the five women given "only a year to live." Each
got a cash award of $10,000 and an annual pension of $600; a maximum of $7,500 for past medical treatment; and the five were given
$15,000 for legal fees and $4,500 for legal disbursements. The settlement also provided for the appointment of three physicians, one
chosen by the company, one by the five women, and the third by the
two physicians. This triumvirate (Drs. Lloyd F. Craver, Edward B.
Krumbhaar and James Ewing) would guide future treatment and,
should at any future time, two of the three agree that any of the
women no longer suffered from radium intoxication, the yearly pen-
sion would stop.[29] The five women withdrew their lawsuit and

waived all claims: Mrs. Q. McD., Miss G. F., and Mrs. A. L., of Orange; Mrs. E. H., of Hillside; and Miss K. S., of Newark.

These five women were the basis for a continuing human interest saga for some years. Believing that they would indeed soon die, some bought otherwise unaffordable automobiles and others invested in various luxuries that pleased them at the time. Mrs. McD., mother of two children, died at New York's Memorial Hospital on December 7, 1929. Next was Miss K. S., on February 18, 1933.[30] A *Newark News* report on July 31, 1930, commenting on the five, stated that Miss K. S. was awaiting her end in the New Jersey Orthopedic Hospital; that Mrs. L. was lame; that Miss F. was able to go to work daily at a Newark bank; and that Mrs. H. had all her lower teeth extracted, "her jaw is slowly being eaten away by the unrelenting radio-activity." Miss F., described as the 22nd victim, died of a sarcoma of the hip and anemia on October 27, 1933; Mrs. H., the 28th victim, died March 31, 1938; and Mrs. L. died November 18, 1946. Mrs. McD. and Mrs. L. were sisters of Miss A. M., the first recorded radium dial painter to die (September 12, 1922).

After the settlement with the five women "doomed to die," a number of other dial painters filed suit against the company.

The U.S. Radium Corp. settled the first two radium-related deaths out of court in 1926 and without assumption of any liability for approximately what the victims' estates would have received under Workmen's Compensation had radium intoxication then been covered by the Act. A law covers only what the law covers, and the general rule regarding industrial accidents at that time in New Jersey was that "where no specific time or occasion can be fixed upon as the time the alleged accident happened, there is no injury by accident within the meaning of the act."[31] When the radium corporation sued its insurance carrier to recover the costs of the claims it had settled, this rule was upheld on appeal: "Poisoning resulting from industrial use of radium is not an accidental injury within the coverage of the particular employer's liability insurance policy." The judge ruled that "radium poisoning is an occupational disease and not an injury by accident."[32] Radium and mesothorium intoxication were made compensable under the Workmen's Compensation Act in 1926,[33] but under the Constitution, a law cannot be retroactive. The company's insurance carriers paid maximum benefits within the limits of coverage.

Suits against the radium company at first claimed that the work was extremely hazardous and that improper safety precautions had been taken for the workers' protection. Later suits added that the company had been negligent in failing to seek out and to treat its former employees. The law was reaffirmed:

> Only fraudulent concealment will stop the running of the time permitted for filing of suit by the Statute of Limitations; in absence of any such fraud, a claim for injuries arising from tipping brushes with tongue to paint radium dials is barred by failure to bring suit within two years (the statutory period) of the causal episode even though plaintiff was ignorant of the harmful potentialities of ingesting radium.[34]

In fact, the company failed from a number of factors—the Great Depression, liability for radium-related deaths, and decline in demand for its products. During the last few years of its New Jersey existence, it manufactured paint. It moved from Orange and its buildings were torn down in 1930.[35] Most of the injured workers got nothing.

Clinical Radium Intoxication

Clinical radium intoxication had a slow, insidiously chronic course, and years or decades of normal health typically elapsed between first exposure to radium and first symptoms. Early signs included tooth resorption, jaw necrosis and a peculiar anemia; later signs included severe bone pain, fractures from relatively minor injury, bone deformities and malignant tumors of the bone and sinuses.

Tooth loss ("Pink Tooth") had an unusual pattern, marked by internal resorption of the dentine portion of the roots, sometimes spreading to involve the crowns or enlarging enough to destroy enamel. Teeth became loose and fell out or broke off, usually at the gum line. Serious bacterial infection often complicated dental extractions, and led to osteomyelitis, bone necrosis, sequestration and sinus formation with chronic extrusion of bone spicules. Ulcerative gingivitis was not rare. Destruction of alveolar crests contributed to this process, but bacterial infections from poor dental hygiene and chronic periodontal disease were also significant. Healing following dental extractions or operations was slow, and sometimes required that all affected teeth be extracted.

Radium osteonecrosis seems to have been a continuing process leading to lesions histologically difficult to distinguish from bone and marrow infarction, but healed poorly and progressed over the patient's lifetime. The greater the quantity of skeletally retained ^{228}Ra(MsTh$_1$) and ^{226}Ra, the more extensive the necrosis.[36,37] Bone changes followed radium exposure by a decade or longer,[38] and as necrosis progressed, symptoms appeared: infection, fractures (often through the shafts of long bones from little trauma), collapse fractures and coxa vara led to crippling spinal and other orthopedic deformities. Fractures healed slowly, but most of them eventually healed, although internal fixation sometimes precipitated necrosis or infection. Sarcoma might develop at any time.

Mild roentgenographic changes reflected more extensive skeletal damage than was suspected, and changes were most prominent in bones subject to pressure and trauma. The earliest sign of radium osteonecrosis was often a single focus in the jaw. When radium osteonecrosis could be diagnosed on roentgenographic grounds, the patient already had suffered irreversible radiation injury.[10]

Roentgenographic signs of radium osteonecrosis resembled those of bone and marrow infarction, and have been well documented.[3,13,19,20,36,39–42] Roentgenographic signs of radium osteonecrosis progressed slowly and healed little if at all. These changes had no consistent relationship to regional blood supplies, and if present in one bone were usually to be found elsewhere in the skeleton. Changes near joint surfaces resembled those of severe osteoarthritis with subchondral infarction, reactive sclerosis and radiolucent areas, the latter farther from joint surfaces and less clearly cystic in outline than in osteoarthritis. Changes in the cortices of long bones included marked irregularities both in cortical thickness and radiodensity, and in some areas the cortex abruptly thinned almost to invisibility. Thickened areas of cortex often contained discrete radiolucent areas where normal trabeculation was interrupted. Cortical bone sometimes appeared laminated, a "cortex-within-cortex" pattern. Diffuse and often patchy areas of sclerosis sometimes obscured the demarcation between cortical and trabecular bone because of increased or decreased mineralization. This diffuse loss of normal trabecular markings did not resemble ordinary osteoporosis, but seemed "moth-eaten," blurred and coarsened. Periosteal and phalangeal tuft changes were too inconsistent to be helpful. Discrete radiolucent skeletal changes sometimes superficially resembled osteolytic metastatic deposits, but lacked smooth borders. When present in the skull, these changes proved difficult to distinguish from normal pacchionian depressions and blood lakes. Changes in jawbones were often obscured or blended with changes caused by root resorption, periodontal disease and osteomyelitis.

Radium Carcinogenesis

The first proved malignant tumors caused by radium were documented when osteogenic sarcomas developed in bones that had been the site of radium osteonecrosis some years after exposure to ^{226}Ra and ^{228}Ra(MsTh$_1$) had ceased.[43] Epidermoid carcinomas of the mucosal lining of the paranasal sinuses and mastoid air cells of the skull are accepted as radium related, and at least some myelomas and leukemias are radium related. Whether radium exposure is also associated with an excess of other malignant tumors is not clear: the statistical base required to detect a general increase in the incidence of all malignancies would exceed the number of documented radium workers whose records are available for review.

Blood Dyscrasias

Mole[44] recently reviewed published material on the New Jersey cases, original histologic material being long lost, and suggests that what Martland consistently termed "leucopenic aregenerative anemia" was either leukemia or a leukemialike disorder. In Martland's day, the diagnosis of leukemia required marked peripheral leukocytosis. Martland, in 1925, wrote, "We believe this to be the first time that fatal, leucopenic, regenerative anemias have been described as due to radioactivity,"[18] and in that year's fuller report,[19] stated flatly that it was not aplastic anemia. In 1926,[45] he attributed the anemia to aged mesothorium, agreeing with Hoffman[22] as to the cause. He consistently maintained this position, and attributed the aplastic anemia with terminal thrombocytopenia and leukopenia of which von Sochocky died to external gamma radiation, not to internally deposited radium.[42] He regarded the marrow changes as the first stage in what he termed radium osteitis,[20] but noted the possibility that myeloid leukemia could develop. R. Philip Custer's 1974 atlas[46] accepts Martland's interpretation of "severe macrocytic anemia simulating pernicious type, associated with megablastomas of the bone marrow" as the first stage of radiation osteitis, to be followed by patchy fibroblastic replacement of marrow associated with an inflammatory reaction; poorly cellular fibrous replacement of marrow spaces; and, in some cases, osteogenic sarcoma. It is clear that neither Custer nor Martland regarded this as leukemia.

Aub et al.,[3] in 1952, reported on 30 symptomatic patients with increased radium burdens: one died of aplastic anemia and one may have died of leukemia, but

> leukemia such as is alleged to have been the cause of death of this patient has not been reported previously in persons with radium poisoning. Indeed, our evidence that this was an instance of true leukemia, rather than a leukemoid response, is not convincing.

Looney et al.[47] found no deaths from leukemia and only one from aplastic anemia among 44 patients given pure ^{226}Ra intravenously; Hasterlik and Finkel[48] reported one death from aplastic anemia and none from leukemia among six patients given ^{226}Ra intravenously; and Spiers et al.[49] found 10 cases of leukemia versus 9.2 expected among 2,940 male and female dial painters, including 4 with chronic lymphocytic leukemia (vs. 3.6 expected), generally regarded as not related to radiation, and therefore no excess. Polednak, Stehney and Lucas[50] found no statistically significant excess of deaths from leukemia among thorium workers, and no deaths from other hematologic disorders. Mori et al.[51] found significantly more erythroleukemia and aplastic anemia among Japanese patients injected with thorotrast than among controls. Both Sharpe[10] and Stebbings, Lucas and Stehney[52] found more myeloma but not more leukemia than expected among dial painters, although both exposure and latent periods were within ranges appropriate for leukemogenesis.[53]

In 1931, Martland wrote to Sir Humphrey Rolleston:

> Although I have been quoted to the effect that the anemias in the radium dial painters were of the aplastic type, I really never did say this. In the dial painters which I autopsied and studied, the anemias during life were only occasionally characterized by hemorrhagic tendencies. At autopsy all of them showed an intense hyperplastic marrow. I believe there is a difference between the effects of internal alpha bombardment and external penetrative radiation by gamma and x rays. External penetrative irradiation undoubtedly produces aplastic or aregenerative types of anemia, although unfortunately the pathological proof of this is meager, very few cases having been

autopsied. Internal radiation by the alpha particle, however, produces regenerative or hyperplastic anemias. . . .

It is interesting to note that in the cases autopsied recently the
mesothorium has disappeared while the radium persists. The lethal
amount of radioactive substances deposited in the bones of some of
the fatal cases has been as low as ten micrograms estimated as radium element deposited over the entire skeleton.[54]

No surviving objective evidence supports the suggestion that
what Martland described as "leucopenic aregenerative anemia"
was leukemia.

Studies of Radium Workers

Interest in the radium workers waxed and waned. The United
States Department of Labor, chiefly through its agent Sven Kjaer,
investigated the industry from 1925 to 1928, and from the late 1920s
through the 1930s, the United States Public Health Service was
involved. Until the 1950s, only symptomatic patients were studied
in any detail, chiefly by H. S. Martland in Newark and by Robley
D. Evans and his group at the Massachusetts Institute of Technology. W. B. Looney, William Norris and Charles Miller did some
early studies, and during the 1950s the Argonne National Laboratory's distinguished group (R. J. Hasterlik, Leo Marinelli, Austin
Brues and A. F. Stehney) began intensive work.

By about 1955, consensus had been reached that all surviving
radium workers could profitably be studied for exposure-response
data, and that such studies would require participation by a variety
of experts. Most of the New Jersey project's efforts were directed
toward individuals with low or undetectable preterminal body burdens of ^{226}Ra and whose only abnormalities, although asympto-
matic, might be anomalous skeletal roentgenographic changes,
many of which proved difficult to distinguish from physiological
skeletal senescence.

The New Jersey Radium Research Project began in November
1957, as a feasibility study and was converted to an epidemiologic
study in March 1958. From 1957 through about 1960, most effort
went into identifying and locating the thousand or so people who
had worked, chiefly between 1913 and 1925, in the New Jersey
radium industry. From 1959 through 1965, the project collected

medical, dental, radiographic, and autopsy material on those willing to cooperate. Active collection of material stopped in June 1967. All of the project material is filed at the Argonne National Laboratory, and a duplicate set of histologic slides and autoradiographs is filed at the Armed Forces Institute of Pathology.

Long-Term Clinical Findings

In 1974, Sharpe[10] reported autopsy findings on 42 long-term survivors, a small enough number but 4.2 percent of all those identified by name as having worked in the New Jersey radium industry, and 8.5 percent of those known to have survived 25 years or longer from their first occupational exposure to radium. Their preterminal burdens of ^{226}Ra ranged from 9.1 μCi to some level that could not be distinguished from natural background radioactivity.

Twenty-four of these 42 long-term survivors had malignant tumors or blood dyscrasias. Women's but not men's lifespans were shortened, probably because of the early deaths among dial painters, so no generalized "shortening of life" emerged from this study. Women radium workers produced proportionately fewer living children than did wives of male radium workers. Deafness and histories of otitis media were more frequent than expected. Jaw necrosis and spontaneous fractures through the shafts of long bones were frequent at preterminal burdens greater than 0.6 μCi ^{226}Ra. Osteogenic sarcoma and carcinoma of the paranasal sinuses and myeloma proved radium-related with long latent periods. Ten of 11 subjects with burdens measurable above background levels of radiation had radium osteonecrosis, as did 6 of 14 whose ^{226}Ra burdens could not be distinguished from background levels. Of 25 subjects whose bones were sufficiently sampled, 10 of 16 with osteonecrosis had cancer, as did 5 of 9 without osteonecrosis.[10,36,37]

Table 5.3 summarizes causes of death among New Jersey radium workers available for review at the time the study stopped data collection. These data have not been corrected when autopsy or other objective evidence indicated that death certificate diagnoses were in error or incomplete.

More New Jersey subjects died of malignant disease and blood dyscrasias than expected, and proportionately more perhaps than Polednak, Stehney and Rowland[55] reported from a midwestern

TABLE 5.3

Summary of Certifications as to Cause of Death, New Jersey Radium Workers

ICD Class		to 1920	1921 to 1930	1931 to 1940	1941 to 1950	1951 to 1960	1961 to 1970	1971 to	Total
I	Infectious and Parasitic	2	4	1	3				10
II	Malignant Neoplasms		5	12	23	31	35	13	119
III	Endocrine and Metabolic				1			1	2
IV	Blood and Blood-Forming Organs		5		1		1		7
V	Nervous System			2			3		5
VII	Circulatory System		6	14	27	27	73	18	165
VIII	Respiratory System	2	4	2	3	1	3	4	19
IX	Digestive System	1	3	3	2	5	5	2	21
X	Genitourinary System		1		2	2	2		7
XI	Complications of Pregnancy		1	1					2
XII	Skin and Subcutaneous Tissues					1			1
XIII	Musculoskeletal System		1						1
XIV	Congenital Anomalies				1				1
XVI	Symptoms and Ill-Defined Conditions						1		1
XVII	Accidents	1	1	6	3	5	11	3	30
	Total	6	31	41	66	72	134	41	391

group comparably exposed. Dealing with small numbers is always hazardous, but New Jersey subjects seem to have had more deaths than expected from cancers in the following primary sites: buccal cavity and pharynx, large intestine, rectum, respiratory system, urinary bladder, bone, "other and unspecified sites," and lymphatic-myeloma. Respiratory system cancers included paranasal sinus tumors and a not unanticipated number of bronchogenic carcinomas. Four of 5 lymphatic-myeloma deaths were from myeloma, and these 4 explain the increase in this category. More subjects than expected died from diseases of the blood and blood-forming organs, but all 7 in this group had anemias, aplastic and the ill-defined aregenerative type described by Martland. These 7 explain the excess, and other processes need not be implicated.

Five deaths from inflammatory conditions of the jaws (4) and mouth (1), 3 during 1921–1930 and one during each subsequent decade, may be regarded as complications of radium-related mandibular or maxillary osteonecrosis and osteomyelitis. Seven died from cirrhosis of the liver, more likely related to infectious hepatitis or to alcohol than to radium.

However, a number of cancers are known, from other sources and for which histologic proof exists, to have been omitted from the death certificates of these New Jersey subjects. Thirteen were omitted from 391 death certificates available from 597 reasonably completely reviewed cases. Hence, the total of 119 malignant neoplasms should be at least 132, and probably more than 132. This is no trivial statistical peccadillo—two of those omitted were osteogenic sarcomas, and one was a cancer of the temporal bone, generally regarded as clearly radium-related. Thus we fear that radium-related malignancies responsible for death in our series have been understated by at least 10 percent and perhaps more.

Review of certifications of death that mentioned *radium* or *radiation* in some form included 15 deaths from cancer or anemia and 11 from other causes. Most (14 of 15) cancer deaths certified as radium-related occurred before 1960, and only 1 was so certified after 1961. The noncancer, nonanemia but radium-related deaths listed were certified before 1960, almost all of them by Dr. Martland himself, and 8 of these unequivocally were radium-related: mastoiditis, inflammatory conditions of the jaws, chronic osteomyelitis and unspecified radiation.

Although the New Jersey Radium Research Project was active during the late 1950s and most of the 1960s, and although many of our subjects died during that period, *radiation* or *radium* in fact appeared on death certificates only when completed by one of the county medical examiners. Review of the hospital records of subjects admitted to quite respectable hospitals when they were actively participating in project studies only exceptionally included notes either as to participation in these studies or as to past radium industry employment. Deaths from external hazards, including ionizing radiation, fall under the medical examiner's jurisdiction, but most such offices are so overwhelmed by homicides and drug overdoses that they lack the resources to pursue occupational and environmental causes of death, much as they would like to do so.

How Much Radiation Did They Get?

The question of just how much radiation the New Jersey workers actually got, considering the insoluble problems introduced by ^{228}Ra(MsTh$_1$) with its short physical half-life and by hard gamma radiation from contaminated workplaces, is perhaps less clear than numbers would suggest. Quite reliable assays of ^{226}Ra can be based on exhaled ^{222}Rn or on whole body counting, techniques used on many living New Jersey subjects, and on direct radiochemical tissue assays. That estimates of lifetime exposures based on these measurements are so problematic proved a major disappointment. The real problem is the need to evaluate radiation exposure by whatever means are available: industrial hygiene reports, radiochemical assay of autopsy or exhumed material, time, place and duration of employment, and comparison with iatrogenic causes.

The radium protection standard remains the only radiologic health standard based on human experience, specifically the radium workers, and many standards for material other than ^{226}Ra have been calculated from it, using the relative biological equivalencies of various radioactive elements to ^{226}Ra. The 1940 standard has served well but may need reconsideration, because the distribution of radium osteonecrosis among subjects whose presumptive preterminal burdens of ^{226}Ra were well below 0.1 μCi suggests that this standard may very well be too high by at least a full order of magnitude.[37] On the other hand, changes in workplace hygiene that followed the early studies of the radium workers have made even this burden unlikely.

Summary

With many caveats and qualifications, data generated from study over seventy-five years of the New Jersey radium workers are consistent. They suggest subtle accumulation of risk over the entire lifetimes of those exposed to radium burdens at and probably below the existing recommended maximum permissible industrial body burden of 0.1 μCi ^{226}Ra. All ionizing radiation is carcinogenic, that due to alpha particles appears to have no threshold and to be linearly proportional in its effect to the accumulated dose. Bearing in mind the uncertainties in evaluating any epidemiologic data, we must also consider such imponderables as the whole biology of human senescence and of the relation of human immune function to carcinogenesis. Not only do we lack any but the most primitive techniques to study these problems, but we may yet need to develop whole new ways to think about them before we can fully assess the impact of seven or eight decades of low levels of ionizing radiation, internal or external.

Acknowledgments

I thank John Paul Decker, M.D., and Andrew F. Stehney, Ph.D., for their thoughtful comments on drafts of this chapter; and recall the memory of four collaborators in the New Jersey Radium Research Project who now sleep in peace—Gerome Bell, H.T.; Hugh G. Grady, M.D.; Carye-Belle Henle, M.D.; and John Raines, M.A.

References and Notes

[1]Alice Hamilton. 1943. *Exploring the Dangerous Trades,* 297–298. Boston: Little, Brown and Co.,

[2]*Radium* refers to ^{226}Ra and ^{228}Ra(MsTh$_1$) with their daughters; specific isotopes and elements are specified when appropriate.

[3]Aub, J. C.; Evans, R. D.; Hempelmann, L. H.; and H. S. Martland. 1952. "The Late Effects of Internally Deposited Radioactive Materials in Man." *Medicine* (Baltimore) 31:221–329.

164 W. D. SHARPE

[4]Petrow, H. G. 1966. *A Study of the Distribution of Ra-226, Ra-228, Pb-210 and Th-228 in Bone and Soft Tissue of Radium Dial Painters.* Ph.D. dissertation, New York University.

[5]Mole, R. H. 1979. "Carcinogenesis by Thorotrast and Other Sources of Irradiation, Especially Other α-emitters." *Environmental Research* 18: 192–215.

[6]Norris, W. P.; Speckman, T. W.; and Gustafson, P. F. 1955. "Studies of the Metabolism of Radium in Man." *American Journal of Roentgenology* 73:785–802.

[7]Rundo, J.; Essling, M. A.; and Huff, D. R. 1976. "Gross Distribution of [226]Ra in Man from External Counting." In *The Health Effects of Plutonium and Radium,* ed. W.S.S. Jee, 409–420. Salt Lake City, Utah: J. W. Press.

[8]Marshall, J. H. 1969. "The Retention of Radionuclides in Bone." In *Delayed Effects of Bone-Seeking Radionuclides,* ed. C. W. Mays et al., 7–27. Salt Lake City: University of Utah Press.

[9]Maletskos, C. J.; Keane, A. T.; Telles, N. C.; and Evans, R. D. 1969. "Retention and Absorption of [224]Ra and [234]Th and Some Dosimetric Considerations of [224]Ra in Human Beings." In *Delayed Effects of Bone-Seeking Radionuclides,* ed. C. W. Mays et al., 29–49. Salt Lake City: University of Utah Press.

[10]Sharpe, W. D. 1974. "Chronic Radium Intoxication: Clinical and Autopsy Findings in Long-Term New Jersey Survivors." *Environmental Research* 8:243–383. Contains a detailed bibliography of reports of the New Jersey Radium Research Project.

[11]Some historians have tried to make this into a male capitalist vs. female laborer issue, but the company's owner and chief chemist both died of radium intoxication, and the truth is that at the time nobody appreciated how dangerous radium was.

[12]Berg, Samuel. 1978. *Harrison Stanford Martland,* 168–190. New York: Vantage Press, has a first hand summary of Dr. Martland's investigation of the radium cases. Dr. Berg was, at the time, a resident and junior attending pathologist at Newark City Hospital.

[13]Blum, Theodor. 1924. "Osteomyelitis of the Mandible and Maxilla." *Journal of the American Dental Association* 11:802–805.

[14]The body of Miss A. M., first dial painter to die, aged 25, and who "used practically to eat the paint," on September 12, 1922, was exhumed in 1927 in connection with a lawsuit against the company. She had jaw necrosis with jugular vein erosion and sepsis, and her death had been certified as due to syphilis. Her body contained 48.4 μCi of [226]Ra. See St. George, A. V.; Gettler, A. O.; and Muller, R. H. 1929. "Radioactive Substances in a Body Five Years After Death." *Archives of Pathology* (Chicago) 7:397–405.

[15]When the AIDS epidemic hit New York City in 1980–1981, hospital pathologists knew that they faced a new disease, but didn't know what it was. It took two or three years to sort it out, and for the horror to set in.

[16]Castle, W. B.; Drinker, Katherine R.; and Drinker, C. K. 1925. "Necrosis of the Jaw in Workers Employed in Applying a Luminous Paint Containing Radium." *Journal of Industrial Hygiene* 7: 317–382.

[17]Cloutier, R. J. 1980. "Florence Kelley and the Radium Dial Painters." *Health Physics* 39:711–716.

[18]Martland, H. S. 1925. "Some Unrecognized Dangers in the Use and Handling of Radioactive Substances." *Proceedings of the New York Pathological Society*, N.S. 25:88–92.

[19]Martland, H. S.; Conlon, Philip; and Knef, J. P. 1925. "Some Unrecognized Dangers in the Use and Handling of Radioactive Substances." *Journal of the American Medical Association* 85:1769–1776.

[20]Martland, H. S. 1931. "The Occurrence of Malignancy in Radioactive Persons." *American Journal of Cancer* 15:2435–2516.

[21]Goldmark, Josephine. 1953. *Impatient Crusader: Florence Kelley's Life Story*, 189–204. Urbana: University of Illinois Press.

[22]Hoffman, F. L. 1925. "Radium (Mesothorium) Necrosis." *Journal of the American Medical Association* 85:961–965. Martland always credited Hoffman with the clinical definition of radium osteonecrosis.

[23]B. B., the patient reported in detail in Glenn, J. A., Jr.; Galindo, Joseph; and Lawrence, C. E. 1960. "Chronic Radium Poisoning in a Dial Painter: Case Report." *American Journal of Roentgenology* 83:465–473, saw *Hazel Flagg*, which she much enjoyed. A 1937 motion picture, *Nothing Sacred*, starring Miss Carole Lombard and Mr. Fredric March, is also based on a dial painter, and is occasionally shown on television.

[24]Bloomfield, J. J., and Knowles, F. L. 1933. "Health Aspects of Radium Dial Painting. II. Occupational Environment." *Journal of Industrial Hygiene* 15:368–382.

[25]Florence Kelley to H. S. Martland, letter dated March 28, 1929, Archives, New Jersey Medical School, Newark. (Hereafter NJMSA)

[26]Schwartz, Louis; Knowles, F. L.; Britten, R. H.; and Thompson, L. R. 1933. "Health Aspects of Radium Dial Painting. I. Scope and Findings." *Journal of Industrial Hygiene* 15:362–367.

[27]Evans, R. D. 1943. "Protection of Radium Dial Workers and Radiologists from Injury by Radium." *Journal of Industrial Hygiene* 25:253–269, is a good summary of the state of radium protection at the time.

[28]National Bureau of Standards. 1941. *Safe Handling of Radio-Active Luminous Compound*. Handbook H27. Washington, D.C.: Government Printing Office.

[29]H. S. Martland to F. B. Flinn, letter dated March 29, 1930: "[O]ver two years ago I refused to examine any living cases to avoid becoming involved in any litigation." (NJMSA)

[30]Sharpe, W. D. 1971. "Radium Osteitis with Osteogenic Sarcoma." *Bulletin of the New York Academy of Medicine* 47:1059–1082, presents medical and social details of this unusually difficult patient.

[31]Liondale Bleach Works v. Riker, 85 N. J. L. 426.

[32]U.S. Radium Corp. v. Globe Indemnity Co., 13 N. J. Misc. 316 178A.271, affirmed in 116 N. J. L. 90, 182A.626 (1935).

[33]P. L. 1926, chap. 31, 62.

[34]LaPorte v. U.S. Radium Corp., 13 F. Supp. 263 (1936).

[35]Waste from radium extracted ores was used as landfill in the then-rural areas of Glen Ridge and Montclair. With the suburban building boom that followed World War II, houses were built on these filled areas, some of which now contain what are regarded as unacceptably high levels of radon. See, e.g., *New York Times*, July 1, 1989, announcing plans to dig up and to haul away some 50,000 tons of "radioactive soil" in Essex County, New Jersey, at a cost of about $53 million.

[36]Sharpe, W. D. 1976. Chronic Radium Intoxication: Morphology of Bone and Marrow Infarcts. In *The Health Effects of Plutonium and Radium,* ed. W.S.S. Jee, 457–483. Salt Lake City, Utah: J. W. Press.

[37]Sharpe, W. D. 1983. "Chronic Radium Intoxication: Radium Osteonecrosis and Cancer in Relation to ^{226}Ra Burdens." *Health Physics* 44(suppl. 1): 149–154.

[38]Looney, W. B. 1958. "Effects of Radium in Man." *Science* 127:630–633.

[39]Barrer, L. A.; Henle, Carye-Belle; Bonda, R.; and Fisher, H. W. 1963. *Atlas of Current Roentgenographic Findings in the New Jersey Radium Cases.* Trenton: New Jersey State Department of Health, NYO-2761.

[40]Hunter, D. 1978. *The Diseases of Occupations,* 6th ed., 889–902. London: Hodder and Stoughton.

[41]Littman, M. S.; Kirsh, I. E.; and Keane, A. T. 1978. Radium-Induced Malignant Tumors of the Mastoid and Paranasal Sinuses." *American Journal of Roentgenology* 131:773–785.

[42]Martland, H. S. 1929. "Occupational Poisoning in Manufacture of Luminous Watch Dials." *Journal of the American Medical Association* 92:466–473, 552–559.

[43]The first deaths, in New Jersey, from occupationally related ionizing radiation occurred among young men at Thomas A. Edison's laboratory in West Orange who, shortly before the turn of the century, worked on the development of a fluoroscope demonstrated at the Columbian Exposition, but that is another story.

[44]Mole, R. H. 1990. "A-Particle Irradiation and Human Leukaemia." *British Journal of Radiology,* in press.

[45]Martland, H. S. 1926. "Histopathology of Certain Anemias Due to Radioactivity." *Proceedings of the New York Pathological Society* N.S. 26:65–72.

[46]Custer, R. P. 1974. *An Atlas of the Blood and Bone Marrow,* 2d ed., 218–219. Philadelphia: W. B. Saunders Co.

[47]Looney, W. B.; Hasterlik, R. J.; Brues, A. M.; and Skirmont, E. 1955. "A Clinical Investigation of the Chronic Effects of Radium Salts Administered Therapeutically (1915–1931)." *American Journal of Roentgenology* 73: 1006–1037.

[48]Hasterlik, R. J., and Finkel, A. J. 1965. "Diseases of Bones and Joints Associated with Intoxication by Radioactive Substances, Principally Radium." *Medical Clinics of North America* 49:285–296.

[49]Spiers, F. W., Lucas, H. F.; Rundo, J.; and Anast, Georgia A. 1983. "Leukaemia Incidence in the U.S. Dial Workers." *Health Physics* 44(suppl. 1): 65–72.

[50]Polednak, A. P.; Stehney, A. F.; and Lucas, H. F. 1983. "Mortality Among Male Workers at a Thorium-Processing Plant." *Health Physics* 44(suppl. 1): 239–251.

[51]Mori, T.; Kato, Y.; Aoki, N.; and Hatakeyama, S. 1983. Statistical Analysis of Japanese Thorotrast-Administered Autopsy Cases. Health Physics 44 (Supp. 1):281–292.

[52]Stebbings, J. H.; Lucas, H. F.; and Stehney, A. F. 1984. "Mortality from Cancers of Major Sites in Female Radium Dial Workers." *American Journal of Industrial Medicine* 5:435–459.

[53]Moloney, W. C. 1987. "Radiogenic Leukemia Revisited." *Blood* 70:905–908.

[54]H. S. Martland to Sir Humphrey Rolleston, letter dated April 2, 1931 (NJMSA).

[55]Polednak, A. P.; Stehney, A. F.; and Rowland, R. E. 1978. "Mortality Among Women First Employed Before 1930 in the U.S. Radium-Dial Painting Industry." *American Journal of Epidemiology* 107:179–195.

[56]Occupational and environmental causes of disease are still not taken seriously, and although the decline in the number of autopsies performed is worrisome, more really useful epidemiologic information is probably lost simply through failure to ask patients appropriate questions.

• CHAPTER 6 •

The Politics of Lead

RICHARD P. WEDEEN, M.D.

This chapter presents an update of the history of lead poisoning to supplement the book entitled Poison in the Pot: The Legacy of Lead, *published in 1984. As a participant in the scientiic and policy debates surrounding lead, Dr. Wedeen focuses on warnings unheeded and opportunities lost. The possibility of eliminating lead poisoning remains mired in the interminable quest for "more data," as if data could decide how to balance wealth and health.*

The story of tetraethyl lead fatalities in New Jersey reached the newspapers in 1923 but was not evident in current medical textbooks until David Rosner and Gerald Markowitz published Dying for Work: Workers' Safety and Health in Twentieth-Century America *in 1987. As a nephrologist, Dr. Wedeen is interested in knowing who knew what and when regarding lead as a cause of kidney disease and how adults came to be so widely ignored in modern descriptions of lead poisoning. The methods of obfuscation of the obvious remain a recurrent theme throughout this book. Vested interests control knowledge as well as policy. The Office of Management and Budget under the Bush administration contended that a hazardous workplace is preferable to none at all because at least the workers are employed ("Wealth Is Health" 1992).*

Lead is the oldest of industrial toxins. Human use of lead began at the dawn of the iron age because it is extracted from ores at relatively low temperatures and is found in great abundance in the company of silver. The signs and symptoms of acute lead poisoning were described two thousand years ago. Vitruvius, the Roman architect, warned his contemporaries about the health effects of the aqueducts he helped design. But lead in water remains subject to never-ending rediscovery. Because more is known about lead than any other environmental toxin, the failure of scientific information to mold public policy is dramatically highlighted. But experts do not constitute common knowledge. Health yields to economic need. And so

New Jersey has had more than its share of hazards from this most venerable of industrial contaminants.

One recent irony concerning lead toxicity came to the U.S. Supreme Court as a sex discrimination case. The suit was based on a 1982 company policy that required premenopausal women to undergo sterilization to be employed in Johnson Controls Inc. automobile battery plants (Greenhouse 1991). On March 20, 1991, the Court ruled that women could not be excluded from jobs under the guise of "fetal protection." While this decision would seem to allow women to be subjected to the same lead poisoning that men encounter in the workplace, the purpose of the ruling is to provide equal opportunity for employment. It is likely that the ruling will provide a major impetus for manufacturers to clean up worksites and make the lead industry safe for both sexes. In other legal news, since Newark would not join the class action suit of Boston, Baltimore, New York, and Philadelphia against the historical suppliers of paint, a leading environmental law firm in New Jersey elected to sue the city on behalf of the young victims of deteriorating lead paint (Shannon 1992).

Politics mediates priorities for science as well as government. The star system of the entertainment industry has found its place in scientific expertise. In lead policy, the stars are Philip Landrigan, M.D., Irving Selikoff's worthy successor at the Mt. Sinai School of Medicine; Ellen Silbergeld, Ph.D., spokesperson for the Environmental Defense Fund and an accomplished neuroscientist; Herb Needleman, M.D., professor of child psychiatry at the University of Pittsburgh; and John Rosen, M.D., professor of pediatrics at the Einstein Medical School in New York. The contributions of these players emerge frequently in both Poison in the Pot *and this sequel. Together with supporters in the National Institute of Environmental Health and Safety, the Centers for Disease Control, and the Agency for Toxic Substance Disease Registry, they have brought the "action" level of blood lead in children down from 40 to 10 $\mu g/dl$ in a decade.*

Needleman is almost single-handedly responsible for the removal of lead from gasoline. He demonstrated the subtle but sure effects of low-level lead exposure on neurobehavioral development in children. Despite the fact that over a dozen subsequent studies have substantially confirmed his findings throughout the world, the lead companies orchestrated a personal attack on Needleman's integrity that resulted in a formal investigation by the University of Pittsburgh. Having an intimate knowledge of the politics of academia as well as the politics of lead, Needleman demanded that the hearings be open to the public, in spite of University policy requiring closed hearings ostensibly to protect the reputation of the accused. He was exonerated of the charge of scientific misconduct by a long, painful, and often humiliating investigation (Putka 1992b). Needleman initiated a class action suit against the University of Pittsburgh and the National Institutes of Health for their roles in supporting the flawed process of adjudicating scientific disputes (Putka 1992a).

The saga of in vivo bone lead determinations described in this chapter also continues with little resolution. In July 1992, the third symposium in four years on in vivo bone X-ray fluorescence measurements was held at the National Institutes of Environmental Health Sciences and was sponsored by Dr. Landrigan's Division of the Mt. Sinai Medical School. As described in this chapter, progress in the field has been paralyzed by the proponent of one form of the noninvasive bone lead measurement (L XRF). In this politically rich environment, where expertise, power, and science merge, none of the scientific luminaries would publicly acknowledge that the emperor has no clothes. Yet none use the technique advocated by this influential expert. The chairman of the symposium calculated that in vivo L XRF is subject to uncontrollable variability. For his efforts he was attacked personally and effectively intimidated. His calculations will not appear in the published summary of the symposium. And throughout the debate among professional scientists, the need to protect the public plays second fiddle to the tunes of self-promotion. Scientific truth seemed highly subjective.

• • •

CONTEMPORARY efforts to control environmental lead pollution reinforce the view that government is incapable of formulating a coherent approach. The societal conflicts are so basic and the stakes so high that effective regulatory policy seems unattainable. When hard choices have to be made, short-term economic needs usually outweigh longer-term environmental consequences. For every policy decision someone pays a price. The question of who pays is the essence of policy development. The decision depends on who is making the cost–benefit analysis.

Blame the Victim

The city of Newark epitomizes the urban decline of the northeastern United States. Nineteenth-century pride in industrial growth gave way to inner-city poverty after World War II. Small businesses that thrived on immigrant labor for over a century were rendered obsolete by advanced technology and communications. In place of the waves of Irish, German, and Italian laborers, southern blacks settled in Newark soon after the war. The promise of employment in the New York metropolitan area faded with the departure of the urban middle class, both black and white, to the suburbs. In the inner city, an underclass of unskilled, underemployed welfare recipients became increasingly isolated from their middle-class suburban neighbors. Real estate taxes climbed as the industrial and business tax base evaporated. In 1989, New Jersey had the highest incidence of AIDS from intravenous drug abuse in the continental United States (Centers for Disease Control 1989); the center of the epidemic was Newark.

Resentment of urban renewal that excluded blacks from construction jobs contributed to racial tensions. The Newark riots of the late 1960s resulted. Fire razed the neighborhood in Newark's Central Ward, where the New Jersey Medical School was to be built in the 1960s and 1970s. In 1988, Newark dealt with deteriorating housing by dynamiting its thirty-year-old federally subsidized developments. Townhouse condominiums for the black middle class replaced the demolished public housing for impoverished blacks. What became of the thousands displaced by this demolition has not been reported.

The dangers of leaded paint to children in urban housing became a major public health concern in the 1960s. Childhood lead poisoning was, however, by no means a new observation. Pica (the ingestion of nonfood substances) for leaded paint had been described in 1776 by Dr. John Fothergill, an eminent London physician and benefactor of America's first medical school, in Philadelphia (Wedeen 1984). Noting several unusual sources of lead poisoning just nine years after Sir George Baker's seminal description of lead poisoning in the "Devonshire Colic," Fothergill described the case of an eight-year-old boy "complaining of pains in his belly and stomach. . . . On examining further," he reported, "I found, also that he had got a trick of being almost continuously wetting his pencils in his mouth, while there was paint on them" (Fothergill 1775). This may be the first reported case of lead poisoning from childhood pica.

In 1852, the Committee on Zinc Paint, established by the Board of Assistant Aldermen of New York City, passed a resolution urging the use of zinc- instead of lead-based paints for "roofs, iron works and places exposed to impure air" (Assistant Aldermen

1852). The committee's efforts had been instigated by the New Jersey Zinc Company, which claimed that zinc paint was necessary to protect painters and paint manufacturers. A testimonial by Edward H. Dixon of New York City, in support of the resolution, stated, "There is no doubt whatever that the poison is slowly and constantly disseminating from walls and painted privies, and noisome places, wherever, sulphurated hydrogen can act upon it" (Assistant Aldermen 1852).

The dangers of leaded paint to children were further recognized in an epidemic of lead poisoning in Queensland, Australia, at the turn of the century (Wedeen 1984). Seventy-five years of study of these children established hypertension and kidney disease in young adults (known as "Queensland nephritis") as a potential consequence of the ingestion of leaded paint in childhood. Between 1922 and 1931 nine countries banned interior leaded paint in housing to protect children, but the United States did not follow their example until 1970 (Rabin 1989).

The recognition of large numbers of lead-poisoned children in Newark in the 1960s as a result of leaded paint finally brought about regulations requiring leaded-paint removal. The Municipal Court of Newark faced its obligation to enforce the city's lead ordinance, Title 14 of 1966. In 1988, having identified elevated blood levels among half of the children of Newark, the city mandated that landlords remove leaded paint from deteriorating housing if any child in the dwelling was found to have an elevated blood lead level. This law seemed to represent a major victory for the lead control forces. The victory was, however, limited. Prevention of lead poisoning played no part in the municipal strategy. The city became involved only after lead poisoning occurred. Fundamental issues of housing for the poor were not addressed, and enforcement of the law created almost as many problems as it corrected. While the lead abatement regulations never resulted in the imprisonment of a nonresident landlord as had been intended, they did result in the imprisonment of a victim of leaded paint.

Newark's lead-poisoning control laws backfired on this family. An army of public health, welfare, and urban renewal officials descended on them. Triggered by an elevated blood lead level found in a nine-month-old infant, state law required the Newark Health Department to take remedial action. The mother was on welfare and the father unemployed. The home had been acquired by default at the death of the original owner. Lead Poison Control officers ordered the parents to remove the interior paint by scraping and sanding, a process guaranteed to cause poisoning of the other children in the home, and the adults as well. In 1989, Newark required "do-it-yourself" lead abatement methods that were specifically forbidden in Baltimore in 1987. Bureaucratic turf remained sacrosanct; the municipalities proved as insular as academic specialties. In Baltimore, under the leadership of Julian Chisolm, Ellen Silbergeld, and Mark Farfel, trained lead abatement workers used "safe houses" to protect families during lead removal and provided interest-free loans to facilitate housing rehabilitation for the poor. Lead removal was not undertaken unless it could be done safely and without costing the homeowners their home. In Baltimore, social workers, rather than the courts, guided the victims of lead poisoning.

In Newark, the judiciary was substituted for the social worker with disastrous results. Each city agency operated on its own agenda. No financial support or technical guidance was supplied to the family. To strengthen the urgency of the lead abatement order, the mother was advised that her children could be taken away on the allegation that exposure to lead is a form of child abuse. Within a month of the mandated amateur lead abatement, two children required hospitalization for acute poisoning caused by the removal process. To finance the court-ordered lead abatement, the mother arranged a new mortgage at 19.5 percent interest. This second mortgage was obtained from the company she had contracted with to replace the old lead-painted windows at a cost ten times the going rate. The father reluctantly removed the paint from the interior walls unassisted but, according to the court, was too slow in completing the task. Unable to pay the $2,400 fine incurred for his slow pace, he was arrested and jailed. When advised of the inappropriateness of incarceration as a method of lead abatement, the municipal judge placed the father on house arrest to permit him to look for a job and to continue his one-man lead removal project. The fine was not waived. Within six months, the family elected to give up their home, hoping to sell it before foreclosure consumed the last of their assets.

The judge, Lead Poison Control officials, and the director of the Newark Department of Health and Human Services maintained that the family was punished because of their unwillingness to comply with the court order. The city saw the suffering of the children brought on by the lead poisoning (and consequent loss of father, income, assets, and home) as evidence of child abuse by the parents. Lead poisoning in Newark was compounded by a program of correction that was blind to the underlying social realities. The insult of blame was added to the injury from lead.

While identifying individual misconduct does not preclude identifying other causal factors, in practice that is exactly what happened. The parents were seen as perpetrators rather than as victims of lead poisoning. Finding and fining the paint manufacturers who profited from leaded paints for centuries after the dangers of the paints were known seemed remote, complex, and impractical. After a year of prodding, city officials still would not join the tort liability suit brought by New York, Baltimore, Boston, and Philadelphia against the paint manufacturers to gain funds for lead abatement (Lubasch 1989).

The perversion of public health goals in Newark is not an idiosyncracy of that beleaguered city but has the earmarks of de facto national policy, "acquiescence to the status quo" (Tesh 1988:162). In Newark, the rhetoric supporting "affordable housing" is belied by policies that create homelessness.

No city or state official asked who should be responsible for safe lead removal. No one assisted the family through the quagmire of city, state, and federal agencies and official misinformation surrounding lead abatement. No one knew how to obtain low-interest loans from the federal Department of Housing and Urban Development (HUD) for lead abatement. It seems likely that these funds never reached the poor of Newark. In May 1989, a dramatic HUD corruption scandal began to unfold in the newspapers. Investigations revealed payoffs to Republican stalwarts from James Watt, secretary of the interior, to Samuel Pierce, secretary of HUD, leading to indictments of HUD staff under the supervision of the Newark regional offices. It was rumored that if HUD funds flowed to Newark at all, they were used to purchase explosives for the demolition of public housing. New Jersey's own low-interest mortgage programs have been described as among the best kept secrets of the state government. In December 1990, HUD and the federal Centers for Disease Control (CDC) announced a renewed effort to rid fifty-seven million American homes of lead paint at an estimated cost of $2.4 billion per year (Hilts 1990). The alphabet soup of federal agencies sharing responsibility for controlling lead exposure—FDA, NIH, EPA, NIEHS, CDC, NIOSH, OSHA, HUD, Superfund, NCTR,

CEH, ATSDR, ERC—attests to the inevitable incoherence of federal policy.

In the 1980s, the rhetoric of individualism undermined community goals and reinforced Draconian municipal policies. The 25 percent reduction in staff and 70 percent reduction in spending achieved by HUD under the Reagan administration, coupled with systematic corruption of housing rehabilitation, left little funding to trickle down to the urban poor. Lead abatement in Newark exemplifies Sylvia Nobel Tesh's observation that "first, and most obvious, economic individualism and political individualism make government regulations perverse" (Tesh 1988:160). The bureaucracy empowered to enforce lead abatement in Newark is characterized by F. B. Smith's description of the superintendents of workhouses in Dickensian London: "So far as I have found, with one exception, they reveal that they were rather pleased with themselves for having gained office and being permitted to order other peoples' lives, and honestly but complacently puzzled that paupers should have allowed themselves to sink into poverty" (Smith 1979).

"A Little Colic"

New Jersey's pride in industrialization peaked with the centennial celebration of 1876. "There is no single industry in our state that gives promise of a better future than that of pottery," proclaimed the Bureau of Statistics of Labor and Industries (New Jersey. Bureau of Statistics [NJBOS] 1879:225; New Jersey State Legislative Documents [NJSLD] 1879). From the first pottery made at Old Bridge in 1800 to the white ware manufacturing centers of Trenton and Jersey City of the mid nineteenth century, ceramics exemplified how industry and art could "restore prosperity and enhance our national wealth" (226).

Official enthusiasm for "ceramic mania" was, however, tempered by consideration of "the diseases of potters, their causes and prevention," which appeared in the eleventh annual report of the Board of Health in 1887 (New Jersey Board of Health [NJBOH] 1887:231; NJSLD 1888) Describing twenty-one potteries in Trenton (the "Staffordshire of America"), David Warman noted that work in these factories was "deleterious to life and health. . . . Those engaged in this industry are more or less subject to the following diseases, viz.: 1. Potters' asthma and potters' consumption. 2. Lead-poisoning. 3. Rheumatism, . . . diseases of the heart, . . . nerve pains or neuralgia. 4. Disorders of the digestive organs, liver and stomach. 5. Anemia. . . ." (98)

Except for pulmonary disease (silicosis and tuberculosis), the afflictions of potters were attributable to lead poisoning. Warman condemned the neglect of cleanliness, inattention to ventilation, and intemperance of the potters. In accord with the thinking of the time, he found "a little colic or constipation, and it may happen, some derangements of digestion," entirely acceptable for these workers. To prevent the more severe cases, "the shops should be freely sprinkled with water and kept scrupulously clean" (112). To prevent pulmonary disease, Warman noted, "The keeping of the mouth closed and breathing only through the nose, and the occasional cleansing and wetting of the nostrils, by a sponge, are of great service" (99).

The failure of state government to require the pottery industry to create safe working conditions stemmed from a reluctance to increase the cost of manufacturing and from the perception that the laborers were responsible for the diseases they acquired. The data painstakingly collected by the Bureau of Statistics of Labor and Industry served to justify the dismissal of sick workers because of their alleged carelessness.

In antiquity, the cost of disease in the workplace was borne by captive slaves condemned to the silver mines of the Aegean. The price of capitulation in war was death in the workplace. In its more modern form, the legal doctrine of the "assumption of risk," the costs of occupational injury and disease were transferred to free workers. Assignment of the risk of injury to the injured effectively relieved employers of responsibility for creating a safe work environment. The workers, the public, and physicians saw this as only natural. All agreed that occupational lead poisoning was due to the carelessness of individual workers. Since only a few lead workers complained of symptoms at any one time, these were deemed either careless or unusually "susceptible," and were fired.

Physicians were central to understanding lead poisoning, but with few exceptions the medical profession remained aloof from the social context of the disease. The culture of medicine kept public health and industrial disease at arm's length (Rosenberg 1987). Science and technology were marshaled to the war on disease, but physicians, ensconced in their institutional citadel, the hospital, catered to those who could afford to pay and to "interesting" cases. A preoccupation with social justice gains no rewards in the medical marketplace or in academic medicine. The hapless, the helpless, and the homeless were left to the almshouse in earlier times and to a punitive social welfare system in the twentieth century (Rosenberg 1987). Industrial diseases were invisible to most physicians (Wedeen 1989). Policing the workplace and environment was not the business of medicine. Practitioners perceived themselves as serving the common good through the cure of disease. Prevention was relegated to public health officials and child welfare advocates. Physicians restricted their role to the admonition of patients for unhealthful behavior, leaving to others the responsibility for dealing with the environmental, cultural, and social causes of disease.

Occupational medicine was the domain of employers whose mandate was to keep production costs down. This usually meant that industrialists too saw occupational injury as the worker's responsibility. To the owners, injury on the job was a consequence of worker behavior rather than the workplace environment (Crawford 1977). Unions acquiesced to the status quo by leaving health in the workplace under the control of the employers.

Conflicts between societal needs and professional priorities remain a source of tension. The medical establishment approaches occupational and environmental issues with caution while embracing organ transplantation and molecular biology with open arms. The imperatives of curative medicine have not been extended to prevention, to the working poor, or to social deviants. Medical ethics does not require accepting responsibility for the environment. Social justice remains beyond the technical curriculum.

Physicians' attitudes toward lead poisoning tend to preserve the status quo. Despite ample evidence of delayed manifestations of lead toxicity, clinical diagnosis still revolves around the classical symptoms: colic, peripheral neuropathy, and encephalopathy. Laboratory diagnosis depends on anemia or elevated blood lead levels, relatively advanced manifestations of toxic exposure. This definition of lead poisoning precludes recognition of the delayed effects of cumulative exposure. It ignores the fact that lead is stored in bone for decades but remains in blood for only a few weeks. Increasing evidence that bone lead stores predict the delayed effects of lead has not generated enough interest to stimulate use of a safe, new, and practical method to measure bone lead stores, even though the technology has been available for twenty-five years. This technique, known as "in vivo tibial K X-ray fluorescence" (XRF), is a noninvasive way to measure lead in bone and may eventually supersede the measurement of lead in blood (Wedeen 1990). Whether acceptance of the new approach, which requires a change in medical thinking, will occur in five or fifty years remains to be seen.

Resistance to using bone lead stores rather than blood lead concentrations for assessing lead exposure has many sources. In addition to medical complacency, both scientific and political controversy surrounds lead poisoning. Genuine differences of opinion arise from the complexity of chronic disease. The reluctance of physicians to accept lead as a newly recognized contributing cause of all-too-familiar medical problems is well illustrated by the role of lead in hypertension. In the last six years, over thirty-five epidemiologic studies have indicated that low-level lead exposure contributes to the development of high blood pressure (Victery 1988). A consensus symposium sponsored by the National Institutes of Environmental Health and Safety (NIEHS), the federal Environmental Protection Agency (EPA), and the University of North Carolina addressed the role of lead in high blood pressure in 1988, but international symposia and publications devoted to hypertension continue to ignore this preventable etiology (Kiple 1987).

Each of the involved medical disciplines, for example, epidemiology, hypertension, occupational medicine, internal medicine, and pediatrics, seems to take a kind of perverse pride in not communicating with the others. Professional advancement depends on recognition by the power structure within each discipline only. Experts outside the circumscribed inner circle can contribute little to career aspirations. Professional status is enhanced by the creation of a private language, a special jargon that is often unintelligible to rival fields. Ignorance by experts on hypertension of the lead/hypertension hypothesis may therefore be viewed as a consequence of the parochialism of medical specialization; a strategy that protects control over research funds and career advancement.

Another explanation for the reluctance of hypertension experts to consider the lead hypothesis is offered by Tesh in *Hidden Arguments: Political Ideology in Disease Prevention Policy*. Tesh finds broad political meaning in the way scientific data are interpreted. In this perspective, an environmental cause of hypertension strikes at the very heart of the lifestyle theory of cardiovascular disease. Hypertension and heart disease experts contend that personal behavior, for example, diet, exercise, smoking, and stress, causes these diseases. The lifestyle theory requires individual behavior modification under the supervision of physician–scientists. An environmental contribution to hypertension, on the other hand, would require government intervening in lead production.

Viewing hypertension as a personal rather than an environmental issue has important implications for preventive actions that are not taken; salt and cholesterol need not be removed from fastfoods if eating is solely an individual responsibility. Individuals, not the tobacco industry, are chastised and receive the brunt of the antismoking crusade. Lead need not be removed from the environment by those who profit from its sale but must be avoided by those who ingest or inhale it. Lead abatement must be accomplished by those who are poisoned rather than by those who profit from lead paint. The excess incidence of hypertension and end-stage renal disease in black males is a lifestyle or genetic issue subject to scientific analysis but not to legislative action to remove lead from the environment.

Identification of environmental factors that require community action is unnecessary if individual lifestyles are the major cause of disease. Those who become sick because of ill-advised behavior are undeserving of financial protection by those who behave properly. Why should those who choose to live wisely pay insurance premium rates to support such deviants? According to this construction, nonconforming victims of AIDS, heart disease, and cancer should not receive benefits from taxes on the earnings of healthy conformists or share in the community protection offered by life or medical insurance.

The prevention policy suggested by the lead/hypertension hypothesis is very different from that suggested by the lifestyle theory. An environmental cause of disease requires fundamental social change; the elimination of lead pollution. Tesh points out that basic assumptions about disease causality are largely unrecognized by those who make them. Such assumptions are rooted in a shared cultural subconscious that determines what questions are important and what answers are acceptable. According to Tesh, the phrasing of questions is as fundamental to policy decisions as it is to the experimental strategies of science. An environmental etiology of chronic disease suggests that medical care costs cannot be reduced by diet and exercise, or by chastising the incorrigible who fail to share the behavioral vision. In terms of economic consequence, blaming lifestyle is far more appealing to physicians, government, and business than is blaming industrial pollution. Moreover, the lifestyle theory has deep cultural roots, being more consistent with the Protestant ethic and American individualism.

Chronic disease induced by long-term lead absorption does not follow traditional medical concepts of causation. The multifactorial nature of chronic disease, with its interactions with age, nutrition, and other diseases, makes cause and effect elusive. It seems likely that only determination of bone lead stores, the body burden of lead, by in vivo tibial XRF can resolve these uncertainties by providing information on the distribution of lead in large populations from which risk ratios can be calculated. Only in the last decade have the experts come to regard lead stored in bone as a hazard (Schutz et al. 1987; Silbergeld et al. 1988). Physicians have come to recognize risk ratios as indicative of causality only in the last two decades.

To address the technical question of whether the high-energy K or the weaker L characteristic fluorescent X-rays from lead should be used to measure bone lead, an international conference on lead in bone, sponsored by the National Institute of Environmental Health and Safety, the EPA, and the University of Maryland, was convened in Columbia, Maryland, in March 1989 (Fowler 1991). The consensus favored the use of K X-rays for determining the distribution of lead stores in the population as a whole. As a proponent of K X-rays for the previous ten years, I received the following letter from the distinguished proponent of L X-rays: "If you are preparing a manuscript for the Maryland meeting, I would urge you to focus on published, peer-reviewed data and not on the opinions of K and L instruments. If you fail to do so, in my view, you may produce injury to yourself and to a very important field that needs to grow." In the heady rush toward social change, this investigator may have lost the distinction between ideology and science. Self-advancement and political advocacy merged. The ends justified the means, and the hint of power behind the scenes was no idle threat. In the academic community, research on lead assumes the risks usually reserved for those exposed to noxious agents.

"The House of Butterflies"

The failure to safeguard the public from environmental lead and workers from occupational exposure is due not only to the complacency of physicians and public officials but also to the attitudes of the wider society. For centuries, a pervasive disinterest reflected shared values that had a powerful economic base. In a remarkable pair of essays published in 1987 in *Dying for Work: Workers' Safety and Health in Twentieth-Century America*, David Rosner, Gerald Markowitz, and William Graebner recount how information about lead toxicity was systematically suppressed for half a century. General Motors, Standard Oil, and the E. I. duPont de Nemours & Corp. effectively controlled research on lead, although their immediate goal was to protect their investment in the "gift from God," tetraethyl lead (Rosner and Markowitz 1987).

Within a year of the discovery of the antiknock properties of tetraethyl lead at the General Motors Research Laboratories in 1922, Du Pont and General Motors formed the Ethyl Corporation to market the additive. The absence of the word "lead" from the new company's name was designed to reduce public anxiety. By October 1924, 138 cases of severe poisoning from tetraethyl lead had been reported, including 13 deaths (Machle 1935). Of the fatalities, 5 occurred at Standard Oil's Bayway laboratories in Elizabeth, New Jersey (Figure 6.1), and 4 at Du Pont's Carney Point, New Jersey, plant (Hamilton et al. 1925). Other deaths occurred at Du Pont's Chambers Works at Deepwater, New Jersey, and at General Motors in Dayton, Ohio. The symptoms of tetraethyl lead poisoning were due to toxic effects on the brain, acute encephalopathy. About 80 percent of those involved in manufacturing the additive experienced hallucinations (Rosner and Markowitz 1987). The *New York Times* referred to the toxic material as "loony gas," while the Deepwater plant was dubbed "The House of Butterflies" by the workers (Figure 6.2).

Recognizing the threat to the company, General Motors contracted with the U.S. Bureau of Mines to investigate tetraethyl lead toxicity, reserving the right of prior approval of publications. The Ethyl Corporation gained the credibility of government for its research but still could prevent release of damaging information. After performing a series of inadequate animal experiments, the Bureau of Mines gave tetraethyl lead a clean bill of health. Speaking for General Motors, vice-president Thomas Midgely, discoverer

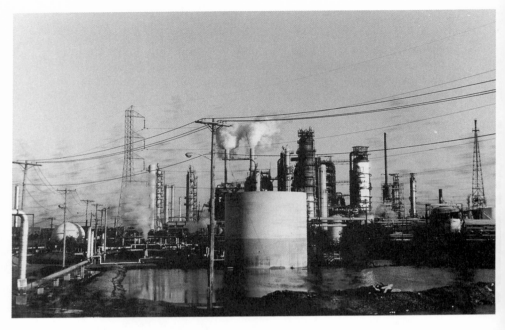

FIGURE 6.1.   Exxon's Bayway Refinery and Chemical Plant, Linden, New Jersey. Site of tetraethyl lead fatalities in 1923. Photo by Lynn Butler, November 1990.

of the antiknock properties of tetraethyl lead, informed the press that the deaths were entirely the fault of the workers. "The minute a man shows signs of exhilaration he is laid off. If he spills the stuff on himself he is fired," Midgely assured reporters (Rosner and Markowitz 1987).

Public health officials, serving simultaneously as paid industry consultants, assured the public that there was no danger from leaded gasoline. Alice Hamilton, a leading expert on occupational lead poisoning, disagreed (Hamilton et al. 1925). But this dissenting voice, even though supported by her Harvard colleagues Joseph C. Aub and David Edsal, and by Yale's distinguished pulmonary physiologist Yandell Henderson, had little impact on a nation enthralled by the automobile (Graebner 1988).

Confident that what was good for General Motors was good for the nation, a major public relations campaign was undertaken. In

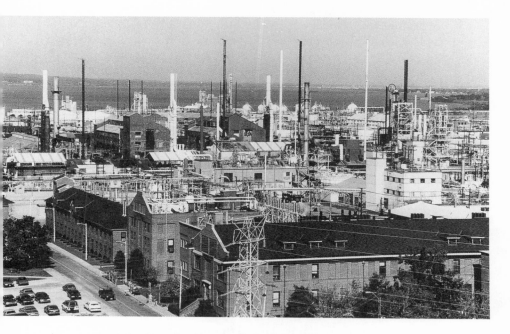

FIGURE 6.2. The Chambers Works, I. E. duPont de Nemours & Company, Deepwater, New Jersey. The "House of Butterflies," where tetraethyl lead was first manufactured, is in the foreground. Photo by Lynn Butler, November 1990.

1925, Robert A. Kehoe, director of the University of Cincinnati's Kettering Laboratory of Applied Physiology, was appointed medical director of the Ethyl Corporation (Graebner 1987). Kehoe was selected by an executive board that included Thomas Midgely and Charles Kettering, director of General Motor's research operations in Dayton. In 1945, with the chairman of General Motor's board, Alfred P. Sloan, the Kettering Foundation created the Sloan–Kettering Institute for Cancer Research in New York. Kehoe held positions simultaneously at the University of Cincinnati, the Kettering Laboratory, and the Ethyl Corporation until 1958.

From this industrial and academic pinnacle, Kehoe influenced lead research throughout the world for sixty years (Kehoe 1987). Despite fundamental chemical differences between organic and inorganic lead, he championed the notion that poisoning from tetraethyl lead was identical to poisoning from inorganic lead. Tetraethyl lead poisoning "bears little resemblance to any clinical types of lead poisoning. . . . Nevertheless, it cannot be doubted that lead is the essential toxic agent in the compound," Kehoe claimed (Kehoe 1925). Inorganic lead was not the cause of organolead toxicity, but Kehoe had control of the research questions. He was in a position to restrict investigation of tetraethyl lead to the Kettering Laboratory, noting that, in the interest of taxpayers, "extensive studies should not be repeated at public expense" (Rosner and Markowitz 1987). Kehoe stressed the danger of lead to children while underplaying the hazard to adults (Fee 1990). He asserted that children were more susceptible than adults, while at the same time assuring that this hypothesis was never actually tested. Kehoe favored the modification of behavior in individual children by education rather than interference with lead production. The relegation of lead poisoning to pediatrics and public health remains an enduring legacy of his service to the Ethyl Corporation. As a result, prevention of lead poisoning in occupational and environmental settings remains outside of the domain of internal medicine.

Although both Aub and Hamilton understood that tetraethyl lead toxicity was fundamentally different from inorganic lead poisoning, the continued confusion today about the two effects still inhibits rational discourse on the subject (Graebner 1988). Organolead produces immediate and striking brain symptoms, inebriation similar to that obtained from model airplane glue. The "high" induced by inhaling such volatile psychotropic solvents is specifically sought by glue and gasoline "sniffers," who not infrequently sustain long-term neurologic or even fatal consequences. Inorganic lead, on the other hand, produces cerebral symptoms that appear only after prolonged exposure, and hallucinations are distinctly unusual. The other classic symptoms of inorganic lead poisoning, colic, paralysis (wrist drop) and anemia, do not accompany tetraethyl lead intoxication.

The clinical characteristics of tetraethyl lead poisoning were, in fact, never released to the public by the Ethyl Corporation (Graebner 1988). The method, quantity, and duration of exposure in the fatal cases were also never made known. Whether absorption was through the skin or by inhalation, whether it occurred during manufacturing or blending remain corporate secrets. Attack rates, incidence, prevalence, dose–response, time course, and intensity of symptoms have never been published. Kehoe did inform the public that tetraethyl lead in the final dilute product for automobiles was safe. In a study of 356 employees, none of whom handled undiluted tetraethyl lead, he reported, "No case of lead intoxication was found among the subjects" (Kehoe et al. 1934). Corporate confidentiality impeded both litigation and the dissemination of knowledge. The same policy proved effective in protecting industry from the costs of cleanup of toxic dusts (for example, asbestos, cotton, silica, and coal) for generations.

Confusion between organic and inorganic lead toxicity assured that researchers would ask the wrong questions. Kehoe maintained that the acute symptoms of tetraethyl lead poisoning were due to the inorganic lead component. But data do not determine what is accepted as proof or how evidence is interpreted. Evaluation of scientific observations is largely subjective. How much evidence is sufficient to warrant the shifting of financial resources is fundamentally a political issue. Science cannot determine policy, but policy does determine what science pursues. No non-corporate-sponsored expert emerged to challenge Kehoe. His evaluation was universally accepted, and his vision was reinforced as necessary by the judicious allocation of corporate largesse. The lead industries sponsored scientists sympathetic to them and disseminated these scientists' views through prestigious international symposia (Graebner 1988). Investigators who were less sympathetic to the industry's view usually redirected their attention to areas in which funding and professional recognition were beyond corporate control. Survival in academic medicine depends on research funds, and research quality is only as good as the funding sources perceive it to be. The scramble for support allows no time for ideological disputes. As a result, occupational disease received minimal attention, and little information was developed to address the health implications of low-level environmental exposure during the phase of explosive growth of National Institutes of Health–sponsored research in the 1960s.

Kehoe was by no means alone in his effort to have biomedical science serve industry. In conjunction with an array of private foundations and public institutions whose members were supported by industry, research in occupational medicine was co-opted for half a century. Physicians and labor acquiesced in the face of powerful economic incentives. Occupational medicine languished and medical scientists focused on molecular biology.

For fifty years, University of Cincinnati research funded by the Ethyl Corporation, General Motors, and the Lead Industries Association showed that lead absorption was harmless unless the classical acute symptoms (colic, wrist drop, encepahlopathy, and anemia) were present. Kehoe and those he sponsored promoted the idea (originally proposed by Aub) that lead stored in bone was inactive. Sequestration in bone was believed to serve a protective function rather than representing a source of slow, continuing release of lead into the blood. High bone lead levels were believed to be good for health. Aub's research at Harvard was also supported by the Lead Industries Association. His theories further obscured the dangers of long-term, low-level lead absorption. The advantage of Aub's view of bone lead was not lost on the Ethyl Corporation. The Cincinnati investigators uncovered no evidence of risk to the public from the release of gasoline residues into the environment (Rosner and Markowitz 1987).

Kehoe brought academic respectability to Ethyl Corporation research. As described by Graebner, the Kettering Laboratory "translated the industries' needs into the language of science" (Graebner 1987). The body of knowledge generated at the Kettering Laboratory in Cincinnati was widely disseminated through industry-sponsored conferences and publications. Since publications, professional leadership, and the training of protégés are the hallmarks of expertise, Kehoe's opinions were widely sought and freely given. University of Cincinnati faculty sat on the major committees concerned with regulating lead in the workplace and the environment. Through Kehoe's considerable influence on generations of occupational health professionals, the blood lead concentration remained the standard for clinical diagnosis. Confusion between organic and inorganic lead toxicity was increased by the use of blood lead measurements to assess both. In 1925, the U.S. Surgeon General could correctly proclaim that no cases of lead poisoning from ethyl gasoline had ever been discovered (Graebner 1988); the right answer to the wrong question. The official pronouncement indelibly merged tetraethyl with inorganic lead in the minds of health professionals. Although inorganic lead was not the cause of the Bayway deaths, the inorganic residue generated by combustion of gasoline presented a real threat to the public in the long term. This threat was obfuscated until the 1960s but led to the banning of lead in gasoline in the 1980s. Fatal poisonings from the antiknock compound were brought under control at production sites without public scrutiny and research was diverted from organic to inorganic lead. Disinformation and public relations paid off.

In the 1960s, Kehoe and his associates presented an abundance of data designed to delay the removal of lead from gasoline. This position was, however, reversed in the 1970s, when the automobile companies began promoting catalytic converters. Initial reductions in gasoline lead were designed to protect these new devices, but later, environmentalists seized the initiative in efforts to protect the public health. Systematic obfuscation of the toxicity of tetraethyl lead had important ramifications for the handling of inorganic lead in the workplace. The hazards of lead to adults were all but forgotten, and lead poisoning became the exclusive domain of pediatricians. Yet recycling lead in secondary smelters remains among the most hazardous tasks in American industry. The classical symptoms of lead colic, wrist drop, and encephalopathy are now distinctly unusual except in this industry. The full eighteenth-century syndrome of lead poisoning can still be found in secondary lead smelters. Recovery of lead from automobile batteries remains the most dangerous of trades. A photograph taken in a battery recovery plant near Birmingham, Alabama, in 1987 illustrates the severity of the problem (Figure 6.3). The floor is covered with several inches of metallic lead powder, enough lead to poison the entire city. The photograph was taken during an Occupational Health and Safety Administration (OSHA) inspection; the workers are wearing respirators, and the lead dust has been sprinkled with water, in 100°F heat. Within an hour, the masks would be off and the lead dust would be airborne.

Most of the employees of the Birmingham smelter sustained acute colic every few months. All of these men were black and eighteen to twenty-five years of age; 10 percent had hypertension. Their blood lead levels were often twice the OSHA upper limit of 50 μg/dl. The company physician stated he did not tell the men of their high blood pressure or that lead might be its cause because high blood pressure is very common in blacks. Workers with high lead levels were rotated to "low-exposure" work areas. In violation of OSHA regulations, the "rotated" workers were required to remove solidified lead adherent to heavy equipment until their blood leads fell to below 60 μg/dl. Some of these men sustained lead cachexia, losing thirty or forty pounds over a few months from the most severe kind of lead poisoning. Such cases were sent home for a few weeks until they stopped losing weight. If their blood lead

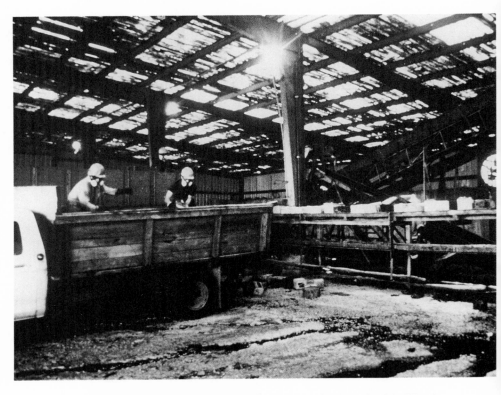

FIGURE 6.3.   Lead-battery recovery plant (secondary smelter) in Birmingham, Alabama. The ground is covered with several inches of wetted-down lead dust.

levels remained elevated, these "susceptible" individuals were dismissed. OSHA's efforts to enforce cleanup in this plant were stymied by interminable litigation. In 1989, after six years, the deadly game between OSHA and the owners was still being played on a judicial chessboard.

Deleaded Gas and Leaded Water

In 1982, the EPA convened an advisory board to revise the "Air Quality Criteria for Lead" as mandated by the Clean Air Act of

1970. This document forms the scientific basis for federal policy on lead in gasoline. Meetings of the board, however, were more akin to adversary proceedings than to scientific deliberations (Hays 1992). A U-shaped seating arrangement was used, with the chair at the apex. To the chair's right were representatives of the Lead Industries Association; executives, lawyers, physicians, statisticians, and investigators whose work was supported by the International Lead–Zinc Research Organization. On the chair's left sat the EPA consultants, biomedical researchers who pursued studies of lead toxicity without benefit of industry support. Those on the right traveled to the meeting place in Cadillac stretch limousines while those on the left were packed into government vans.

The hope that science can provide objective truth from which public policy can be formulated received little encouragement from these proceedings. Observations presented by the EPA consultants were regularly challenged by the lead industries' representatives seeking, they claimed, a "balanced" presentation. The body of information accumulated under Kehoe's influence over sixty years cast doubt on newer evidence of the harmful effects of low-level lead exposure. Kehoe's message that inorganic lead posed no threat to the environment was reinforced by the National Institute for Occupational Safety and Health's (NIOSH) "Criteria for a Recommended Standard for Occupational Exposure to Inorganic Lead," released in 1978 after six years of public hearings (Mendeloff 1988). In what might more properly be described as a double standard, NIOSH accepted blood lead levels up to 60 μg/dl for workers, although 40 μg/dl was the upper limit for children at the time. The limit for children was lowered to 25 μg/dl by the CDC in 1984, and to 10 μg/dl in 1991.

Lead industry spokesmen on the EPA Scientific Advisory Board insisted that dubious German studies, initially interpreted as showing that lead is essential for good health, be incorporated into the NIOSH air criteria document; a topic termed "the essentiality of lead." At the insistence of industry, a summary of the discredited work was included in the final document (USEPA 1986). The lead industries promoted further spurious controversy by supporting the retraction of another paper that showed that low-level lead absorption diminished intelligence in children. The psychologist who reinterpreted her own work with the support of the lead industry was strongly criticized by the independent scientists. The emotional intensity of the controversy over statistical interpretations proved too much for the psychologist at the center of the storm. She condemned her critics as "reprehensible," "irresponsible," and "libelous," and broke into tears.

Equally contentious were challenges to Needleman, whose data on the neurobehavioral effects of low-level lead in children had stimulated research on environmental lead as no other findings had (Needleman et al. 1990). Industry attacks on Needleman were regular features of the EPA hearings. Needleman represented a special threat to corporate interests because his work provided insight into the risk from "low-level" lead absorption (Needleman et al. 1990). The six-point median reduction in IQ of children with elevated tooth lead concentrations reported by Needleman at first glance seemed trivial. No physician could make the diagnosis of lead poisoning by examining a single victim of this low-level lead effect. The loss of IQ points means, however, that the intelligence test scores of the 5 percent of children with minimally elevated lead levels are reduced from "normal" to "subnormal" (IQ below 80). These children perform poorly in school because of behavioral as well as intellectual difficulties. They have diminished attention spans and show hyperactivity, indicators of future antisocial behavior. Equally important, the IQ scores for the 10 percent of children who would have been expected to be classified as exceptionally bright (IQ above 125), are reduced to average levels because of low-level lead absorption. Their intellectual resources are lost to the nation as well as to themselves.

The lead industry demanded that the EPA form a special panel to reexamine Needleman's data. It appears that no scientific data had previously been subjected to such intense hostile scrutiny in the United States in the absence of an accusation of fraud. Science as a process amenable to "falsification" took on new meaning with this panel. Described by one observer as a "hanging jury" (Marshall 1983), the panelists hoped not only to cast doubt on Needleman's data but on his integrity as well. The controversy was widely reported in the press and recounted in all its contentious detail in the authoritative journal *Science* (Marshall 1983).

A less tenacious investigator might have been intimidated by such vitriolic attacks. But in reality, the lead companies' campaign to discredit Needleman was a lost cause almost before it began. His findings were quickly reproduced throughout the world and ultimately provided the major rationale for removing tetraethyl lead from gasoline (Davis and Svendsgaard 1987). The prompt world-wide confirmation of Needleman's findings established the adverse effect of low-level lead absorption on IQ and behavior in children beyond reasonable doubt (Baghurst 1992).

But opposition to Needleman proved no less tenacious than Needleman himself. In 1991, the gauntlet was again thrown down. With the psychologist who was shaken up at the 1982 EPA Scientific Advisory Board meeting leading the attack, Needleman was now charged with "scientific misconduct" and reported to the National Institutes of Health Office of Scientific Integrity for disciplinary action. A lawsuit was filed against the U.S. government for participating in a cover-up for protecting Needleman's "flawed" data, his 1979 paper. Low-level lead effects had achieved notoriety, and Needleman would forever have to defend his credibility. (Palca 1991).

Policy goals had become indistinguishable from scientific findings, with the result that advocates on both sides were vulnerable to accusations of bias. It is reasonable to accept the psychologist's claim that she was simply defending a tenable, if unpopular, interpretation of very complex data. But the fine points of statistical analysis were lost among the huge financial, academic, and political stakes surrounding lead. In this polarized environment, giving aid or comfort to the lead companies, regardless of reason, is construed as evidence of bias. Politics overwhelms science, and professionalism, the power of expertise, is the biggest loser.

The battle over the "essentiality" of lead and the IQ effect delayed release of the EPA "Air Quality Criteria for Lead" for almost three years (USEPA 1986). Effects in adults had played little part in the debate on lead in gasoline because the data showing that lead produces kidney disease in adults had been obtained from individuals with presumed high-level occupational exposure. The chronic kidney effects were, therefore, deemed irrelevant to the low-level exposure produced by gasoline residues. However, the kidney findings stimulated an intensive examination of the relationship between environmental lead, low-level lead exposure, and hypertension. Sixteen new analyses were published in 1985 and 1986 showing that low-level lead contributes to high blood pressure in adults. A discussion of hypertension was therefore added to the EPA document before its release. Lead nephropathy in adults thus bolstered the EPA effort to lower lead in gasoline. Had it not been for the regulatory delays engineered by the lead industry, the data on adult hypertension would have been collected too late for incorporation into the policy debate.

The final EPA "Air Quality Criteria for Lead" had the mark of a profusion of authors who were in fundamental disagreement with one another. It was five volumes in length, comprehensive but almost incomprehensible; a minor victory for the lead companies. But for low-level lead exposure, absence of evidence could no longer be misrepresented as the absence of an effect. The causal relationship and the importance for policy making could be debated, but the association of low-level lead absorption with hypertension and diminished intellectual ability had been clearly documented.

The EPA also has responsibility for regulating lead in drinking water. The architect of ancient Rome, Vitruvius, recognized that water can dissolve lead from pipes, but his advice was honored more in the breach than in observance. For centuries, scientific observations were confounded by the variable corrosive properties of water and the tendency of lead pipes to become coated with calcium and, therefore, to leach less lead after several years. In 1848, Samuel L. Dana sparked a heated debate over the use of lead pipes in Boston's water supply. In an appendix to his translation of Tanquerel des Planche's landmark monograph on lead poisoning, Dana urged the use of tinned copper pipes instead of lead pipes. He recommended "joints by screw couplings of pure tin, for even the solder, used to unite these, may not be wholly harmless" (Dana 1848:12). In a rambling, typically bureaucratic response, the Boston Water Commission rejected Dana's plea for lead-free pipes and accepted the advice of Harvard's Eben N. Horsford, who asserted that "water can be served from leaden pipes, connected with iron mains, without detriment to health" (Hale and Curtis 1848). Horsford argued with some justification, but little relevance, that colic did not result from drinking water and that lead was always present in human tissues anyway. Dana considered 25 μg/l of water (the current EPA standard is 15 μg/l) too much, while Horsford considered it but a trace (Hale and Curtis 1848). Once again, a Harvard professor's advice prevailed when it coincided with the needs of commerce.

The legacy of the Boston Water Commission's decision still haunts the EPA. Although today water accounts for only about 20 percent of the lead absorbed by most individuals, the exposure to lead in water is both universal and cumulative. In infants, believed to be most vulnerable to the neurobehavioral effects of lead, 50 percent of the body lead burden derives from water (Agency for Toxic Substances and Disease Registry 1988). Recognition of new adverse effects of lead at ever lower exposure levels perpetuates the controversies surrounding this ancient disease. Increasingly sensitive chemical measurements and computer-intensive statistical analyses necessitate the continuous evolution of the concept of lead poisoning. In 1988, the EPA acknowledged the adverse biologic effects including enzyme, neurologic, and reproductive defects; diminished body stature; and hypertension at blood lead concentrations between 5 and 15 μg/dl. No lower limit (i.e., threshold) for toxicity was identified. This was a concept of lead toxicity that was very different from that promulgated by Kehoe and the Ethyl Corporation for half a century. Lead in drinking water creates a background of exposure with health effects comparable to those created by exposure to cosmic radiation. But unlike background radiation, exposure to lead from water is entirely preventable.

In 1985, the EPA proposed reducing permissible lead in drinking water from 50 to 20 μg/l and estimated that forty-two million Americans consume water containing lead above this limit (USEPA 1988). The EPA estimated the mean concentration of lead in tap water to be 29 μg/l, indicating that many homes were far above the proposed maximum of 20. Of the lead in drinking water, 4 percent arises from municipal water systems while 96 percent is leached from household interior plumbing, primarily from lead solder connecting copper pipes. Lead solder was outlawed by federal statute in 1986, but enforcement was left to the states and has, consequently, been virtually nonexistent.

In 1988, the EPA reduced the recommended maximum contamination level of lead in water supplies to 5 μg/l (USEPA 1988). EPA regulations are directed at the municipal water supply systems, leaving it to the homeowner to protect water from the tap. The major public health effort is left to the individual. Government chooses not to regulate drinking water at the most important site, the private home, because no one is prepared to foot the bill. With similarly limited vision, the EPA in 1989 demanded recall of lead-lined water coolers from schools but assumed no responsibility for water coolers in office and work settings. The drinking water and water cooler regulations serve to protect the bureaucracies from litigation more than to protect the public from lead. After 150 years, Dana's goal for eliminating lead in drinking water has yet to be achieved.

The Glare of Glaze

Despite innumerable laws and vast bureaucracies devoted to controlling lead exposure, blatant industrial poisoning still occurs. No one objects very effectively. Outsiders are unaware of the problem, and lawyers are kept busy. Lead poisoning in the workplace and among inner-city children is a familiar tale that lacks the drama of today's news. Congressional hearings on lead in gasoline and water are dutifully reported on the back pages whenever the regulatory agencies must adapt to the changing interpretations of long-established scientific data. Lead becomes just another toxic scare of the week. It fails to grip the imagination.

Journalists are more attentive when the threat is perceived to be from housewares they themselves use. The danger of lead poisoning from dinnerware as told by an articulate Air Force lieutenant colonel rivets the attention of the news media. "Our near fatal experience as victims of lead poisoning caused by Italian coffee mugs now dates back almost a decade," Don Wallace stated at the opening of the House Subcommittee on Oversight and Investigations hearing "Lead in Housewares," on June 27, 1988. This former Vietnam fighter pilot had been forced to retire from an outstanding military and diplomatic career in 1979 because of lead poisoning from Italian ceramic coffee cups. Wallace and his wife, Fran (who had also been lead-poisoned), subsequently dedicated themselves to eliminating dangerous lead glazes from the marketplace (U.S. House of Representatives 1988).

In his master's degree thesis in industrial hygiene, Wallace documented the leaching of lead into acidic liquids that occurs following repeated washing of previously safe dishes in automatic dishwashers. He further showed that, like dishwashers, microwave ovens cause deterioration of lead glazes and that lead underpainting can diffuse in dangerous quantities through lead-free glazes. Using their personal savings to pay for the research, the Wallaces demonstrated that federal Food and Drug Administration (FDA) monitoring of imported ceramics was astonishingly ineffective. "We have concluded," Don stated, "that a significant worldwide public health problem exists" (United States House of Representatives 1988).

To deflect the embarrassment of this private demonstration of public inefficiency, the FDA commissioner awarded Don Wallace a special citation in 1988. The *Washington Post* produced a series of investigative reports on lead in imported housewares that was picked up by smaller newspapers all over the country. Television reporters in the United States, Canada, Italy, and China interviewed the Wallaces, and *Newsweek, Time, People,* and *Harrowsmith* magazines photographed the attractive couple with their glamorous but hazardous ceramics. Suddenly, lead wasn't boring anymore. In 1985, having read *Poison in the Pot* (Wedeen 1984), Don contacted me. He was struck with the similarity between the diagnostic dilemma presented by King George III, described in the book, and that presented by his wife, Fran. Fran had been told she had acute intermittent porphyria for two years before Don came upon the correct diagnosis of lead poisoning in the library. I gave the Wallaces a letter I had received offering to transfer a patent to me for a lead-glaze test kit if I would manufacture the kit. The Wallaces picked up the offer, got the FDA to confirm the accuracy of the method, and within one year were distributing it worldwide through their corporation, Frandon Enterprises. They used the income from the test kit to do more testing and to confront the FDA with its failure to control lead glazes in imported dinnerware. In 1985, the FDA had recalled a single shipment of improperly glazed ceramic ware. In 1987, there were twenty recalls of imports from Spain, Portugal, Italy, and the Netherlands. The House of Representatives Oversight Hearings followed. Chairman John D. Dingell generated a surge of interest in unrecognized sources of lead poisoning and in vivo tibial XRF, culminating in the 1989 "Lead in Bone" conference at the University of Maryland (Fowler 1991).

The Wallaces accomplished what no mass of scientific reports on industrial lead poisoning and pica, or federal guidelines could do. They captured the public imagination in a way that armies of learned experts or less articulate victims could not. Political pressure was mobilized in the United States in 1988 as it had been in Devonshire, England, in 1767, when contaminated cider threatened the local economy and middle-class consumers. Within one year of the congressional oversight hearings, the FDA lowered fortyfold the national standards for leachable imported glazes. The Wallace's success in changing government policy supports Tesh's penultimate argument in *Hidden Arguments:* "There is no science uninfluenced by politics" (Tesh 1988:177). The Wallaces brought the scientific evidence into the legislative hearing room, reinforcing Tesh's final plea, "to get the politics out of hiding" (177).

An Alternative

The final link of the toxic circle for lead is waste disposal. After all the buildings have been cleaned, unnecessary production stopped, and use of lead curtailed, where is the discarded lead to go? Like nuclear wastes, lead waste simply will not go away. Lead in the earth's surface is free to move from place to place in time and geographic space. There is no plan for its disposal.

Disorganized federal policy surrounding lead should not be mistaken for an absence of policy. Ineffectiveness is not a chance event but a disingenuous way to assert the intent to clean up while avoiding the actual effort. The requirements for effective environmental policy to eliminate lead poisoning in this society are worth examining as an alternative to this bureaucratic footwork. Silbergeld has proposed an approach to preventing environmental contamination with lead that would dispense with self-contradictory and counterproductive regulatory gestures (pers. comm. 1991). She sees three fundamental needs: (1) the need to reduce current use, (2) the need to correct past contamination, and (3) the need to plan for lead-waste disposal. Silbergeld notes that in both biologic and environmental systems, lead accumulates steadily in unstable storage "sinks." Bone is the "sink" in humans; soil is the "sink" in the environment. It is in these repositories where success or failure of environmental solutions must be measured.

A comprehensive lead policy would have to be administered by a single federal agency with the mandate to achieve blood lead levels below 10 μg/dl and water lead concentrations below 5 μg/l. The mean blood lead level in the United States approximates 12 μg/dl (Mahaffey et al. 1982). Implementation of this policy could be accomplished if new lead production required a federal permit. Fees for permits could be used to support research on lead abatement and environmental protection. Silbergeld warns that methods for disposal of lead residues generated by solid waste incinerators should be worked out before, rather than after, incinerator proliferation. The cost of contaminating food, air, water, and soil should be made to exceed the profit derived from these practices. Financial incentives for lead mining should be diminished by eliminating depreciation allowances and other tax benefits. Voluntary reductions of lead in food containers (for example, tin cans, lead glazes) should be replaced by mandatory controls.

Silbergeld envisions social action arising from scientific evidence that a specific toxin causes chronic disease. Her proposal defies political clichés and implies that reductionist science can stimulate preventive health policy (Tesh 1988). The prospects for her plan, unfortunately, remain very much in doubt. Money rather than knowledge appears to determine policy. Knowledge of the need to protect health gained over two millennia has been consistently overwhelmed by the force of economic necessity. But the unique role of toxic tort liability claims in the United States may offer an opportunity to reverse the economic imbalance by persuading insurance companies to intervene in the prevention of toxic exposure in the workplace. The courts may be the final battleground for controlling lead in the environment. Neither dedicated scientists nor regulatory agencies can be as compelling as the cost of liability insurance. Until recently, workers' compensation laws have precluded suits that would tax the insurers. The situation was changed substantially by the Johns–Manville asbestos rulings, which allowed tort actions outside of the constraints of compensation law. The door of third-party litigation may now be open to clean up the lead industries.

References

Agency for Toxic Substances and Disease Registry. 1988. *The Nature and Extent of Lead Poisoning in Children in the United States: A Report to Congress.* Atlanta Georgia United States Department of Health and Human Services.

Assistant Aldermen. 1852, April 22. *Report and Resolution of the Board of Assistant Aldermen of the City of New York on Zinc Paints.* Document no. 7. New York: McSpedon and Baker.

Baghurst, P. A.; McMichael, J. A.; Wigg, N. R.; Vimpani, G. V.; Robertson, E. F.; Roberts, R. J.; and Tong, S. 1992. "Environmental Exposure to

Lead and Children's Intelligence at the Age of Seven Years." *New England Journal of Medicine* 327:1279–1284.

Bowman, K. M., and Howard, P. 1935. "Encephalitis Due to Exposure to Tetraethyl Lead: Report of a Case." *Archives of Neurology Psychology* 34:2327.

Centers for Disease Control. 1989. "Update: Acquired Immunodeficiency Syndrome Associated with Intravenous Drug Use—United States, 1988." *Morbidity and Mortality Weekly Report* 38:165–170.

Chadwick, E. 1965. *Report on the Sanitary Condition of the Labouring Population of Great Britain, 1842.* Ed. M. W. Flynn. Edinburgh: University Press.

Crawford, R. 1977. "You Are Dangerous to Your Health: The Ideology and Politics of Victim Blaming." *International Journal of Health Services* 7: 663–680.

Dana, S. L. 1848. *Lead Pipe, Its Danger: A Rejoinder to the Reply of Professor Horsford to the Argument in the Appendix to Tanquerel.* Lowell, Mass.: Bixby.

Davis, M., and Svendsgaard, D. J. 1987. "Lead and Child Development." *Nature* 329:297–300.

Fee, E. 1990. "Public Health in Practice: An Early Confrontation with the 'Silent' Epidemic of Childhood Lead Paint Poisoning." *Journal of the History of Medicine* 45:570–606.

Fothergill, J. 1775. "Observations on Disorders to Which Painters in Water Color Are Exposed." *Medical Observations and Inquiries* 5:394–405.

Fowler, B. A., organizer. 1991. "International Workshop on Lead in Bone: Implications for Dosimetry and Toxicology." *Environmental Health Perspectives* 91:3–88.

Graebner, W. 1987. "Hegemony Through Science." In *Dying for Work: Workers' Safety and Health in Twentieth-Century America,* ed. D. Rosner and G. Markowitz. 140–159. Indianapolis: Indiana University Press.

———. 1988. "Private Power, Private Knowledge, and Public Health: Science, Engineering, and Lead Poisoning." In *The Health and Safety of Workers: Case Studies in the Politics of Professional Responsibility,* ed. R. Bayer, 15–71. New York: Oxford University Press.

Greenhouse, L. 1991. "Court Backs Rights of Women to Jobs with Health Risks." *New York Times,* March 21, p. 1, sec. B.

Hale, N., and Curtis, T. B. 1848. *Report of the Water Commissioners of the Material Best Adapted for Distribution Water Pipes; and on the Most Economical Mode of Introducing Water into Private Homes.* Boston: J. H. Eastburn.

Hamilton, A. B.; Reznikoff, P.; and Burnham, G. M. 1925. "Tetra-ethyl Lead." *Journal of the American Medical Association* 84:1481–1486.

Hays, S. P. 1992. "The Role of Values in Science and Policy: The Case of Lead." In *Human Lead Exposure,* ed. H. L. Needleman, 267–286. Boca Raton, Fla: CRC Press.

Hilts, P. J. 1990. "U.S. Opens Drive to Wipe Out Lead Poisoning Among Children." *New York Times,* December 20, secs. A and B.

Kehoe, R. A. 1925. "Tetraethyl Lead Poisoning." *Journal of the American Medical Association* 85:108–110.

———. 1927. "On the Toxicity of Tetraethyl Lead and Inorganic Lead Salts." *Journal of Laboratory and Clinical Medicine* 12:554–560.

Kehoe, R. A.; Thamann, F.; and Cholak, J. 1934. "An Appraisal of the Lead Hazards Associated with the Distribution and Use of Gasoline Containing Tetraethyl Lead. Part 1" *Journal of Industrial Hygiene* 16:100–128.

Kehoe, R. A. 1987. "Studies of Lead Administration and Elimination in Adult Volunteers Under Natural and Experimentally Induced Conditions over Extended Periods of Time." *Fd Chem Toxic* 25:421–493.

Kiple, K. F. 1987. *The African Exchange: Toward a Biological History.* Durham, N.C.: Duke University Press.

Lubasch, A. H. 1989. "New York Sues Paint Makers over Lead." *New York Times,* June 9, sec. B.

Machle, W. F. 1935. "Tetra-ethyl Lead Intoxication and Poisoning by Related Compounds of Lead." *Journal of the American Medical Association* 105:578–585.

Mahaffey, K. R.; Annest, J. L.; Roberts, J.; and Murphy, R. S. 1982. "National Estimates of Blood Lead Levels, 1976–1980: Association with Selected Demographic and Socioeconomic Factors." *New England Journal of Medicine* 307:573–579.

Marshall, E. 1983. "EPA Faults Classic Lead Poisoning Study." *Science* 222: 906–907.

Mendeloff, J. D. 1988. *The Dilemma of Toxic Substance Regulation: How Overregulation Causes Underregulation at OSHA.* Cambridge, Mass.: MIT Press.

Needleman, H. L. 1992. "Salem Comes to the National Institutes of Health from Inside the Crucible of Scientific Integrity." *Pediatrics* 90:977–981.

Needleman, H. L.; Schell, A.; Bellinger, D.; Leviton, A.; and Allred, E. N. 1990. "The Long-Term Effects of Exposure to Low Doses of Lead in Childhood: An 11 Year Follow-up Report." *New England Journal of Medicine* 322:83–88.

New Jersey State Legislative Documents. 1879. *New Jersey Bureau of Statistics of Labor and Industries of New Jersey: Embracing Its Operations from April 1 to Oct. 31, 1878. First Annual Report (1879).* Vol. 2, document no. 55. chap. 8, "Industries: Pottery, Flax, Hemp and Cranberry," 223–254.

———. 1888. *Eleventh Annual Report of the Board of Health of the State of New Jersey and Report of the Bureau of Vital Statistics (1887).* "Exposures and Diseases of Operatives: The Diseases of Potters, Their Causes and Prevention." By D. Warman. Vol. 3, document no. 27, 97–116.

Palca, J. 1991. "Get-the-Lead-Out Guru Challenged." *Science* 253:842–844.

Putka, G. 1992a. "Pittsburgh Professor Sues School, NIH, to Block Inquiry into Lead-Poison Study." *Wall Street Journal,* April 2, sec. B.

———. 1992b. "Professor's Data on Lead Level Cleared by Panel." *Wall Street Journal,* May 27, sec. B.

Rabin, R. 1989. "Warnings Unheeded: A History of Child Lead Poisoning." *American Journal of Public Health* 79:1668–1674.

Rosenberg, C. E. 1987. *The Care of Strangers: The Rise of America's Hospital System.* New York: Basic Books.

Rosner, D., and Markowitz, G. 1987. " 'A Gift of God'?: The Public Health Controversy over Leaded Gasoline in the 1920s." In *Dying for Work: Workers' Safety and Health in Twentieth-Century America,* ed. D. Rosner and G. Markowitz, 121–139. Indianapolis: Indiana University Press.

Schutz, A.; Skerfving, S.; Christoffersson, J. O.; and Tell, I. 1987.

"Chelatable Lead Versus Lead in Human Trabecular and Compact Bone." *Science of the Total Environment* 61:201–209.

Shannon, A. F. 1992. "Class Action Against Newark Cleared to Force Lead Paint Cleanup." *Star Ledger,* February 28.

Silbergeld, E. K.; Schwartz, J.; and Mahaffey, K. 1988. "Lead and Osteoporosis: Mobilization of Lead from Bone in Postmenopausal Women." *Environmental Research* 47:79–94.

Smith, F. B. 1979. *The People's Health 1830–1910.* New York: Holmes and Meier.

Tesh, S. N. 1988. *Hidden Arguments: Political Ideology in Disease Prevention Policy.* New Brunswick, N.J.: Rutgers University Press.

U.S. Environmental Protection Agency. 1986. Environmental Criteria and Assessment Office. *Air Quality Criteria for Lead.* Vols. 1–4. EPA-600/8-83/028aF, Research Triangle Park, N.C.: EPA.

———. 1988. *Drinking Water Regulations: Maximum Contaminant Level Goals and National Primary Drinking Water Regulations for Lead and Copper, Proposed Rule.* Pt. V, 40 CFR 141, pts. 141 and 142, Federal Register, August 18, pp. 31,516–31,578.

U.S. House of Representatives. 1988. *Lead in Housewares: Hearing Before the Subcommittee on Oversight and Investigations of the Committee on Energy and Commerce, June 27, 1988.* serial no. 100–134. Washington, D.C.: Government Printing Office.

Van de Vyver, F. L.; D'Haese, P. C.; Visser, W. J.; Elseviers, N. M.; Knippenberg, L. J.; Lamberts, L. V.; Wedeen, R. P.; and DeBroe, M. E. 1988. "Bone Lead in Dialysis Patients." *Kidney International* 33:601–607.

Victery, W., ed. 1988. "Symposium on Lead–Blood Pressure Relationships." *Environmental Health Perspectives* 78:

Warren, J., ed. 1988. *The Role of the Primary Care Physician in Occupational and Environmental Medicine.* Washington, D.C.: Institute of Medicine, National Academy of Medicine.

"Wealth Is Health." 1992. Editorial. *Nation* (April 27): 1.

Wedeen, R. P. 1984. *Poison in the Pot: The Legacy of Lead.* Carbondale: Southern Illinois University Press.

———. 1989. "Were the Hatters of New Jersey 'Mad'? *American Journal of Industrial Medicine* 16:225–234.

———. 1990. "In Vivo Tibial X-ray Fluorescence." *Archives of Environmental Health* 45:69–71.

• CHAPTER 7 •

Tainted Gold:
Chromium Contamination in
Hudson County

HELENE A. STAPINSKI

The case studies end with the story of chromium landfill in Hudson County, New Jersey, by Helene A. Stapinski, a newspaper reporter for the Jersey Journal, a local newspaper, at the height of the chromium story. Stapinski received the North Jersey Press Club Memorial Journalism Award for public service in 1991 for her coverage of the chromium debacle. Stapinski's unraveling of the chromium story in Hudson County made her a participant in the local conflict. She documented the inability of government to address effectively public perceptions and community concerns. Indeed, it now appears that in May 1987, six years after the chromium story became public knowledge, the New Jersey Department of Environmental Protection itself used chromium slag for landfill in Liberty State Park, in the shadow of the Statue of Liberty (Figure 7.1), and failed to inform the public of the blunder (Rosenfeld 1991).

The lack of scientific data for chromium is in sharp contrast to the situation regarding lead. The biologic effects of chromium are virtually unknown. Extrapolation from massive occupational exposure to the effects of chromium landfill is difficult and faulty. While chromium is a known pulmonary carcinogen in the workplace, low-dose effects in the environment have not been studied. Renal damage from certain chromium compounds in experimental animals is well known, but no case of renal failure from environmental or occupational exposure can be found in the medical literature. The absence of evidence cannot be considered evidence of absence, however. It merely proves that the investigation of chromium toxicity has a low priority.

Outside of Hudson County, little attention has been paid to the state-government-endorsed use of chromium slag for landfill for most of this century. The people of the county have received no relief from the anxiety caused by the scientific uncertainty about low-level chromium's effects. In the absence of scientific data and in the face of public concern, government is forced to make a policy decision to take action or not. In Jersey City by the end of 1992, all residential sites identified as chromium contaminated had been cleaned up at a cost of 30 million dollars (Pofeldt 1992). Throughout 1991 and 1992, the state had carried out the site-by-site cleanup, with truckloads of contaminated soil transported daily to unidentified locations outside the city. Another environmental disaster of our age unfolded quietly, noted in the local press, with an occasional report in a national newspaper. While neighborhood coalitions have spoken out of their fears, no countywide grass-roots leadership has emerged to represent the citizens. And so government and science play out their appointed roles in this never-ending drama, which is punctuated by news releases of new contaminated sites discovered and new medical tests performed—to no one's satisfaction.

• • •

The Gold Coast

THE twelve towns and cities that make up Hudson County in northern New Jersey have always sat in the shadow of Manhattan. The skyscrapers across the Hudson River have sometimes beckoned, and sometimes intimidated, the county's residents and politicians. But there was a time when Hudson—Jersey City in particular—had its own identity and claim to fame: industry. Unbeknownst to many of its people at that time, Hudson County would find that its strength would some day be the source of many of its worst problems.

Before Hudson County became the bedroom community for hundreds of professionals beginning in the 1970s, it was an industrial mecca. Jersey City, New Jersey's second-largest city and the Hudson county seat, was known for two things: political corruption

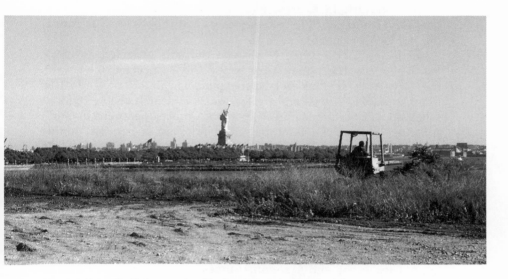

FIGURE 7.1.　Bull-dozing (without protective clothing) chromium-contaminated landfill behind the Statue of Liberty. Chromium site no. 19, Jersey City, New Jersey. Photo by Lynn Butler, October 1990.

and industry. Billboards advertised "Jersey City has everything for industry." As one of the leading manufacturing centers on the Atlantic coast, Jersey City produced pencils, cans, medicine, electrical machinery, steel, cigarettes, soap, and perfume, among other goods. Together with neighboring Kearny, Jersey City also established itself as one of the biggest chromate producing areas in the country. For seventy years, Hudson's chromate-producing companies thought nothing of selling their waste as landfill. It wasn't until the companies left town and the New Jersey Department of Environmental Protection (NJDEP) was formed, in 1970, that anyone thought much about the yellowish green slag that lurked underneath houses, schools, and playgrounds.

　　The discovery of chromium contamination took place just before the development boom in Jersey City, which was to become one of the brightest jewels on the Hudson County "Gold Coast." During the 1960s and 1970s, industry had begun to desert Hudson County, leaving in its place abandoned factories and high unemployment rates. Companies such as American Can Company in Jersey City,

Western Electric in Kearny, and Tootsie Roll in Hoboken took a bow. Thousands of blue-collar workers lost their jobs. The future did not look promising.

But Jersey City's prime waterfront property attracted developers. They saw the potential of Jersey City's spectacular view of the New York skyline and its inexpensive, abundant land. The Manhattanites—artists and professionals in search of low rents—followed. Corporations moved their back-office operations to Hudson, and some even relocated from Manhattan because of the cheaper office space. In the late 1970s, the county's smokestacks, ill-smelling chemical plants, and tired-looking factories were all ready to be traded in for townhouses, shopping malls, and outdoor cafes. "Condo" was about to make its way into everyone's vocabulary. It was around this time that Hudson's chromate production past became a chromium contamination problem.

In the summer of 1979, Thor Engineers was hired by Grace Retail Corporation to conduct a study of Grace's property on Route 440 in Jersey City. A soil and foundation investigation was done because Grace planned to build a trucking terminal on the site. The parcel of land was near the Roosevelt Drive-In movie theater, a dinosaur of the 1950s still operating on the congested industrial highway.

When Thor crashed its mighty shovel into the soft, yellowish green soil at the drive-in site, it was obvious that some strange substance had been used as landfill. The site was immediately referred to the United States Environmental Protection Agency (EPA) and the NJDEP for further inspection.

Meanwhile, a hidden force began to rock the foundations of the Valley Fair supermarket, also located on Route 440. The floor of the nearby Stage Restaurant began to separate from the rotting concrete below. Everyone was soon in agreement that something on Route 440 was very wrong. What they did not know was that other sections of Hudson County—one of the most densely populated counties in the United States—was the victim of one of the worst cases of chromium contamination in the world. Other cities throughout the United States, such as Baltimore and Corpus Christi, were suffering from similar problems. But none would prove to be as large as Hudson's.

The symptoms were not widespread yet, but the poison was already underground, ready to close grammar schools, destroy businesses, and seep into the lives of people living on the Hudson

River Gold Coast. The county with the best view in the world was about to become the county with the worst toxic waste problem in the state.

Chromium's History in Hudson County

From 1905 to 1976, three Hudson County plants manufactured chromate chemicals from chromite ore to produce their major product—sodium dichromate. (See Table 7.1 for the history of these companies.) The three companies changed hands a number of times but always operated from the same sites in Hudson County irrespective of the formal name. Mutual Chemical Company of New Jersey opened its plant in 1905 on Route 440. It evolved over the years to Mutual Chemical Company of America, Allied Chemical and Dye Corporation, Allied Chemical Corporation, and finally, Allied–Signal Incorporated.

In 1924, Natural Products Refining Company began operating its plant on Garfield Avenue in Jersey City. In 1954, Pittsburgh Plate Glass Company acquired Natural's portion of the site and continued operations. Pittsburgh transferred title of the site to its subsidiary, Columbia Southern Chemical Corporation. In 1960, the two companies merged. Then, in 1968, Pittsburgh Plate Glass changed its name to PPG Industries, Incorporated.

In 1916, Martin Dennis Company opened its plant on the Belleville Turnpike in Kearny. Diamond Alkali Company acquired the business in 1948, then changed its name to Diamond Shamrock Corporation in 1967. Stock was later transferred to Occidental Petroleum Corporation, and Diamond changed its name to Maxus Energy Corporation.

Over the years, sodium dichromate was made into pigments used for paints, ceramics, and printing inks. It is a necessary ingredient in the ink on all government money. The substance acts as a corrosion control in metal systems (for example, the chrome on cars). It also serves as a wood preservative and is used in the manufacturing of chemical catalysts and for textile mordants and dyeing. Chromic acid, a byproduct of sodium dichromate, is used in electroplating; potassium dichromate, another byproduct, is used in photographic processing (McKee 1984).

TABLE 7.1

Allied-Signal's Corporate History

1905 Mutual Chemical Company of New Jersey opens plant
1908 Mutual Chemical Company of New Jersey changes its name to Mutual Chemical Company of America
1954 Allied Chemical and Dye Corporation acquires stock
1955 Allied Chemical and Dye Corporation dissolves Mutual
1958 Allied Chemical and Dye Corporation changes its name to Allied Chemical Corporation
1981 Allied Chemical Corporation changes its name to Allied Corporation
1985 Allied Corporation acquires The Signal Companies, Incorporated, and changes its name to Allied–Signal Incorporated

PPG Industries' Corporate History

1924 Natural Products Refining Company opens plant
July 1954 Pittsburgh Plate Glass Company acquires Natural Refining Company's portion of the site
December 1954 Pittsburgh Plate Glass Company transfers title to its subsidiary, Columbia Southern Chemical Corporation
1956 Columbia Southern Chemical Corporation transfers title back to Pittsburgh Plate Glass Company
1960 Pittsburgh Plate Glass Company merges with Columbia Southern Chemical Corporation
1968 Pittsburgh Plate Glass Company changes its name to PPG Industries, Incorporated

Occidental's and Maxus's Corporate History

1916 Martin Dennis Company opens
1948 Diamond Alkali Company acquires the site
1967 Diamond Alkali Company changes its name to Diamond Shamrock Corporation
1983 Diamond Shamrock Corporation changes its name to Diamond Shamrock Chemicals Company
August 1983 New Diamond Corporation acquires Diamond Shamrock Chemicals Company
September 1983 New Diamond Corporation changes its name to Diamond Shamrock Corporation
1986 Diamond Shamrock Corporation transfers title to Diamond Shamrock Chemical Land Holdings, Incorporated, an indirect subsidiary; Diamond Shamrock Corporation sells all outstanding stock of Diamond Shamrock Chemicals Company to Oxy-Diamond Alkali Corporation, a company owned by Occidental Petroleum Corporation
1987 Diamond Shamrock Corporation changes its name to Maxus Energy Corporation
1987 Diamond Shamrock Chemical Land Holdings, Incorporated, changes its name to Chemical Land Holdings, Incorporated

A high-grade chromite ore, containing chromium, is the basic raw material processed at all chromate production plants in the country. Chromium is contained in the ore in its trivalent state as chromium iron oxide. In this form, the chromium is inert and is not soluble in either water or acid. To produce water-soluble chromate chemicals, the trivalent chromium must be changed to the hexavalent form. Therefore, the ore is pulverized, mixed with soda ash and lime, and roasted at 1,100 to 2,250°C. (McKee 1984). After leaching, the end product is a deep yellow solution that is saturated with sodium chromate. The sodium chromate is then converted by acidification and crystallization into the marketable product—crystalline sodium dichromate.

The residue left over the leaching process contains enough chromium to be reprocessed. The solid material remaining after the second leaching is called "secondary residue" or "waste mud." This waste mud is produced at a rate of approximately 1.5 times that of the product. Between two and three million tons of that waste have been buried and used as landfill throughout Hudson County (McKee 1984).

The companies that produced the waste buried much of it on site. The remaining slag was used for backfilling of demolition sites, preparation of building foundations, and filling in wetlands.

Chromium's Effects on the Body

Discovered in 1797, chromium is now familiar as the gleaming surface on automobile fenders.[1] The potential for serious poisoning from compounds of the metal was recognized in the mid nineteenth century by physicians who used chromic acid to cauterize certain skin lesions (Major 1922). As early as 1877, chromic acid was used to induce experimental acute kidney disease in rabbits. In 1885, perforations of the nasal septum were observed in workers engaged in chromic acid production, and in 1980, a cancer was reported at the site of a nasal "chrome hole" acquired from chromic acid exposure twenty years earlier (Langard 1990).

The dangers of corrosive compounds of the metal were described in an annual report from the New Jersey Department of Labor in 1916.

The ore after it has been calcined becomes poisonous, and, consequently, is harmful to health when breathed; and, furthermore,
causes painful sores if it comes in contact with the flesh and is not
immediately washed off. Numerous instances have come to the notice of the Department of workers who have suffered painful sores of
the fingers and legs; and in some cases have parts of the nostrils
destroyed from continuous exposure to air laden with this poisonous
dust. (New Jersey. Department of Labor [NJDOL] 1916:80; New Jersey State Legislative Documents [NJSLD] 1917)

The annual report explained in detail the engineering and personal hygiene measures needed to protect workers from these hazards and noted additional dangers from chromate that entered the
body: "It also acts upon the digestive tract by swallowing the dust,
upon the pharynx by inhalation, and upon the kidneys by blood
absorption" (81). In 1924, chromium poisoning was specifically recognized as a compensable disease by the New Jersey legislature
(Gelman 1988:231). But knowledge of the hazards of this metal
were learned only with difficulty by state officials responsible for
public health.

Lung cancers acquired as early as 1911 in workers in the German
alkali–chromate industry were reported in the 1930s. But despite
New Jersey officials' recognition of the causal relationship of chromium to lung cancer, effective measures to protect workers were
never instituted. A steady stream of reports subsequently confirmed
the worst fears about chromium and lung cancer. From chemical,
chrome-plating, welding, and paint-manufacturing plants throughout the world, the relative risk of lung cancer was found to be
increased up to fortyfold in chrome industry workers, an extraordinary incidence that could not be attributed to smoking (Langard
1990). The carcinogenic potential of chromium was decisively confirmed in experimental animals (Agency for Toxic Substances and
Disease Registry 1989).

The vast number of chemical forms of chromium makes it difficult to be sure which compounds are most toxic. It is nevertheless
agreed that the hexavalent, soluble form is far more carcinogenic
than is the trivalent, insoluble form. Hexavalent chromium is
highly reactive with tissue and, in contrast to trivalent chromium,
is readily absorbed into the body and the cells. Skin irritation and
sensitivity reactions from hexavalent chromium are the most common toxicities in industry.

Although acute kidney disease from hexavalent chromium was

recognized in the nineteenth century, the massive accidental absorption that leads to fulmanent renal failure is rare in humans. Whether a more insidious, slowly progressive, chronic renal disease results from continuous low-level exposure remains controversial (Wedeen 1991). Kidney disease is usually cited as one of the dangers of exposure to chromium, but chronic renal failure from either occupational or environmental exposure has never been reported. In the absence of evidence to the contrary, it is prudent to assume that even low-level chromium exposure simply represents less of what is seen at occupational exposure levels. Although such caution is reasonable, measuring toxic effects at environmental exposure levels is quite difficult, expensive, and time consuming. Because of uncertainties surrounding the toxicity of the different chemical forms of chromium and because of the lack of information on low-level toxicity, it is difficult to use biologic monitoring (i.e., blood or urine chromium concentrations) to predict adverse health effects. As long as those who distribute research funds place a low priority on understanding environmental pollution, the answers to these questions will remain unknown. At present, the health effects of nonoccupational exposure to chromium in the environment remain entirely unknown.

Workers and Community
Face Chromium Exposure

Until the 1987 death of Hudson County resident Frederick Trum of lung cancer, after prolonged exposure to chromium dust at the St. Johnsbury trucking terminal in Kearny, it was thought that only workers in the chromate-producing industry were in danger. An analysis of bone tissues revealed that Trum, a Harrison resident who worked at the terminal for ten years, carried high levels of chromium in his body. "When the doctor opened up his body, he was horrified," said Trum's widow, Florence. "Every bone in his body was yellow. Yellow from chromium" (Trum 1989).

In addition to lung cancer, Trum suffered from a rare bone infection. In the roof of his mouth when he died was a hole left when doctors surgically removed a lump the size of an egg. His teeth had rotted away by that time; his nasal passages were lined with polyps. He suffered from a perforated nasal septum, a problem often linked to chromium exposure. Although the sixty-year-old smoked a pack of cigarettes a day, doctors blamed his death on chromium.

According to Trum's wife, the truck terminal was covered with a yellow watery liquid whenever there was a heavy rain. The cafeteria where Trum and his co-workers ate lunch contained the largest amounts of yellow liquid and dust. Chromium that is buried underground leaches into the water and eventually makes its way to the surface, where it dries and can be inhaled. This leaching process appears to have taken place at the terminal.

Chromium typically creates a bright yellow green tint when it dissolves in water. Trum's wife often noticed that her husband's work boots were covered in a yellow crust. Workers from chromate factories often find the same yellow crust on their boots. Joe Szatmary, a retired chemical company worker employed next door to the Mutual Chemical chromate factory on Route 440, remembers the yellow tracks the workers would leave behind. "The men had red handkerchiefs tied around their necks to wipe their brows because the coke fires were so hot from cooling the chrome," he remembered (Stapinski 1990). Workers roasting the chromium ore at extremely high temperatures to produce the sodium chromate would take a break from time to time to get a beer. "When they walked away on the snow, you could see the yellow tracks they left behind," recalled Szatmary (Stapinski 1990).

Aloysius Sebian was a plant manager at the Diamond Shamrock facility, the source of the chromium buried at the St. Johnsbury site where Trum later worked. During a federal court case in Newark in 1986 regarding a chromium-contaminated development site in Jersey City, Sebian said he thought that chromate workers were the only ones in danger of suffering health effects from chromium exposure. In his deposition, Sebian said,

> Well, in those days, we did not consider it a hazard or anything. We just operated. We wanted to recover all the chromium we could. . . . The normal problem with the septum of your nose being eaten out by chrome. That was, at the time, wasn't considered serious. For example, before I went in the service, by working in the lab and occasionally going out in the plant . . . I had a perforation in the septum of my nose (Sebian 1986)

Workers at the Diamond Shamrock plant were given two bars of Octagon soap along with their weekly paychecks to prevent skin irritation due to contact with chromium (Sebian 1986).

Based on health studies commissioned by the companies producing chromium in the United States in the 1940s (including the two Jersey City companies and the Kearny company), the chromate industry knew that chromium was a hazard. According to a 1948 study, 21 percent of all deaths in the chromate industry were due to cancer of the respiratory system. The ratio was sixteen times higher than the expected ratio of 1.3 percent. The crude death rate for cancer of the lung was twenty-five times the rate expected in normal people. In five of the plants studied, the death rates for lung cancer in workers fifty years old or younger ranged from twenty to seventy times that for a comparable industrial group (Machle and Gregorious 1948).

Effects of chromium on the liver and kidneys have not been studied in detail. However, cases of acute hepatitis, liver necrosis, and congested liver are documented (World Health Organization [WHO] 1988). In the kidneys, acute nephritis and acute tubular necrosis have been observed after massive absorption of chromium.

Respiratory effects other than lung cancer are documented as well. Hexavalent chromium can sensitize the respiratory tract, resulting in allergies. Although little information is available on the effects of chromium on reproduction, it has been shown that hexavalent chromium can cause genetic damage in experimental mammals. Trivalent chromium too causes genetic damage in very high doses. Compounds of hexavalent chromium penetrate biologic membranes easily, so they can interact with parts of the cell, including genetic materials (WHO 1988).

Although chromium is regarded as dangerous in its hexavalent form, it is an essential requirement for the body in its trivalent form. The glucose tolerance factor, which is bound organically by a trivalent chromium compound, acts with insulin in removing glucose from the bloodstream. A safe intake of total chromium (hexavalent and trivalent combined) is 50 μg per day (WHO 1988). The EPA has not derived an acceptable daily intake of hexavalent chromium by inhalation, so no safe levels are established. The NJDEP has decided, however, that any levels under 75 parts per million of total chromium found in soil in residential areas need not be covered or excavated.

Few studies have been done on people other than chromate workers exposed to chromium. When Tokyo experienced its chromium crisis in the 1970s, a crisis similar to but not as large as Hudson County's problem, tests on residents were conducted. The

NJDEP has copies of those health studies but has had difficulty translating into English. In January 1990, the NJDEP announced that it planned to test one hundred residents and workers from Hudson County who might have been exposed to chromium. The New Jersey Department of Health did its own studies on children and adults at Public School 15 in Jersey City, which was contaminated with chromium. Ear, nose, and throat tests were conducted on 160 men, women, and children. Although elevated levels of chromium were found in the urine of the children and the adults living closest to the school, the Department of Health reported that no health effects related to exposure were found (New Jersey. Department of Health [NJDOH] 1989).

NJDEP officials said that chromium inhaled by the students and staff was chromium dust tracked in on their shoes from the contaminated vacant lots in the surrounding neighborhood. Parents were concerned with the contamination in the surrounding area, but after the school was reopened, they were still worried that the chromium was leaching its way into the school basement. At a meeting with the NJDEP, the president of the School 15 Parents Council said that the agency's shoe-tracking theory was absurd. She noted that one of the highest concentrations of chromium was found on the rug in the principal's office. "I'm sure Mr. Bill Smith didn't play in those lots," said Fakira Brown (1990).

The Public School 15 neighborhood is one of several communities in Jersey City that was contaminated with chromium when two to three million tons of waste mud were mixed with an undetermined amount of soil and used as landfill. More than 170 sites throughout Jersey City, Kearny, Bayonne, Weehawken, and Secaucus were polluted with fill. While many of the sites—particularly those in Kearny—are industrial sites, about three dozen residential sites are known to contain chromium-tainted fill. All are located in Jersey City.

In Jersey City, the three residential communities most affected by chromium are the Bergen–Lafayette section, the downtown area, and the Greenville section, which includes the industrial Route 440 properties. One known site is in the city's Journal Square area, and one is in the Heights' neighborhood. The people who may have been affected by chromium come from all walks of life because of the long time span of chromium dumping. Until the 1960s, Bergen–Lafayette and Greenville were primarily middle-class white neighborhoods. But the demographics began to change as white residents moved to the suburbs and the African-American community began settling in that part of the city. Downtown, once occupied by Italian, Polish, and Irish families, is now a mix of those ethnic groups, with the addition of Latinos who immigrated there in the 1950s and 1960s. The young urban professionals and artists came in the 1970s and 1980s. These newest arrivals, many of whom came before the real estate market skyrocketed, were attracted by Hudson's proximity to New York and its low rents. Composed of people from many ethnic backgrounds, this group includes WASPS, a new ingredient in the city's diverse ethnic and racial population.

The downtown sites were the first residential areas found to contain chromium. In 1983, Earl "Tex" Aldredge of the Jersey City Hazardous Waste Task Force identified chromium at a development where townhouses were planned. Aldredge discovered that the Ninth Street site was filled with chromium-tainted soil in 1974 by Anthony Ambrosio and Sons Construction Company of Jersey City under commission by the Jersey City Redevelopment Agency. Countless other sites around the city were filled with chromium by Ambrosio and other contractors after PPG Industries and Mutual gave the chromium-tainted soil away as cheap landfill. Contractors used chromium fill because it kills rats on site. One downtown site believed to be most heavily contaminated is the Gregory Park apartments, one of the city's largest housing developments. The two twenty-two-story buildings are believed to have been built on top of eleven thousand tons of chromium waste. Some of Gregory Park's three thousand residents have complained of heaving asphalt and cracking concrete for years. Chromium is known to erode concrete and asphalt, causing foundations to crack.

Ambrosio, responsible for hauling much of the chromium waste buried at sites throughout the city, was cleared of any wrongdoing by U.S. District Judge H. Lee Sarokin in 1987. During his deposition in a suit regarding the Ninth Street property, Ambrosio stated it was common practice for contractors to pick up soil from the PPG Garfield Avenue site. According to Ambrosio, the soil was regarded as clean fill and was purchased for twenty cents a cubic yard.

Ambrosio said of the contaminated fill: "The city of Jersey City used quite a bit. The county of Hudson built roads with this material. The city was taking it every day, using it, filling potholes or whatever they were doing with it." Indeed, many of the contaminated sites throughout Jersey City are city-owned lots. "If anybody

had told me it had any chemicals in it, I would not have bought it,"
Ambrosio said (Ambrosio 1985).

Because the Ninth Street site was slated for luxury development,
the city's Redevelopment Agency cleaned the site at a cost of
$700,000 to make room for the new townhouses in the gentrifying
neighborhood. Eventually, PPG and Clif Associates, a construction
firm that bought the tainted land from PPG and proceeded to sell
the contaminated soil on site as "clean fill," reimbursed the city.

Sarokin, who ruled on the landmark case in March 1987, placed
total blame on PPG and Clif. "It is undisputed," said Sarokin, "that
as early as 1954, PPG was aware that there were potential health
hazards associated with the processing of chromium ore. . . . PPG
knew or should have known that the chrome might present environmental risks." Clif Associates, he asserted, either knew of the
hazard or should have known. "Nothing less than reckless indifference to a known risk will justify punitive damages," said Sarokin
(Sarokin 1987). Although PPG paid the damages, it did so "in a
spirit of compromise and without admitting liability in any way,"
according to the company's attorney (Sarokin 1987). But Sarokin's
landmark decision set a precedent for future chromium plaintiffs.
PPG claimed it never sold the fill as part of the property but simply
turned the land over to the construction company.

The Chromium Producers

PPG did not produce all the chromium waste on Garfield Avenue;
Natural Products helped. Many Bergen–Lafayette residents fondly
remember the mountains of yellow green sludge that they sledded
on as children. Szatmary, the retired chemical worker, recalls that
mountain. "It was about 75 feet high. A little cart would drive
round and round to the top of the pile and dump some more"
(Stapinski 1990).

In 1954, PPG acquired Natural Products' portion of the site, continuing operations there until 1964. From 1954 to 1963, various
contractors, including Lawrence Construction Company, affiliated
with Clif Associates, removed waste mud from the facility. PPG
allowed approximately forty tons of chromate waste per day to be
taken from their site free of charge. In July 1964, Clif Associates,
headed by Lawrence's principal, Fred Fishbein, purchased the site

from PPG. Since by 1987 Fishbein was deceased, his office manager, Allyn Molyneux, was called to testify during the Ninth Street proceedings. Molyneux, an employee with Lawrence and Clif for thirty years, had no idea that there was chromium-contaminated soil on the Garfield Avenue property. "I wouldn't have known a chemical if I had seen one," Molyneux testified (Molyneux 1986). When the floor started to heave in the Lawrence Construction offices, Molyneux thought it to be a common occurrence on construction sites. Chromium soil, in addition to killing plant life and rats, destroys concrete foundations, causing floors to shift and buildings eventually to fall. In 1991, a number of companies continued to operate on the contaminated land owned by Clif. The piles of chromium are long gone—their contents buried long ago in vacant lots and under schools and playgrounds. But traces of chromium are still to be found on the Garfield Avenue property.

Allied–Signal, originally Mutual Chemical Company, operated its plant on Route 440, across the road from the site where the Roosevelt Drive-In was built. Until a 1989 "sweeping," the thirty-four-acre drive-in site resembled an alien landscape, not unlike a scene from one of the many horror movies that once played there. Barely any vegetation survived; large yellow green ponds swirled around the giant, abandoned movie screen. The strangely haunting screen, which was removed in 1989, was the only object on the site that reminded a visitor that she was still on Earth.

From 1905 to 1953, the commercial area known today as Route 440 was the site of Mutual Chemical, which churned out a million tons of chromium waste (NJDEP 1989). The slurry was pumped across the highway to the drive-in site. Szatmary remembers the wooden bridge that was built to hold the pipe that transported the slurry. "You could hear the loud gears clanging so that the pump could suck the fluid up through the pipe," he recalled (Stapinski 1990). Operations ceased when Allied acquired Mutual. However, the company continued to give waste away as fill. Aerial photographs taken in December 1953 show a pile of material, assumed to be chromate waste, stored at the eastern edge of the Roosevelt Drive-In site. This thirty-foot mountain of waste covered five to ten acres. Allied made the waste available to construction contractors for use as fill in building projects.

While Mutual was still in operation, a diking system was used to control the material and confine it to the property to prevent it from washing into the waters of the Hackensack River and Newark Bay.

But when Mutual was dissolved in 1954, the diking system was abandoned. As a result, today, approximately 12,600 gallons of chromium-contaminated groundwater flow into the Hackensack River each day (Hunter/Environmental Science and Engineering 1989).

Jersey City's groundwater is believed to be tainted with chromium. Samples taken at the drive-in site in 1983 revealed hexavalent chromium concentrations from 4.3 to 30 mg/l. The maximum limit, according to New Jersey's Groundwater Quality Standards is .05 mg/l. Jersey City does not use its groundwater; its drinking water is piped in from Boonton, New Jersey. Residents often fish and crab in the Hackensack River and Newark Bay, however. The NJDEP has not taken any measures to prevent flow of chromium into the river or to warn Jersey City fishermen not to eat whatever they catch from the bottom of the contaminated river.

In Kearny, the chromium story began in 1916, when the Martin Dennis Company opened its facility on the Belleville Turnpike, now bordered by a toxic stretch of polluted streams and garbage dumps. In 1948, Diamond Alkali Company took over the company; then in 1967, it changed its name to Diamond Shamrock Corporation. In 1986, Diamond Shamrock sold its stock to a company owned by Occidental Petroleum Corporation, and in 1987, Diamond Shamrock changed its name to Maxus Energy Corporation. Diamond Shamrock owned and operated the Kearny plant from 1948 to 1976. Sebian, the plant manager who testified in the Ninth Street proceedings, said that his company knew of the health effects associated with chromium: "We were well aware that close contact with fumes or dust was a health hazard. . . . We knew from studies that the Germans did that there was a possible cancer problem" (Sebian 1986). While Diamond Shamrock was in operation, Disch Haulers in Kearny removed 300,000 tons of chromium waste from the facility, which equaled nearly half the amount the company produced. In an in-house letter surrendered to the NJDEP in 1989, Maxus attorneys stated that "Disch Construction had an oral agreement with Diamond Shamrock Chemical Corporation in Kearny to provide twenty-four-hour, seven-day service to remove residue from the plant" (NJDEP 1989). Lee Pot, a Bayonne hauler, may have also transported chromium waste from the Diamond Shamrock plant to various sites throughout the county, including the second-largest chromium site in Hudson County, the Bayonne Exxon site.

The Kearny Diamond Shamrock site was also a regular source of fill for the Kearny Water Department. "They would occasionally come in and ask if they could have a truck or two when they were doing some pipework," said Sebian (Sebian 1986). The engineers put the chromium fill near the pipes, believing the high alkaline and chrome content would protect the pipes from corrosion. Sebian said he recommended the chromium-laced fill only as subfill, not as regular fill. However, he was not the one who made up the contracts for disposal of the waste. The operations manager or someone higher up made those deals. "At first we used the residue to fill in around our own property and in the neighboring plants," said Sebian (Sebian 1986). One of those plants was probably the St. Johnsbury Trucking Terminal where Frederick Trum later worked.

"In those days, our concept of anyone living on a site never existed," said Sebian. "We had no idea that anyone would use this in a residential area. We never advocated it" (Sebian 1986). Near the Belleville Turnpike, the Jersey City water line from Boonton once operated. The line is surrounded by chromium-contaminated fill. The pipeline has not been used since 1957, but the Jersey City Water Department is considering rehabilitating it as a backup water line. Jersey City officials contend that chromium in the area will be cleaned up before the water line is put into operation.

Maxus Energy Corporation is now a Dallas oil company. Maxus agreed in 1990 to spend $51.5 million to treat or remove chromium-tainted fill at twenty-six industrial and commercial sites throughout Kearny and Secaucus. The landmark agreement with the NJDEP, which freed stockholding Occidental from any liability, marked the first time a private company took full responsibility for chromium waste in Hudson County. In addition, Maxus agreed to pay the NJDEP a $2.5 million settlement stemming from allegations that it violated the Spill Compensation and Control Act. That money would go toward the Spill Fund, which provides money for government cleanups.

Residential Contamination in Jersey City

Because all the residential areas in Hudson County known to be contaminated with chromium are located in Jersey City, much of the media attention given to the chromium crisis has centered on that city. Residents at greatest potential risk live in the Bergen–Lafayette area, the neighborhood with the largest number of identified sites. For years, it is surmised, residents there have been exposed to airborne hexavalent chromium. Children have grown up with chromium, playing in contaminated dirt lots, attending contaminated schools, and later setting up their own homes in the same contaminated neighborhoods. The 1,100 children who attend Public School 15 are only a small number compared to the total 35,000 population in Bergen–Lafayette. In 1988, the community formed a grassroots coalition to deal with chromium contamination. In Tokyo, as in Jersey City, the Japanese government developed its plan to clean chromium there only after intense pressure from dozens of citizens groups (Bureau of Environmental Protection, Tokyo 1980).

In Jersey City, the only residential areas cleansed of chromium are the private development sites where expensive condominium projects have been built. But chromium still plagues some of these sites. Developers like to characterize their chromium woes as distant memories rather than grim realities. In 1987, two chromium-tainted sites where railroad tracks and warehouses had once stood were cleaned to make way for the ten billion dollar Newport development on the Hudson River waterfront, a complex including a shopping mall, luxury apartments, and office buildings. Sam Lefrak, the largest residential landlord in New York City, creator of Lefrak City in Queens and the residential buildings at Battery Park City, was the father of Newport. Lefrak will not admit that chromium once existed on his Newport site. "The only place I have chrome is on my car," Lefrak declared (Rosenfeld 1989).

Despite Lefrak's attempts to downplay the problem, chromium crept into the Newport picture again in 1990. The lifeline from New York City to Newport is the PATH train system. Operated by the Port Authority of New York and New Jersey, this subway is a vital link in the development's success. Newport paid for a multimillion dollar overhaul of the station; in return, the Port Authority renamed the Pavonia Avenue station "Pavonia/Newport." When chromium was found at the station in 1989, both the NJDEP and the Port Authority downplayed the problem. Jersey City resident and PATH commuter Gina Franklin took a sample of the yellow material dripping from the ceiling of the station and sent it to International Testing Laboratories, Incorporated, in Newark. The results: 120 parts per million of total chromium, considerably higher than the NJDEP's 75 parts per million limit of safety. A newspaper reporter from the *Jersey Journal* took his own sample, and tests revealed similar results. The NJDEP, calling the tests unscientific, brushed them aside. After conducting its own tests, the NJDEP declared the station safe. But yellow stalactites hanging from the station columns continue to grow and drip.

At Society Hill, the $150 million condominium complex on Newark Bay, a chromium cleanup was paid for and executed by the developers, K. Hovnanian Companies. When Hovnanian tested its ninety-acre property in 1984, high concentrations of chromium were found on the northern twenty-six acres, which is connected to the Roosevelt Drive-In site. A clay wall (one method of containing chromium) was built on the Hovnanian property to separate the contaminated land from the place where the townhouses were built. Ten thousand Hudson residents and others throughout the metropolitan area entered a lottery held in the fall of 1989 to win a chance to buy an inexpensive "dream house." With a severe lack of affordable housing in the county and the entire region, it was no surprise that droves of people turned out for the lottery. What most of the twelve hundred lucky winners were unaware of was that they would be living next door to the Roosevelt Drive-In site—the second-largest chromium dump in the world, second only to one in eastern Europe. NJDEP officials, though determined to have other residential sites in the city cleaned, said the drive-in site was too large for excavation. In other words, Society Hill residents would live next to the biggest chromium dump in America forever. One lifelong Jersey City resident who won the lottery and planned to move into the development with his two daughters quickly dismissed any possibility of danger. "I've been in that drive-in a thousand times," said Jersey City detective John Salmon. "I played in that drive-in. I'm not dead yet. I'll probably die one day, but what are you gonna do? Just live with it" (Stapinski 1989d).

Some lottery winners who grew up in Jersey City voiced similar opinions. Having grown up around toxic waste, they believed, would somehow make them and their children impervious to any future harm. Others, more concerned with possible health hazards, flooded the NJDEP and local newspapers with calls. "Is it safe?" they asked. The best answer anyone could give was "probably," since no health studies existed to support any other determinations. Dozens of families moved into Society Hill. Some residents, after learning of the highly contaminated drive-in site, were more concerned that the property values of their new homes would swiftly decline. They asked Hovnanian to include language in the contract stating that the company would be responsible for any damages due to chromium—structural, health, or otherwise. Hovnanian refused and instead included a clause in the contract releasing the developer from any responsibility linked to hazardous waste. In fact, when interviewed, Hovnanian officials said they didn't think it was necessary to warn buyers of the nearby contamination (Stapinski 1989c).

The only other residential parcel of land to be cleaned was the Ninth Street site. When the Redevelopment Agency cleaned the site in the early 1980s, it neglected to remove high concentrations of chromium waste from the abandoned firehouse next to the site. After years of complaining, a family living in one of the newly built townhouses finally got the city's attention and showed them the yellow crystals creeping up the wall of the firehouse next to their house. In 1990, the city hired contractors, partly paid for by PPG, to demolish and clean the firehouse for $450,000. The firehouse was demolished because the city feared that another public school, School 37, on the other side of the firehouse, would become contaminated. Parents feared that children from the school would wander near the firehouse and be exposed to the chromium. The city did not want another School 15 on its hands.

Public and Private Agendas

While private developers made some attempts to rid their properties of chromium, the city and the state stood by for years and watched as chromium destroyed property values. In a 1990 radio interview, Jersey City mayor Gerald McCann said the worst problem associated with chromium was the decline in property values. He blamed the New York media for the city's problem, claiming that they were owned by New York developers eager to destroy their Jersey City competition. Regardless of whose fault it was, affordable housing projects that could have been built on abundant, city-owned, vacant land in the Bergen–Lafayette area could not even be considered until the chromium there was removed. And until the waste is unearthed, the chromium will continue to leach to contiguous parcels of land, contaminating more and more of the city.

Two grass-roots organizations—the Interfaith Community Organization, made up of residents from both Bergen–Lafayette and downtown; and Citizens Concerned about Chromium, composed of many parents from School 15—began to attack the chromium issue in the late 1980s. An anonymous group calling itself the Chromium Underground distributed leaflets and spray-painted warnings on the sides of buildings and on sidewalks contaminated with the toxic waste. "If we don't do anything about it, nobody will," said ICO member Ellen Wright (1989). She and eighty other ICO members traveled to Trenton in the summer of 1989 to discuss the chromium problem with then-NJDEP commissioner Christopher Daggett. Although Daggett promised the ICO members that chromium would be removed from the residential sites in Jersey City, many members remained skeptical.

The residents' mistrust of government officials had a basis in past experience. In 1985, the NJDEP commissioned a million-dollar study of the county's chromium problem. Five years later, the residents still had not witnessed the NJDEP's removal of a single ounce of the substance. In the last weeks of 1989 and the last days of Governor Thomas H. Kean's administration, the NJDEP announced its eighty-million-dollar plan to remove chromium from thirty-one residential sites and ship it to a federally approved commercial landfill out of state. After presenting the plan to about one hundred residents at a meeting at Jersey City City Hall, the NJDEP was told by the residents that it was simply doing too little too late.

For years, Tex Aldredge led the city's fight against chromium, pestering the state for some concrete answers. Tex would travel from one potential site to another, conducting a simple chromium test using a set of portable test tubes. After pioneering the crusade and uncovering dozens of contaminated sites, Tex finally gave up the fight. Suffering from kidney problems and chrome holes in his skin, Tex left the city's board of health in 1989 and moved back to Texas. He was the first in what was to become a long line of chromium-crusading alumni in Hudson County. Almost a year later he observed that "the politicians in Hudson County are still playing tiddlywinks" (Aldredge 1989). "You're talking about people's lives, children's lives. Politicians are only concerned about money. But children ain't money. They're human beings." Lou Manzo, the city's chief health inspector, took over Tex's battle. Manzo closed chromium-contaminated School 15 in May 1989. The state Department of Health knew about the chromium problem in the school for three years but never notified parents or officials of the potential danger.

Manzo, an outspoken critic of the state's plans and some city officials' positions (including Jersey City mayor Gerald McCann's ideas), was called, among other things, a headline hunter. Along with county health officer Diana Crowder, Manzo kept the media and the public up to date on the chromium problems plaguing the city. If Manzo had never closed School 15, one county official said, the children would never have been tested for chromium. The School 15 crisis made the national news, putting Jersey City chromium and the NJDEP in the spotlight. The Democratic candidate for governor, James Florio, visited the school during his campaign, thereby thrusting the chromium problem into the political limelight. Florio was elected, his stance on the environment contributing to his successful bid. In his first month in office, Florio appointed an environmental prosecutor whose primary function was to search out and bring to justice those companies that left their stain on the Garden State.

Meanwhile, Manzo, because of his political opposition to Mayor McCann, was fighting to keep his job with the local board of health and was faced with the city curbing his responsibilities—among them chromium. In 1990, Crowder was fired from the Hudson Regional Health Commission because of budget cuts. Sources said, however, that she was removed because of her adversarial relationship with the NJDEP. With Aldredge and Manzo out of the picture, Crowder's departure left Hudson County without a health official knowledgeable about chromium. The Hudson Regional Health Commission, by eliminating Crowder's position and firing another chromium investigator, freelance chemist and occupational physician Ronald Ross, removed itself from the chromium forum altogether, leaving the NJDEP to lead the way.

Both Crowder and Manzo blamed the NJDEP for the long delay in cleaning up the city and the rest of the county. The NJDEP, in part, blamed Manzo because he stood in the way of what they called "interim remedial measures." Manzo called their plan, which involved covering over the sites with asphalt, a Band-Aid solution. Surprisingly, several NJDEP officials blamed the NJDEP itself. Bureaucracy was a common enemy of local environmentalists and of the bureaucrats themselves. "Bureaucracy" was constantly getting in the way of progress. And there was nothing the bureaucrats could do about it. After several years of study, the NJDEP's plan in

1983 was to have the chromate-producing companies and their successors clean up their own mess. The NJDEP then launched a new study to determine just how to go about the cleanup. PPG took a step in the right direction in 1990 when it excavated one hundred tons of chromium slag from an industrial site in Jersey City as part of a pilot program to recycle the pure waste into stainless steel ingots. The process, however, works only with pure slag and cannot be used for most of Hudson's chromium, which is mixed with soil. One of the main problems associated with chromium in Hudson County is that most of the soil was buried when no environmental laws were in place. In 1980, after high chromium levels were detected at the Roosevelt Drive-In site, the area was listed on the NJDEP Hazardous Discharge Bond Act. Under the Spill Compensation and Control Act, Allied and the other companies involved were required to take measures to clean up Hudson County. The combined uncertainty about the location of and types of chromium wastes and proper remediation measures made it difficult to prepare a cleanup plan.

What the NJDEP orders and what is actually done are two very different things, however. In April 1991, the state agency ordered Allied to pay $9.7 million in penalties and for a cleanup study for sites in Jersey City and Bayonne. Allied refused and filed suit against the NJDEP. A year earlier, the agency ordered PPG to pay for the $80 million residential cleanup. PPG filed a suit that claimed that the agency's findings were "arbitrary, capricious, unreasonable and without factual or legal foundation" (PPG 1990). PPG disputed the NJDEP's findings that anything over 10 parts per million of hexavalent and 75 parts per million total chromium was unsafe. The company teamed up with Allied and Maxus and hired the Industrial Health Foundation (IHF) to study the chromium problem and present its own findings. The IHF found that levels as high as 75 parts per million hexavalent and 1,000 parts per million total chromium were safe. The NJDEP refused to negotiate and threatened to sue PPG for triple damages. In July 1990, PPG gave in. The Pittsburgh-based company agreed to pay $80 million to remove hazardous levels of chromium from all residential sites linked to their company. They also agreed to pay $2.5 million in fines to the NJDEP. Autumn 1990 was chosen as the time to begin the cleanup. The leaves fell and the Jersey City streets were soon covered with snow, but the only sites cleaned were the Ninth Street firehouse and the industrial experiment site.

In the winter of 1991, PPG started digging. As the list of sites continued to grow, excavation began at some sites along Grand Street in Jersey City. The long process of waking the county from its toxic nightmare had begun.

Tests, Tests, and More Tests: Foreign and Domestic Solutions

In five large volumes of their remedial investigation, the NJDEP explained the seriousness of the chromium problem in Hudson County. The study, conducted by Environmental Science and Engineering of Gainesville, Florida, examined in detail forty-eight representative sites in Jersey City, Kearny, and Secaucus. The state concluded that hexavalent chromium is dangerous and that the concentration of trivalent chromium must be at least two hundred times higher than that of hexavalent to elicit an equally toxic response. It further stated that eating tainted soil, vegetatbles grown in tainted soil, or shellfish from contaminated bodies of water; or having skin contact with or breathing in chromium dust can be hazardous to health (Hunter/Environmental Science and Engineering 1989).

All this information, which was generally known several years earlier, was released in March 1989. Other obvious conclusions were made. For example, houses built on top of chromium or where chromium had leached may have to be demolished. The study then broke down each contaminated site into level of contamination. For example, the family living near a highly contaminated site on Pacific Avenue knows that levels there are above normal and may cause their children to develop asthma. But when the chromium would be removed was still a question. The NJDEP announced that further studies concerning commercial and industrial sites would soon be commissioned.

It is no coincidence that heightened awareness of Hudson's chromium problem came at the same time as the surge in development. But some say the timing could not have been worse. Some local health officials have theorized that the state's reluctance to move on the chromium issue was tied to the Republican governor's push for development. In 1985, Governor Kean's Waterfront Development Office was established in Jersey City. Manzo believed that the governor's popular "New Jersey and You, Perfect Together" campaign and the state's elaborate waterfront development plans never could have taken hold if half of Hudson County were turned upside down in hazardous waste excavation. Indeed, the 1980s was Hudson County's shining decade. "The DEP downplayed a lot of the chromium problems," Manzo said, "because who would have developed in this area?" (1989).

Baltimore, undergoing its own waterfront revitalization, signed an agreement with Allied in 1989 to clean chromium from its Inner Harbor. Allied had used secondary residue from its chromate production plant there as fill near the Baltimore Harbor. Leachate from the fill drained to the harbor through storm sewers, disrupting aquatic life at the bottom of the harbor. A containment and treatment system consisting of cutoff trenches and leachate collection is being planned.

The Tokyo problem, much closer in size to Hudson County's problem, involved 573,700 tons of chromium residue. More than 60,000 tons were dumped into the Pacific Ocean, and several hundred thousand tons were buried at 170 sites throughout the city. In 1973, the Tokyo Metropolitan Government recognized the problem and began a study. After two years, the government's expert committee decided that it was necessary to completely remove the waste from the sites, which included parking lots, homes, factory sites, roads, schools, and parks. A special landfill for the containment of the waste was designed, and in 1980, excavation began. By 1983, the cleanup was finished. The landfill, designed to limit chromate migration, was first filled with sand mixed with a slow-release reducing agent. Sheet piling was then installed around the edge of the landfill, and a clay liner was placed inside. Waste from around the city was mixed with the reducing agent and placed in the landfill. Preliminary health tests revealed elevated incidence of skin, respiratory tract, and digestive disorders in residents in the immediate area of the contaminated fill (Bureau of Environmental Protection, Tokyo, 1980).

In his 1984 study, NJDEP site manager Thomas McKee recommended that Hudson County follow the same plan as Japan did in dealing with its chromium problem. Twelve years have passed since the first discovery of chromium in Jersey City, however, with only a handful of sites cleaned and a few more covered over. In the summer of 1989, the state began covering contaminated residential areas with asphalt to prevent chromium dust from becoming airborne, where it can be breathed in by neighborhood residents. Local health officials, including Manzo, and local residents objected to the plan because they feared that the NJDEP would cap the sites and walk away from the problem. In 1989, with the new McCann administration in office and with Manzo silenced, the NJDEP pursued its cover-up plan. Sensing the residents' fears, McCann secured a written statement from the NJDEP commissioner guaranteeing that excavation of residential sites would take place. No timetable for excavation was given in the letter, however. "The only feasible alternative for cleanup of chromium contamination at these lots is excavation and removal," the letter from Commissioner Daggett reads. "The Department is committed to the excavation and removal of all chromium-contaminated residential sites in Jersey City. However," he continued in true bureaucratic style, "it must be recognized that excavation and removal at these residential properties can only occur subject to a full public review process and only after resolution of transportation issues and the location of an acceptable disposal or internment facility" (Daggett 1989).

While the letter was being signed by Daggett, workers were revving up their steamrollers for their ride across Bergen–Lafayette. Once those sites were covered, like the Kearny and Secaucus sites had been earlier in the summer, Hudson County's chromium fate would be sealed forever, residents thought. Once Daggett stepped aside for the new commissioner, Judith Yaskin, residents hoped that the new Democratic administration would come through on a few promises. The PPG agreement was signed, but more and more sites turned up every day as Florio, the new governor, struggled with a severe budget crisis. The NJDEP underwent a reorganization, with Yaskin stepping down and Scott Weiner taking over, delaying the chromium removal even further.

Large industrial areas that were contaminated were either fenced in or left alone, since there were not enough people to complain about them. Or, as NJDEP explained, exposure was minimal. As late as 1989, the largest site—the drive-in site—was open to any curious child or bored teenager who drove past. Two homeless men, impressed with the wide-open space and absence of police, took up residence on the site in 1990. By then, Allied had mopped up the property and installed a plastic lining over much of it. Until 1989, the NJDEP had a plan to contain all the city's chromium on that one site. A containment device similar to the one used in Tokyo would have been installed. But this metal container was to be the size of two football fields. Even at that mammoth size, the container would not have held all the city's chromium waste. The two or three million tons of slag that were produced were mixed with an undetermined amount of soil and buried throughout the county. A few sites even turned up in Newark. The actual amount of chromium-tainted soil is unknown. Because the chromium is leaching to other areas, the number of chromium-contaminated sites will only increase as time goes by. For obvious reasons, the drive-in vault plan was scrapped. For one, nearby residents and Society Hill developers were not happy with the idea. In addition, new federal regulations, which reclassified chromium as a hazardous waste, prohibited the NJDEP from creating a chromium landfill in the densely populated county.

Meanwhile, students at contaminated School 15 returned to classes in late fall 1989 while local health officials tried to determine the extent of the chromium problem there. In August, the state Department of Health and NJDEP told parents that it was safe for their children to return to the school. "It's like the mayor in the movie *Jaws* telling people it's safe to go back in the water," said Manzo (1989).

Chromium-tainted crystals growing on the school's basement walls—similar to the crystals growing on the walls of homes and businesses in the neighborhood—still could not be explained to the parents' satisfaction. The NJDEP's reasoning for why the crystals tested positive for chromium was that the simple calcium formations on the basement walls caught some particles of chromium dust that were present in the air, which traveled in on the shoes of the children and staff.

During that same summer, David Hoffman, the owner of a hardware store located down the block from the school, was forced to close up shop when the Department of Health warned him of "potential exposure" due to chromium leaching into his store from a contaminated vacant lot next door. His landlord was forced to evict the rest of her tenants and was left with an empty, vandalized building (Stapinski 1989a).

Mildred Napolitano, a single mother with two teenaged children, lost her homeowner's insurance because of chromium leaching from the tainted playground next door. Her son, Neil, was forced to live with relatives elsewhere because high levels of chromium (above .5 $\mu g/l$) were found in his urine. Neil once played in La-Pointe Park next door, and his bedroom window faced the tainted site. Gregory Park residents wonder whether eleven thousand tons of chromium buried beneath their high-rise apartments were the reason their parking lot, which resembled a roller coaster, buckled. Society Hill lottery winners moved next to the drive-in site with no cure in sight. Newport residents are safe in their condominium towers until their commute via the contaminated PATH station each day. Frederick Trum's co-workers worry that they will suffer the same painful death from years of exposure to chromium at the St. Johnsbury Trucking Terminal.

Manzo, who was elected to the county Board of Chosen Freeholders while still fighting to get his city job back, just shakes his head when he says it's been over a decade and hardly any chromium cleaning has been done. "If the chromium had been a problem in a more prominent area of New Jersey like the suburbs or the Jersey Shore, it would have been rectified a long time ago. There's no doubt in my mind" (Manzo 1989).

Aldredge, the first chromium pioneer in Hudson, voiced his frustrations with the politicians along the tainted Gold Coast. "You don't spend money to take care of development until you take care of where the people live," said Tex (1989). "They all say, 'To hell with the ordinary man whose child is being exposed to chromium.' But how the little kid who won't live to see his twenty-first birthday because he's got chromium poisoning?"

Becky Linstrom and her family live in downtown Jersey City, across the street from one of the most highly contaminated residential sites in the city. In 1989, she gave birth to a healthy baby boy. However, doctors have no idea what effect chromium has on women or children. "It makes me angry because I think of all the prenatal care I've taken," said Linstrom while still pregnant with her son, Benjamin (Stapinski 1989b). "Perhaps some politician's decision not to clean this up will have an effect on how healthy my newborn baby will be. If this was the governor's mansion, the chromium would be gone. But our homes are just as sacred as anyone else's."

Notes

[1]The section on the medical history of chromium was contributed by Richard P. Wedeen, M.D.

References

Agency for Toxic Substances and Disease Registry. 1989. *Toxicological profile for chromium*. U.S. Public Health Service. ATSDR/TP-88/10, 1989.

Aldredge, E. 1989. Interview with the author.

Ambrosio, A. 1985. Deposition in the Jersey City Redevelopment Agency v. PPG and International Fidelity suit; Office of Schwartz, Tobia and Stanziale; October 17; Montclair, New Jersey.

Brown, F. 1990. Interview with the author, January 11.

Bureau of Environmental Protection, Tokyo Metropolitan Government. 1980. *Measures for Treating Soil Contamination Caused by Hexavalent Chromium in Tokyo*.

Daggett, C. 1989. Letter to Gerald McCann, mayor of Jersey City, August 15. New Jersey Department of Environmental Protection, Trenton.

Gelman, J. L. 1988. "Workers' Compensation Law." *New Jersey Practice*, vol. 38. St. Paul, Minn: West.

Hunter/Environmental Science and Engineering. 1989. Feasibility Study for Chromium Sites in Hudson County, New Jersey. Prepared for the State of New Jersey Department of Environmental Protection, Trenton, New Jersey.

Langard, S. 1990. "One Hundred Years of Chromium and Cancer: A Review of Epidemiological Evidence and Selected Case Reports." *American Journal of Industrial Medicine* 17:189–215.

Machle, W., and Gregorius, P. 1948. "Cancer of the Respiratory System in the United States Chromate-Producing Industry." *Public Health Service* 63.

Major, R. H. 1922. "Studies on a Case of Chromic Acid Nephritis." *Johns Hopkins Hospital Bulletin* 372:56–61.

Manzo, L. 1989. Interview with the author.

McKee. T. 1984. *Chromate Chemical Production Industry: Waste Treatment Past and Present*. Trenton: New Jersey Department of Environmental Protection.

Molyneux, A. 1986. Deposition in the Jersey City Redevelopment Agency v. PPG and International Fidelity suit; Offices of Pitney, Hardin, Kipp and Szuch; November 19; Morristown, New Jersey.

Pofeldt, E. 1992. "Residential Chromium Sites Clean." *Jersey Journal*, November 9, p. 2.

New Jersey. Department of Environmental Protection. 1989. *Hudson County Chromium Exposure Directive*. Trenton, New Jersey, 12.

———. Department of Health. 1989. *Medical Evaluation of Children and Adults of the Whitney Young, Jr., School, Jersey City, New Jersey*. Trenton, N.J.: Environmental Health Service Division of Occupational and Environmental Health.

New Jersey State Legislative Documents. 1917. Vol. 3, doc. nos. 14–23 inclusive. *Annual Report of the Department of Labor (1916)*. Doc. no. 15:3–103.

PPG Industries, Incorporated. 1990. Civil Appeal Case Information Statement, Superior Court of New Jersey, Trenton, May 31.

Rosenfeld, D. 1989. "Rosy Future Predicted for Gold Coast." *Jersey Journal*, July 21, p. 17.

Rosenfeld, D. 1991. "DEP Dumped Chromium Soil in Park." *Jersey Journal*, August 12, p. 9.

Sarokin, H. L. March 17, 1987. Judge's decision in the Jersey City Redevelopment Agency v. PPG and International Fidelity, Newark, New Jersey.

Sebian, A. 1986. Deposition in the Jersey City Redevelopment Agency v. PPG and International Fidelity suit; Offices of Pitney, Hardin, Kipp and Szuch; November 10; Morristown, New Jersey.

Stapinski, H. 1989a. "Chromium Closes a Hardware Store." *Jersey Journal*, August 3, p. 1.

———. 1989b. "Chromium Contamination Casts Long Shadow over Couple's Life." *Jersey Journal*, December 28, p. 8.

———. 1989c. "Developer Disclaims Toxic Hazard." *Jersey Journal*, November 2, p. 10.

———. 1989d. "A Lottery Winner Shrugs at Chromium Danger." *Jersey Journal*, November 2, p. 10.

———. 1990. "Retired Chromium Worker Tells When and Where It Was Dumped." *Jersey Journal*, June 25, pp. 1, 4.

Trum, F. 1989. Interview with the author.

Wedeen, R. P. 1991. "Chromium-Induced Kidney Disease." *Environmental Health Perspectives* 92:71–74.

World Health Organization. 1988. *Chromium: Environmental Health Criteria 61.* Geneva: United Nations Environment Programme, International Labour Organisation, and World Health Organization.

Wright, E. 1989. Interview with the author.

• CHAPTER 8 •

"A Prejudice Which May Cloud the Mentality": An Overview of the Birth of the Modern Science of Occupational Disease

CHRISTOPHER C. SELLERS, M.D., Ph.D.

Christopher C. Sellers, a physician with a doctorate in American Studies from Yale, traces the historical origins of the discipline of occupational medicine. Beginning with the Progressive Era (circa 1912), when faith in the progress of American civilization was unbounded, Sellers examines the distortions of medical practice that can occur when corporations control medical care for their employees. He examines the social and economic forces that subverted disease prevention in the workplace. Uncertain goals were further diffused by divided authority and genuine ambivalence. Jealousies among physicians and government health officials fed institutional inertia. A long tradition of blaming the injured for physical "accidents," and of simply ignoring occupational disease, resisted change. The medical profession remained aloof. Only in the 1970s did a new breed of occupational health physicians emerge. Paid by third-party insurance carriers, government, or universities, the new breed were not "company" physicians. By not being corporate employees, they held conflict of interest at bay and aspired to prevent occupational disease.

New Jersey played a leading role in the development of state health departments and occupational medicine programs in the United States. From its inception in 1866, the New Jersey State Sanitary Commission pressed for state intervention in public health in the occupational setting as well as in the community at large.

The commission's chairman, Ezra Mundy Hunt, traveled to England with his close friend, the eminent Massachusetts physician John Shaw Billings, where they met Sir Joseph Lister in 1876 (Alewitz 1986:13). As Hunt came to understand the new concept of contagion, the germ theory, he saw that public health legislation was essential for controlling the spread of infections in densely populated cities. The specificity of diagnosis provided by bacteriology promised similarly objective methods for defining noninfectious diseases. Hunt was elected president of the Medical Society of New Jersey in 1865 (24). In 1877, he became secretary of the New Jersey Board of Health, which he had been instrumental in creating, and in 1882 was elected tenth president of the American Public Health Association (Alewitz 1986; Kober 1921). In 1878, he helped form the Bureau of Vital Statistics. The health of workers remained a central concern to Hunt even as the demands of office drew his attention elsewhere.

In 1885, Hunt headed a committee for the American Public Health Association that awarded the Lomb Prize to George H. Ireland for an essay entitled "Preventable Causes of Disease and Death in American Manufactories and Workshops, and the Best Means and Appliances for Preventing and Avoiding Them" (Ireland 1886). While encouraging industrial development in New Jersey, Ireland noted that manufacturers "find it profitable to their pockets, as well as contributory to the health of their operatives, to erect their buildings in moderate sized towns, or in the suburbs, rather than in the heart of the great cities themselves" (139). Ireland described how factory design could reduce accidents, fires, and noxious dusts. He urged avoidance of "naphtha and benzine" because of the fire hazards (146), described the ergonomics of chair construction, and promoted noise abatement in the workplace well before these issues found many proponents.

Although Hunt influenced the development of public health in the United States, Ireland's recommendations accumulated dust on the library shelf. Insight into what needs to be done was far removed from effective policy. Knowledge that indicates that costly investments are required for health protection had to be relearned again and again, not only by the corporations, but by the medical community as well. The resources necessary to establish definitive dose–response relationships were rarely available for the practical tasks at hand. Information on toxicity was regularly rediscovered. These toxic circles were not broken by occupational medicine textbooks or government reports but by legal actions: workers' compensation and tort liability provide their own economic imperatives. As long as the corporations paid the piper, physicians danced to corporate tunes. As the responsibility for occupational medicine shifts to state government and university clinics in the 1990s, reemphasis on environmental conditions in the workplace can be anticipated.

• • •

Today, it is difficult to imagine any effective program against industrial disease that does not rely at least in part on measurement and control of atmospheric chemicals. Especially since World War II, when both the American Standards Association and the newly formed American Conference of Governmental Industrial Hygienists (ACGIH) endorsed numerical estimates of the maximum safe concentrations for several industrial chemicals, atmospheric regulation has played a central role in efforts to monitor and maintain factory health (Paull 1984:231). When the federal government became more involved in the field in 1970, it too acknowledged a pivotal role for atmospheric controls. The new Occupational Safety and Health Administration (OSHA) made the ACGIH safe concentration estimates, called "threshold limit values" (TLVs), into the cornerstone of its first rules on workplace chemicals (Ashford 1976). The ACGIH standards even achieved international recognition, as many other countries followed the example of OSHA (Vigliani et al. 1977; Toyama 1985:87–89; Salter 1988:53–54). No wonder the methods for preserving industrial health available around 1920, which included few atmospheric measurements and no quantitative safety estimates, now seem unimaginably primitive, unscientific, and unsuccessful. In this chapter, however, I mean to argue for the attractiveness of at least some aspects of this earlier system.

In no way do I question whether the type of knowledge that took hold in this country after 1920, involving quantitative correlations between atmospheric chemical levels and disease, was more scientifically sophisticated or more useful than much earlier knowledge in the field. Rather, I wish to focus upon the institutional and rhetorical changes that accompanied this new kind of knowledge. The new epistemological emphasis arrived in this country hand in hand with a new community of experts, centered in the public health schools, in company medical clinics, and in state divisions of industrial hygiene. Particularly disturbing is the strategy by which many in this community came to justify their activities: they began to invoke a mutually exclusive distinction between the science and the politics of occupational disease. In the way they employed this demarcation, the call to "science" became increasingly an autocratic assertion of one's own expertise rather than a preface to public argument. This mode of justification has retained a central place in the rhetorical armor of today's industrial health professionals.

Only a closer look at the roots and historical role of this self-definition will allow us to move beyond glib criticism toward at least an outline of a suitable alternative. To begin with, we need to better understand the deep dependence of both the pre- and post-1920 American conceptions of a science of occupational disease on the actual means for occupational disease control available in each era. Changes in possible and actual health interventions in the workplace by physicians, government officials, and company owners and employers correlate closely with the changes in occupational disease science between these two eras. This historical contrast between scientific styles parallels the pre-1920 differences between American and European scientific approaches. In fact, the intellectual origins of the new form of knowledge lay in Europe, in the context of relatively longstanding and elaborate national systems for monitoring and controlling occupational disease (Kober 1921; Teleky 1948; Rosen 1958). In Germany from 1886 onward, Karl Lehmann performed animal experiments closely correlating air levels of particular industrial chemicals with pathological effects (Lehmann 1886). By 1912, Britain's Thomas Legge and Kenneth Goadby had investigated the minimum toxic dose of lead dust in the laboratory (Legge and Goadby 1912:31–32). In America, a regulatory system for occupational illness as extensive as those in Germany and Britain developed somewhat later. Only following World War I, when such a system had appeared, did Americans feel compelled to fully embrace this kind of laboratory investigation and its products. Only then did they also adopt a justificatory strategy invoking a clear distinction between science and politics.

The earliest American textbooks on occupational diseases appeared in the latter part of the Progressive Era, after the election of Woodrow Wilson in 1912. During this time, medical and scientific compilers of this knowledge expected it to retain a convincing prescriptive power for those without scientific training. The knowledge itself remained closely tied to either preventive or curative interventions in the separate realms of factory inspection and the clinic. Between then and the mid twenties, however, controversies arose over the application of medical knowledge in the factory, centering around a crucial element in the emerging American system of regulation—the company physician. Responding to the resultant problematic status of this knowledge, postwar researchers in the new public health schools and in expanded government investigations seized upon the integrated laboratory-oriented methods pioneered by the Europeans. The new epistemological norms the Americans adopted for their scientific work shifted it from practical toward more theoretical questions; they also began to address their work increasingly to each other and to a specialized audience of physicians and hygienists, rather than to laypersons. They thereby came to feel justified in locating their work on the scientific side of a newly discovered boundary between science and policy. Yet the impartiality they claimed for this new knowledge, in contrast to the ideologically manipulable knowledge of the earlier era, actually laid the groundwork for a new form of policy prescription. Exemplified by their estimates of safe concentration levels, forerunners of the TLVs, it relied more upon the authority of expertise than the art of persuasion.

Control of Occupational Disease During the Late Progressive Era

Writings on occupational causes of illness in the United States appeared long before the Progressive Era. Texts on the diseases associated with particular vocations appeared sporadically throughout the nineteenth century (McCready 1837; Rohe 1885). In the latter third of the century, sanitarians in New York City and elsewhere published reports on their investigations of factories (Galishoff 1975:135–138; Rosen 1988:391–425). Their efforts led to the establishment of the first state factory inspection bureaus in New Jersey in 1885 and in New York and Massachusetts, both in 1886 (Price 1919 165–166; Galishoff 1975:137). The early inspection bureaus, though they concentrated on protecting child and women laborers, also enforced laws regulating dust and ventilation. Similarly, mining and railroad companies recognized particular health hazards associated with their industries many years before the turn of the century and began hiring their own physicians to treat employees (Hazlett and Hummel 1957; Derickson 1988).

In the Progressive Era, however, both the volume of writing and the forms of intervention on behalf of industrial health multiplied dramatically. Many of the diverse and rapidly changing activities through this period with regard to occupational disease must remain beyond the scope of this chapter. To understand the distinct social apparatus that had evolved to contend with maladies specific to the workplace, however, we need to look briefly at the ways in which knowledge about occupational disease came to be collected and applied in this country around 1914. Both government and industry used a number of strategies for monitoring and remedying occupational maladies by this time, including curative and preventive means.

Factory inspection bureaus were seen as a necessary adjunct of government in the more industrial states. In 1914, thirty-three states had factory inspection bureaus. Though not all of these agencies had clear legal authority to act against chemical causes of occupational diseases, twenty-two enforced laws against injurious dusts, and fifteen against poisonous gases, fumes, and vapors (Thompson 1914:136, 140). Some of the laws required the presence of specific devices to remove dust or fumes. Others relied upon the judgment of inspectors about whether the dust in a particular factory was "excessive" or the preventive methods already in use were "suitable" (Andrews 1911:123–134). Invariably, inspectors carried out the laws by simple visual observation and purely qualitative decisions. Even when officials such as C. T. Graham-Rogers, medical inspector of factories for New York, made more precise measurements of atmospheric dust or chemical concentrations, they almost always invoked these figures in a qualitative way, as an argument for the presence of a "poison" (New York. Bureau of Factory Inspection 1913a:36–37). Neither laboratories nor expert personnel for measuring atmospheric dust or chemical concentrations seemed practical or necessary.

Graham-Rogers was the first of only a handful of physicians employed in state factory inspection. By 1915, only Illinois, Massachusetts, New York, and Pennsylvania had medical factory inspectors (Price 1915:96). Graham-Rogers's training allowed him to make occasional use of another investigative technique that soon became a much more integral part of occupational disease control than quantitative measurements: the physical examination. In his capacity as a government factory inspector, Graham-Rogers usually examined either children, to determine their fitness or age, or the victims of occupational disease (New York. Bureau of Factory Inspection 1913b:74,82). Outside the government, companies themselves began to make more use of the physical examination of factory workers, partly because of new government demands. Three states passed laws by 1914 requiring periodic physical examinations for those employed in lead industries (Committee on Occupational Hygiene 1914:528). Others ordered exams for those who worked in compressed air ("Protection for Compressed Air Workers" 1914:549). When states required physical exams, they allowed companies to make independent arrangements for carrying out the law. Whether a company physician or a private practitioner performed the exams, he or she had to report any lead poisoning discovered to the labor department or the health department.

These laws became part of a growing government mechanism to monitor illnesses of the workplace. Between 1911 and 1914, largely on the initiative of the American Association for Labor Legislation, fifteen states passed laws requiring all physicians to report any cases of occupational disease to the state labor or health department (Committee on Occupational Hygiene 1914:525). This attempt to enlist the aid of private practitioners and company and academic physicians in a government-based program of surveillance had mixed success. Through the reports that did arrive in state agencies sometimes supplied factory or medical inspectors with leads for their investigations, relatively few physicians sent in reports. Private practitioners in particular showed little awareness of occupational disease. Their apathy reflected the dearth of instruction about this kind of malady in the medical schools, as well as the frequent difficulty of distinguishing between occupational and other causes of disease.

At the same time, without government prodding, some physicians began to devise forms of practice directed more specifically toward wage earners, in which the diagnosis and treatment of job-related disease became a central concern. In a few medical schools, professors sponsored clinics devoted solely to occupational disease (Kober 1921:393–394). Some unions, such as New York's Cloak and Skirt Makers' Union, began to sponsor their own clinics ("Garment Workers' Union" 1913:313). Efforts by the employers themselves against occupational disease probably had the most widespread impact on the health of the working population in this period, however. Some of the earliest attempts of companies to supervise the health of their employees fell under the auspices of "welfare work." Systematic medical examinations became part of paternalistic programs to care for the workers' broader needs, often to wean them away from trade unions (Andrews 1916:825; Nugent 1983:579–581). In 1911, Theodore Sachs convinced some Chicago employers to sponsor physical examinations of their workers for tuberculosis, which was known at the time to be more prevalent in certain industries (Sachs 1914). From then on the company physical exam became a major weapon in a broad progressive crusade against tuberculosis. Many workers viewed these initiatives with mistrust and suspicion (Gompers 1914:54–58).

The advent of workers' compensation further propelled the spread of physical examinations in industry. Montana passed the first state workers' compensation law in 1909, and by 1914, twenty-four states had enacted similar laws (National Industrial Conference Board [NICB] 1917:5; "Standards for Workmen's Compensation Laws" 1914). In the wake of these laws, company officials found the physical exam useful as a way of providing evidence that could later combat any false compensation claims. But occupational diseases played for the most part only a negative role in the compensation system at this time. Early compensation law covered only accidents, and a diagnosis of occupational disease generally served to invalidate a claim (Bale 1986:444–521). Still, diagnoses of these diseases could now serve a useful purpose for companies threatened with compensation suits by providing evidence against worker claims. For these reasons many more establishments hired their own physicians and set up their own factory clinics. Yet the early members of the American Association of Industrial Physicians and Surgeons, founded in 1916, had little awareness of their predecessors and considered industrial medicine a "new specialty" (Mock 1919b: 1, 3–5; Selleck and Whittaker 1962: 57–69). The new industrial physicians increased the overall number of physical exams given to workers and probably devoted greater attention to job-related illness than did the average private practitioner. By 1921, membership of the AAIPS stood at 449. Quantitatively, they and their nonmember colleagues constituted the most extensive new intervention in the area of occupational disease during the Progressive Era (Selleck and Whittaker 1962:442).

Between the turn of the century and 1914, the social mechanism to both detect and prevent or treat work-related illness thus encompassed numerous government agencies as well as several groups of physicians. Physical examination constituted the main mode of information gathering in the clinics, and visual inspection, occasionally along with laboratory analysis of air, dust, or other material, served a similar role in the factories themselves. For the most part, however, the information from physical examinations about workers' bodies remained in the clinics among physicians, while the information on factory environments, from observation and analysis, remained within the inspection bureaus. Even Graham-Rogers performed physical exams and sampled factory air at different times and places, and he never systematically correlated the two kinds of information, according to his labor department reports.

During the Progressive Era, clinical and environmental knowledge did come together in the numerous studies of working environments unassociated with any legal regulatory or medical treatment functions. David Rosner and Gerald Markowitz have written about the diverse group of reformers, muckraker journalists, social scientists, lawyers, and physicians who carried out these studies, and the "social survey" format they employed (Rosner and Markowitz 1985:507–524). Publishing articles in popular magazines such as *Harpers'* and *The Survey*, and in social science journals, this group often devoted attention to the home environment of particular groups of workers as well as to conditions and diseases of the factory, and usually emphasized industrial accidents over poisonings (Maclean 1908–9; Clark and Wyatt 1910–11; Sanville 1910; McFarlane 1911; Palmer 1911). Only rarely did these studies closely examine the connection between the dust or fume exposure they reported and actual cases of disease.

Those investigations that did concentrate exclusively on occupational disease and its environmental causes usually depended on government sponsorship. The national Bureau of Labor and its successor, the Bureau of Labor Statistics, supported both John Andrews's investigation of the phosphorus match industry and Alice Hamilton's of the lead industries from 1909 onward (Andrews 1910; Hamilton 1912, 1913, 1914). Unlike investigators in the twenties, however, Hamilton and Andrews aimed only to establish the significant presence of lead or phosphorus poisoning in the industries they studied rather than to extensively map the relations between increasing exposure and disease. Their fundamentally qualitative goal meant that their reports on the factory environment and their clinical case histories could remain spatially and conceptually separate within their reports, except for common references to particular tasks within the factory. In contrast to Graham-Rogers, neither Hamilton nor Andrews found laboratory measurements or physical examinations necessary for their purposes. They relied largely on interviews, hospital records, and direct observation.

Their assumed audience for these industrial disease studies inclined them to this qualitative approach. Hamilton and Andrews wrote their reports primarily for the laypersons who then had power over the factories and the inspection laws: company managers, factory inspectors, and politicians and the public. They did not discern a coherent expert community in a position to both appreciate and effectively interpret a more quantitative or interventionist approach. The authors of the earliest American textbooks on occupational disease, which appeared during this period, also stressed forms of knowledge that would remain comprehensible for a lay audience. W. Gilman Thompson's *The Occupational Diseases: Their Causation, Symptoms, Treatment and Prevention,* which appeared in 1914, constituted the first textbook length attempt in this country to compile the knowledge appropriate to the new public and private arrangements for controlling occupational disease. Within a couple of years, other textbooks joined Thompson's volume, most notably George Kober and William Hanson's *Diseases of Occupational and Vocational Hygiene* in 1916. Not surprisingly, given the medical training of the authors and the growing role of physicians within the existing system for controlling occupational disease, these texts aimed at physicians, whether in the public health, private, or academic medical communities. Simultaneously, however, they each claimed in their preface or foreword to speak to a diverse crowd that included many other groups engaged in efforts to control job-related illnesses. Thompson, Kober, and Hanson all expressed the hope that those without technical backgrounds, such as employers, social workers, labor leaders, and employees, would consult their texts (Thompson 1914: v; Kober and Hanson 1916: xvii).

Along with addressing laypersons concerned about worker health the authors of these new textbooks meant to foster greater attention to occupational disease within the wider medical and public health communities. They faced an uphill struggle in many corners of these professions. The eighth edition in 1915 of the most famous medical textbook of the era, William Osler's *Principles and Practice of Medicine,* devoted only 7 of 1,225 total pages to industrial chemical disease (Osler and McCrae 1915:393–395, 402–407). Whether out of ignorance or fear of the "reformer" label, physicians generally paid scant attention to any industrial factors in their patients' illnesses (Edsall 1909:1873–1874; Hamilton 194?:115). Public health officials' enthusiasm for bacteriology led many of them to deemphasize the most typical occupational maladies, which had chemical causes. J. Scott MacNutt's *Manual for Health Officers,* published in 1915, devoted only 4 of some 600 pages to industrial hygiene (MacNutt 1915:434–437).

Reviews of the Thompson, and Kober and Hanson textbooks suggested that these communities preferred to view occupational disease as more of a public health than a clinical medical problem at this time. Thompson, who organized his text predominantly around clinically identifiable diseases, received a particularly scathing critique in the *Journal of the American Medical Association:* "There are so many indications of carelessness in thought and diction that the book falls far short of the front rank" ("Book Notices" 1915). The same journal praised the Kober and Hanson volume, which more evenly balanced clinical and factory inspection perspectives by including sections organized by disease and by industry, for "a commendable tendency to stick closely to known facts" ("Book Notices" 1917). In the *American Journal of Public Health,* Kober and Hanson also received a generally positive assessment (Armstrong 1916). In this era, occupational disease seemed much more amenable to a combination of preventive and curative approaches than to purely clinical treatment.

These textbooks reflected key stylistic features of knowledge about occupational disease in this period. Both texts recognized the separateness of the two major zones for intervention in occupational diseases at the time. Thompson, for instance, gave diseases double descriptions, ones appropriate to both medical and factory inspection perspectives. Following a section on maladies resulting from "impure air," grouped together on the basis of an environmental cause for which he gave little technical or other definition, he included short chapters devoted to poisonings by specific gases, distinguished by their different arrays of clinical symptoms. In both texts, quantitative analyses of factory environments involved only the substances used in manufacturing processes, and ignored the atmospheric concentration that better approximated chronic worker exposure. When the authors did offer quantitative information about atmospheric contents, they, like Graham-Rogers, took the figures simply as evidence for the simple presence of a substance (Kober and Hanson 1916:541). Clinical laboratory results played a minor role at this point in the diagnostic procedures these writers recommended for chemical diseases. The author of Kober and Hanson's lead-poisoning chapter discounted the medical usefulness of "stippling"—or speckling—of red blood cells, which was detectable only with a blood sample and a microscope; it "does not possess the diagnostic value which some attribute to it." He suggested reliance on clinical observations, such as the blue green "lead line" across the gums in identifying lead poisoning (97).

The lack of quantitative information on either the factory environment or the clinical manifestations of disease allowed for only rough correlations between these two types of data, and little consideration of safe concentration levels. Only rarely did these texts closely evaluate estimates of safe atmospheric exposure levels from the German and English literature. In discussing European studies of carbon monoxide, the author of Kober and Hanson's chapter on the subject even expressed skepticism about the validity or merit of such estimates.

> Gruber says that the limit of toxicity is 0.02 per cent. A volume of air containing 0.01 per cent may cause distress, headache, nausea, and other phenomena. Others say that symptoms will not be produced until 0.05 per cent of the gas is present. The point of toxicity will vary in individuals. This has been accurately proven by Haldane in humans and in animals. (45)

Clearly, the safe exposure level did not seem a crucial or a useful figure in these schemes of knowledge about occupational disease.

Whether the target was a public who could press for new laws, the manufacturers themselves, or doctors and public health officials, both texts reflected similar general requirements for knowledge about occupational disease. Valid knowledge of these maladies consisted of "facts" or "data" that met only minimal formal requirements. This information could be unproblematically collected, disseminated, and used, without any necessary special training. Most important, however, knowledge about occupational disease had to be, in Thompson's words, both "effective" and "reliable" (Thompson 1914:xvii). The need for effectiveness meant that this knowledge was not simply what we would call "objective." It had to touch the moral fiber of a reader or listener and compel him or her toward a particular line of action. Essentially, this knowledge had to have ethical implications for its intended audience. Thompson put it this way:

The employer, when presented with such data, may be convinced of the extent and seriousness of the disease hazards as they concern his industry; and if practical and reasonable suggestions for betterment are simultaneously issued, he is almost certain to be convinced, at least, of the economic value of the suggestions, and may put them into effect for greater efficiency if not for humanitarian reasons. (xvii)

Though avowedly scientific, this knowledge had to remain comprehensible to physicians and laypersons alike; it was obliged to stir them not just to greater awareness but to social betterment.

This understanding of scientific knowledge about occupational disease accorded well with contemporary institutions and practices. We have seen how the means for gathering information about job-related illnesses remained closely linked to responsibilities for treatment or regulation. Even those who undertook government studies without any regulatory power often made personal efforts to see that the prescriptions dictated by their facts became translated into actions. Following his study of the phosphorus match industry, Andrews successfully lobbied for legislation placing a prohibitive tax on that industry's product. Hamilton personally presented the results of her studies, along with her recommendations for improvement, to company managers or owners (Sicherman 1984:168). Practically no one in the United States studied the problem of industrial chemical waste without a view toward making immediate changes, either in particular factories or in the behavior of sick or threatened workers themselves.

Some historians have portrayed the Progressive Era as a time of overweening belief in "science," when claims to scientific practice came to dominate the rhetoric of professions like medicine, forestry, and management, and became a familiar cry in the political arena (Haber 1964; Hays 1969; Nash 1973; Montgomery 1979; Vogel and Rosenberg 1979; Warner 1985). Others have remarked on the moral fervor that pervaded the era, from the settlement houses to Theodore Roosevelt's progressive political crusade of 1912 (Mowry 1946:237–283; Blum 1967:149–150; Davis 1967). However incongruous this combination may seem to our modern understanding, it becomes more comprehensible in the light of the contemporary norms for knowledge about occupational disease. This knowledge, accessible to laypersons yet fully scientific in its time, had to serve at once as fact and as prod to the economic or humanitarian aspirations of its audience. For those involved in this era's system for recognizing and combating occupational disease, facts, to make sense, took shape from values. The "is" remained explicitly inseparable from the "ought."

The Growth of a Community of Experts

In the ten years between 1915 and 1925, several new institutions arose for the study and control of work-related disease. World War I stimulated increased federal interest in research into occupational disease, as well as a new organizational structure for government research efforts. Before the war, responsibility for federal research in industrial disease remained split between the Bureau of Labor Statistics and the field studies office within the Public Health Service (PHS). The wartime surge of government interest in this research, partly a response to new American munitions and chemical industries, led to centralization of these efforts within the PHS (Young 1982:68–106). At the Bureau of Mines, investigations of chemical weaponry gave way during the postwar years to research into industrial chemical effects, often in cooperation with the PHS's new Office of Industrial Hygiene and Sanitation.

Another important institutional event occurred in 1918, when Harvard established the nation's first Department of Industrial Hygiene (Curran 1970:156). By the early twenties, the new public health schools and some medical schools had created a niche for laboratory and clinical research into occupational disease within the universities. Harvard, with an entire department devoted to industrial subjects, became the academic center for the new forms of science that developed in the twenties. Other schools sponsored similar but more limited research, often within different departmental divisions. The Johns Hopkins School of Public Health included significant research on industrial disease in its Department of Physiological Hygiene. The medical school at Yale resorted to a similar strategy, though the University of Pennsylvania's School of Hygiene followed the Harvard model more closely (Yale University School of Medicine 1917:41; University of Pennsylvania 1920:10, 18; Fee 1987:124–126, 172–176). In addition, these and other public health and medical schools became centers for formal instruction on industrial health topics (Kober 1921:390–393).

Coupled with the emergence of these new research efforts, new audiences for the research also coalesced. Within the medical profession, physician groups created local forums where the new specialists could present their work. In 1917, the College of Physicians of Philadelphia established its Section on Industrial Medicine and Public Health, which invited experts to give lectures to its members and interested members of the public. The New York State Society of Industrial Medicine, formed in 1921, not only sponsored lectures but in 1923 began its own journal. State and local medical societies welcomed discussions of industrial topics at their general meetings. Texts of many of these lectures found their way into society proceedings or transactions (Zielger 1921; Utley 1922; *Transactions of the College of Physicians of Philadelphia* 1917). On the national level, two new journals also appeared in 1919 devoted partly or solely to industrial topics: *Modern Medicine* (soon to become *The Nation's Health*) and the *Journal of Industrial Hygiene*. The American Medical Association in 1922 added responsibility for industrial medicine to its section devoted to public health.

Public health professionals joined physicians in establishing new outlets for discussions of industrial health issues during this period. The supranational Conference of State and Provincial Health Authorities of North America, a group of public health officials, created its Committee on Industrial Hygiene in 1919. Throughout the twenties and thirties, the new committee promoted activities within state and local health departments on job-related illness. In consultation with the PHS's Office of Industrial Hygiene, it also undertook periodic surveys of state and local activities regarding industrial health.

Changes in the compensation system demanded new attention to occupational disease, both among company physicians and many private practitioners. Harry Mock could report that in 1919 only Massachusetts provided workers' compensation for such diseases, but by 1923, seven other states had passed legislation granting coverage, particularly for work-related chemical disease (Mock 1919a:678; NICB 1923:242). Anthony Bale found that this wave of legislation arose as an attempt to stave off the efforts of the American Association for Labor Legislation and others to enact a general health insurance system for workers (Bale 1986:529–596). In its wake, medical involvement in compensation decisions became more of a necessity. Unlike accidental injuries, whose cause, extent and effects were often obvious, industrial diseases were often more subtle entities, requiring the diagnostic skills of a physician.

Almost all state compensation boards could appoint physicians to carry out official physical exams, and an increasing number of states hired permanent medical directors or advisors (23). Long-term physician appointments helped ensure that claim decisions would reflect constant diagnostic criteria. Yet with the growing numbers of claims, the requirements of the compensation boards for an efficient and consistent appraisal of cases helped convince many that explicit standardized principles of diagnosis were necessary as well for the major industrial chemical diseases (Committee on Medical Questions 1923:38; Hatch 1923; Sayer 1923). The compensation system thus began to exert pressure on the form that medical knowledge should take.

Not until 1919 did the first studies reveal the extent to which companies had begun to hire their own physicians. In a PHS survey of industrial clinics, 118 of the 170 plants questioned paid a physician for services, either part-time or full-time (Selby 1919b:22). The widening coverage of the compensation acts probably led even more companies to hire their own physicians and thereby broadened the audience for new occupational disease research. No reliable comparative figures are available to indicate any trends. In 1927, however, a study of the Philadelphia area by the Philadelphia Health Council and Tuberculosis Committee in cooperation with the Philadelphia Association of Industrial Medicine revealed that of 873 firms employing more than 25 people, 473 reported some form of medical service (*Proceedings* 1927:188). If a 1926 study by the National Industrial Conference Board was representative, then around half of these firms with medical service gave physical examinations to prospective and actual employees (NICB 1926:25).

The growth in the numbers of company physicians and the increasing use of the physical examination met with considerable resistance in some quarters. Angela Nugent Young has written on the controversy over the physical exam during this period (Nugent 1983). Many labor leaders believed the technique to be an invasive and all-too-manipulable evil. When Andrews wrote some twenty labor leaders in 1915 to ask them where they stood on the issue, "without exception a vigorous protest against medical examination came with every reply" (Andrews 1916:825). More than anything, labor worried that management might unjustly exploit the exam to deny jobs to prospective or actual employees. The abolition of physical exams became a major union demand in the labor–management struggles of the late 1910s (Nugent 1983; Brody

1965:101; Sellers 1991). The shadow of this conflict extended into the programmatic statements of company physicians from progressive times onward, and it came to haunt those occupying the new academic posts in industrial hygiene as well (Kerr et al. 1916; Selby 1919a).

New Modes of Research and Self-Justification

During the time that workers battled the exams and that new research positions began to open up while new forums and audiences appeared, industrial hygiene researchers themselves began to revise their strategies for pursuing knowledge about industrial chemical disease. New textbooks began to appear in the mid twenties that propounded a reappraisal of the kind of knowledge considered scientific as well as the social role of that knowledge. No textbook more fully embodied the changes than Hamilton's first book, *Industrial Poisons in the United States,* published in 1925 (Hamilton 1925).

Hamilton's role as advocate of the new approach might at first seem surprising. After all, she had been one of the major architects of the earlier form of knowledge. Yet the trajectory of her career symbolized as well as anything else the institutional changes that made a new kind of science possible. In 1919, she received an appointment as the nation's first professor of industrial medicine at Harvard, and thenceforth she left her field studies almost entirely behind. Within her new academic abode, she joined with Cecil and Philip Drinker, David Edsal, and other Harvard colleagues in their attempts to convert industrial hygiene into a more coherent and prestigious scientific pursuit. Her 1925 book was the first book-length scientific compendium to emerge from the nation's only academic department devoted strictly to research and teaching in occupational health.

In a striking departure from the pre-1920 textbooks, Hamilton included no direct mention of the audience to whom she addressed her writing, in the preface or elsewhere. With the arrival of organized forums and recipients for knowledge about chemical disease within medicine and public health, she could now assume who her readers would be. She only alluded to the new situation in a detached manner, when she noted an "enormous increase in the interest of the medical world in industrial toxicology of late years" (Hamilton 1925:vii). She now wrote scientific texts almost exclusively for physicians and other technically trained professionals. Hamilton would continue to compose articles on her work for popular magazines throughout her long career, but these would have a different character. In 1925, her textbook gave clear witness that the science of industrial disease native to the Progressive Era, with its potential audience of both laypersons and physicians, had now quietly met its demise.

The topography she offered for her subject matter bore only modest resemblance to that of the earlier texts. Rather than attempting to encompass all diseases thought to have some causal relation to particular occupations, she restricted herself to "industrial poisons"— the chemical diseases. Her maneuver reflected a growing sensitivity toward disciplinary boundaries in her field. As the public health schools like Harvard had begun to undertake research and teaching on industrial health, they partitioned the subject into tentative specialty areas whose full content they left to the discretion of the new faculty. At Harvard, Hamilton called her particular pursuit "industrial toxicology." She handed over the dust diseases to Philip Drinker, with his interest in "ventilation and illumination," while Cecil Drinker and others in "applied physiology" took responsibility for investigating fatigue and other nonchemical industrial complaints (Curran 1970:159). Hamilton hoped by her textbook to definitively establish the boundaries of her specialty and to further consolidate it as a discipline. Not only did she confine herself to chemical health effects, she also asserted from the beginning that she would stress "chronic, not acute" forms of poisoning (Hamilton 1925:1). This last objective did not result in much practical difference between the pre-1920 texts and her own, but it did mark a programmatic shift.

Hamilton's attempt to carve out a coherent area of specialty accompanied a new self-consciousness about the proper form of scientific investigation of industrial chemical disease. "There are already some studies of poisonous trades in the United States which for thoroughness leave nothing to be desired," she could now write (Hamilton 1925:vii). She had in mind a particular study of manganese poisoning conducted by Edsal and Drinker in 1919 (Edsal et al. 1919–20). The "thoroughness" of their work, investigating mysterious ailments at a New Jersey factory, inhered mainly in the several types of information they were able to collect and assemble into a single integrated understanding of industrial manganese poisoning. They brought together data on "the incidence in a large group of workmen, the conditions under which poisoning occurred, the mode of entrance, and the clinical manifestations, of early stages of poisoning as well as of later stages" (Hamilton 1925:vii).

Hamilton used her praise of "thoroughness" to designate a new exemplar for research in occupational disease. To meet its standards, investigators would have to design studies incorporating techniques that for the most part had remained in separate realms before the war. Quantitative studies of working environments would have to be combined with clinical laboratory data to study how a chemical entered the body, and this information would have to be synthesized with results of physical exams. Preferably, large numbers of subjects and both short and extended terms of exposure would be involved. Obviously, all investigations did not have to meet these standards. Yet their very presence relegated those that did not to a place of lesser importance and even lesser epistemological status. The new scientific exemplar, with its more extensive correlations of data from the clinic and factory environment and its more comprehensive and interventionist scrutiny of the relation between exposure and poisoning, promised greater certainty in scientific judgments about the chemical causes of disease (Sellers 1991).

In concert with her promotion of new scientific practices, two scientific concepts gained more prominence in Hamilton's text than they had in the earlier ones. One related directly to the increasing dependence on clinical laboratory data as a necessary link between information on atmospheric concentrations and complexes of signs and symptoms. The notion of "chemical absorption" began to receive greater attention, as researchers began to notice that many workers could tolerate high levels of poisonous chemicals in their bodies without showing clinical signs of poison. The writer on the diagnosis of lead poisoning in Kober and Hanson's text could assert that the classic lead line "is in itself of no greater weight in the diagnosis of lead poisoning than is the fact that the patient's history shows that he is working in a lead process" (Kober and Hanson 1916:98). For Hamilton, this condition had become a matter of greater concern: "It is evident that if the line be present the worker is absorbing lead, although for the moment perhaps not beyond his capacity to excrete it, but it is impossible to say when he may pass beyond the limits of his tolerance" (Hamilton 1925:95). As medical scrutiny and concern shifted toward chemical absorption, this concept began to evolve into a separate clinical category, an intermediate stage between health and disease.

For Hamilton in 1925, the maximum safe concentration level also occupied a more central place in the available knowledge about chemical disease than it had for pre-1920 writers. The new methodological standard duplicated the combinations of knowledge by which European authors had derived the earliest such figures. Not only did American researchers now undertake similar calculations, but an independent estimate of the safety limit became an obligatory task for Hamilton as textbook author, when the appropriate data on a chemical was available. She offered figures for lead, mercury, ammonia, carbon monoxide, and benzene, among others (Hamilton 1925:55–57, 234, 319, 381–380, 480–481).

Alongside the new notions about the best scientific methods for studying chemical disease, Hamilton expressed a new self-consciousness about her own role as a scientist in the field. She elaborated this role as a critical stance toward the evidence offered by industrial physicians.

> Mental reservations may have to be made. One must always remember in a study of this kind the existence of a prejudice which may cloud the mentality of some first-class men. Apparently it is impossible for some physicians to treat industrial diseases with the detachment and impartiality with which they approach those diseases which are not confined to the working classes. For a striking example of this the reader is referred to a bulletin issued by the Bureau of Labor Statistics. . . . Not only is there the widest divergence of views presented, but the physician who was retained by the men shows so strong a sympathy for them as to quite dull his critical sense, and the physicians for the companies accept evidence which is on the face of it one-sided, and then indulge in moral observations on the character of workingmen and the evils of trades-unionism. (Hamilton 1925:vi)

For the first time in an American textbook about occupational disease, we see a plea for the necessity of an objective attitude toward the study of workers' health. Hamilton's appeal to impartiality

only became possible with the emergence of more elaborate methodological standards for research, ones that could more effectively
guarantee constant results under any social circumstance. Still, as
Hamilton's own example suggests, the need for the new standards
and the kind of objectivity they could make possible originated at
least partly in social crisis. Only after interventions within the system for controlling industrial disease had become controversial, in
the context of a struggle between labor and management did those
responsible for producing knowledge about the subject attempt to
construct a self-consciously objective science. Here, objectivity had
a specific meaning: the evaluation of evidence only on the basis of
agreed-upon scientific standards, without regard for the economic
ideology of the particular physician who reported it or the social or
economic position of his or her patients.

Hamilton's new expression of an objective ideal applied not only
to her own role as researcher but, in a modified fashion, to the
physician who treated patients in the factory: "Let him be careful
never to sacrifice his own intellectual integrity nor adopt the standards of the non-medical man to whom the proper working of the
plant is of first importance. His task is to safeguard the health of
the patients who are entrusted to him" (Hamilton 1925:541–542).
The physician's "intellectual integrity" had little to do with a sympa-
thy for the working class, even though, apparently on the workers'
behalf, it might lead him into conflict with the plant managers.
Rather, Hamilton referred to the physician's steadfastness to the
standards of diagnosis, judgment, and treatment that he or she
had acquired through professional training. Presumably, researchers such as Hamilton were responsible for these standards. In con-
ceiving of the pursuit of worker health as an objective undertaking,
Hamilton also asserted a pivotal role for her own kind in developing the standards upon which the research community could
agree. She further assumed that the main responsibility for intervening on behalf of worker health should rest with those who
followed these standards, assuring the disinterestedness of their
actions—namely, properly trained physicians. Her plea for an objective approach toward industrial health thus constituted an argument for the centrality of expertise in the study, prevention, and
treatment of occupational disease. She thereby affirmed the new
system of knowledge and regulation that was emerging within the
interstices of the older one.

The Widening New System
and Its Consequences

Reviews of Hamilton's book suggested that she and her Harvard colleagues were creating a science of occupational disease much more acceptable to the medical community than Thompson's version was, but at the expense of the public health movement's support. Both the *Journal of the American Medical Association* and the *American Journal of Medical Sciences* had glowing words for the new textbook ("Book Notices" 1925; P. 1925). In the *American Journal of Public Health*, however, Emery Hayhurst decried the narrowness of Hamilton's focus on pathology, symptoms, and case reports, and her neglect of "trade processes, chemical, laboratory, clinical, social, actuarial, and economic aspects." The balance of his criticism seemed weighted against the author's partial abandonment of the factory inspector perspective and her turn toward a form of knowledge "of more use to the student perhaps than to the busy practitioner" (Hayhurst 1925:907–908).

Hamilton's textbook captured many of the newer currents in the contemporary system of knowledge about industrial chemical disease, which were to become even more pronounced as the twenties progressed. In 1926, shortly after her work appeared, the PHS's Office of Industrial Hygiene established an even more elaborate and synthetic exemplar for research with its tetraethyl lead study (Leake et al. 1926). The office included significantly more workers in its investigation than were involved in the manganese study. By including physical scientists on its research team, the office also became able to undertake more extensive quantitative studies of the working environment. In subsequent field studies, office researchers continued to follow the methods they had established in the tetraethyl lead study, and they began to calculate safe concentration levels as well (Greenberg 1926; Bloomfield and Blum 1928; Neal et al. 1937). They soon extended the same research practices into the area of dust diseases (Sayers et al. 1935).

Compensation law may well have had an impact on the move to more standardized scientific practices, but the precise form these standards took most likely had some influence on legal thinking as well. When workers in New Jersey filed a total of 110 different claims for compensation for benzene poisoning in 1927 and 1928, the state compensation commission used a set of three "postulates" as a "standard and guide" for decision making on claims:

1. The claimant must demonstrate an exposure to benzol poisoning. 2. The claimant must present symptoms of benzol poisoning. 3. The claimant must demonstrate a change in his blood picture. (Kessler 1929)

These three kinds of information, all of which were necessary for a "positive diagnosis" and full compensation under the law, paralleled the array of knowledge in the manganese study. Law followed science in asserting the need to know about chemical exposure and absorption as well as clinical disease. The compensation system thus evolved its own hybrid system of medicolegal logic.

Finally, the new scientific standards of both method and attitude accompanied the emergence of new forms of government intervention in the workplace. New or expanded divisions and bureaus of industrial hygiene emerged within state departments of labor and health. New York increased the personnel with scientific training in its Division of Industrial Hygiene from one doctor in 1922 to four doctors and two engineers in 1924 (New York. Industrial Commissioner 1923:40, 1925:110). Connecticut began its Division of Occupational Diseases in 1928, which included both a physician and an "industrial hygienist" on its staff by 1930 (Connecticut State Department of Health 1929:207, 1931:241). In that year, a survey by the Conference of State and Provincial Health Authorities of North America revealed that these two states conducted the most extensive industrial hygiene activities in the country, but twelve other states reported special groups devoted to industrial hygiene work, evenly distributed between departments of health and labor (Proceedings 1930:106). A clear division of responsibilities arose between researchers in the public health schools and federal agencies, and these new state officials in the field of industrial hygiene.

The state industrial hygienists investigated problems of occupational disease in specific factories, usually at the request of employers but also at the invitation of the regular factory inspectors (McBurney 1927; Connecticut State Department of Health 1929:207; Flexner 1939:9–10, 19–22). The industrial hygiene organizations in both Connecticut and New York preferred to offer recommendations to factory owners or managers, though they could legally order preventive measures in collaboration with their respective inspection bureaus. With engineers as well as doctors on their staffs, they could carry out physical examinations, atmospheric chemical analyses, and clinical laboratory work. Though their capabilities reproduced the array of knowledge in the investigational exemplars of the time, state industrial hygienists became increasingly reliant upon the conclusions of the researchers about maximum safe atmospheric concentrations and the proper diagnostic use of laboratory tests or X-rays. More and more, they could thereby turn away from visual observation and physical examinations toward environmental and clinical laboratory tests to arbitrate the safety of working environments. While the New York Division performed 1,512 examinations in 1921, it conducted only 70 in 1931, many of which were for the Compensation Bureau rather than for inspection purposes (New York. Industrial Commissioner 1922:110, 1932:123). Connecticut's Bureau of Preventable Diseases performed some physical examinations in the mid twenties to follow up official reports of occupational disease (Connecticut State Department of Health 1925:93). After 1928, however, the reports of the new Division of Occupational Diseases rarely mentioned physical examinations, though they included extensive quantitative environmental analyses (Connecticut State Department of Health 1931:427–433).

To understand how this new complex of experts, knowledge, and rhetorical defenses operated, let us dwell for a moment on the role of safe concentration estimates within it. These estimates preserved the combination of fact with imperative in the knowledge of Thompson but now in a technical form suitable to a professional audience of state and company industrial hygienists and physicians. For their expert audience they addressed an unsentimental professional obligation to promote safety, and for much of this audience and the public they seemed to belong to the realm of objective science. The standardized methods that some researchers such as those at the PHS developed to calculate these estimates reinforced such perceptions, along with the political and cultural authority of the new research community. PHS investigators regularly set their estimates at the highest atmospheric concentrations associated with no clear cases of poisoning (Russell et al. 1933:32, 55; (Dreessen et al. 1938:89, 91, 1941:58–59).) This method itself, however, contained numerous decisions that today seem more appropriate for policy makers: PHS's safe concentration levels did not include a safety margin and ignored cases of chemical absorption. Despite its pretenses otherwise, the researchers' science/policy distinction actually served to disguise and protect their policy prescriptions.

The state Industrial Hygiene Division became the final leg in the circuit of specialized study and intervention that constituted a new system of knowledge about industrial disease. By 1940, thirty-one states sponsored industrial hygiene work, according to the Conference of State and Provincial Health Authorities of North America (*Proceedings* 1940:86). By this time, as well, the ACGIH had crystallized from a seminar for industry hygienists as well as state and local public health officials sponsored by the PHS's Division of Industrial Hygiene. It had begun work on establishing the first set of what were to become the threshold limit values—essentially safe concentration levels on which the ACGIH's Threshold Committee could reach agreement. Not only did the ACGIH make use of Hamiltonian appeals to objectivity, its estimates largely duplicated those of Hamilton and her colleagues. In twenty-eight of thirty-eight cases, the organization's 1946 listing of threshold limits followed the 1940 recommendations of a group of mostly Harvard and Yale academics, including Hamilton. Six ACGIH estimates were lower and only four were higher (Bowditch et al. 1940; Subcommittee on Threshold Limits 1946). The consensual and numerically precise appearance of the TLVs reinforced their proponents' claims to objectivity and expertise, on which the prescriptive power of the estimates now almost entirely depended. These efforts brought the system of knowledge that emerged in the twenties to full fruition. The same patterns of investigations, attitudes, and practices dominated the field of industrial health for another quarter of a century.

Conclusion

Sheila Jasanoff has written about how both sides in modern controversies over occupational risks usually attempt to draw boundaries between the parts of their arguments that are science and those that are policy, and thus subject to interest-group pressures (Jasanoff 1987). This strategy, which is not just a rhetorical ploy but a gesture closely tied to one's professional identity, had its origins in the sweeping changes of the twenties. It began with the birth of a new system for producing and using knowledge in the field of occupational disease. As research institutions grew separate from regulatory ones, and as groups of trained experts emerged within the regulatory agencies, a new type of knowledge and a new stance toward knowledge evolved, in close relation. As objectivity came to seem opposed to the "cloud" of economic interest, researchers began to invoke "science" in a different and more characteristically modern way.

For the progressives, the science of occupational disease had been a democratic knowledge, which would rally public support and the commitment of factory owners to improve the factory environment. From the twenties onward, claims to science served increasingly as defenses of expertise by bolstering arguments for closing particular decisions and rationales to lay scrutiny and debate. The new system did better assure the reliability of what was known about occupational diseases, and chemical diseases in particular. The more elaborate standards for knowledge may thus have better guaranteed that the prescriptions of its bearers would be heeded. On the other hand, the new requirements also ensured that this knowledge would remain accessible to a limited audience only. Except for occasional flurries of unavoidable public attention, such as that surrounding the silicosis deaths at Gauley Bridge, West Virginia, knowledge about industrial diseases remained largely sealed within the same community of experts until the challenges of the sixties (Cherniak 1986; Rosner and Markowitz 1991).

Today, the basic scientific methods, disciplinary boundaries, and institutions from the twenties remain in place, despite our greater scientific sophistication. Appeals to a more scientific or objective knowledge still form a cornerstone of debate on occupational and environmental health issues, as well. Barry Castleman and Grace Ziem, for instance, can argue effectively that present TLVs are not objective, since interested corporations had undue influence on the decisions about them (Castleman and Ziem 1988). At the same time, the conventional notion of scientific objectivity has become problematic, subject to assault from such diverse corners of our culture as the sociology of science and feminism. Some recent writers have carried these criticisms into the health arena, through attacks on the kinds of intellectual and institutional partitions that arose in the twenties in the field of industrial chemical disease. Sylvia Tesh, after analyzing the attempts of scientists to assess the toxicity of Agent Orange, concludes that Hamiltonian objectivity about such socially embedded issues is impossible: "Science, because it does not exist without scientists, necessarily requires value-filled human decisions at every step" (Tesh 1988:5).

To meet such a critique, researchers and physicians in the field of occupational disease need to fundamentally revise their intraprofessional conception of their role. A new form of self-justification must avoid Hamilton's belief that scientific standards will somehow be capable of completely suppressing pressures and influences from conflicts external to the expert community. At the same time, this self-understanding must grant the standards more objectifying power than do many recent science critics, who portray scientific judgments as mere transparent reflections of external conflict. Somehow, scientists and physicians in this field need to develop a way of explicitly acknowledging how even their scientific judgments are influenced at once by the standards of the research community and by economic and other social interests. Of course, such an acknowledgment may threaten their credibility among parts of the public and the scientific world where simpler notions about objectivity still hold sway. Still, this more realistic understanding will not only counter many of their critics, it may even aid these professionals toward a surer pursuit of their given tasks.

Recognizing the social and political roots of Hamiltonian objectivity can help us orient ourselves toward this pathway of ideological revision. In a field so potentially contestable as that of occupational disease, it is not surprising that a particularly insistent rhetoric about scientific impartiality emerged. Yet the immediate relevance of this knowledge to many workplace controversies makes a more balanced appraisal of its status and role all the more necessary, for industrial health professionals as well as labor and management. Though the full shape and practical implications of the revision remain unclear, we must hope that it proceeds apace.

Acknowledgments

The author wishes to thank William Cronon, Frederick Holmes, Steve Sturdy, Nancy Tomes, John Warner, and the editors of this volume for providing comments and suggestions on earlier drafts of this chapter.

References

Alewitz, S. 1986. *Ezra Mundy Hunt: A Life in Public Health.* Trenton: New Jersey Historical Commission, Department of State.

258 C. C. SELLERS

Andrews, J. 1910. "Phosphorus Poisoning in the Match Industry in the United States." *Bulletin of the Bureau of Labor* 86:31–146.
———. 1911. "Scientfic Standards in Labor Legislation." *American Labor Legislation Review* 1:123–134.
———. 1916. "Physical Examination of Employees." *American Journal of Public Health* 6:825–29.
Armstrong, D. B. 1916. Book Review. *American Journal of Public Health* 6:1122.
Ashford, N. 1976. *Crisis in the Workplace: Occupational Disease and Injury.* Cambridge, Mass.: MIT Press.
Bale, A. 1986. "Compensation Crisis: The Value and Meaning of Work-Related Injuries and Illnesses in the United States, 1842–1932." Ph.D. diss., Brandeis University.
Bloomfield, J. J., and Blum, W. 1928. "Health Hazards of Chromium Painting." *Public Health Reports* 43:2330–2347.
Blum, J. M. 1967. *The Republican Roosevelt.* Cambridge, Mass.: Harvard University Press.
"Book Notices." 1915. *Journal of the American Medical Association* 64:362.
———. 1917. "Book Notices." *Journal of the American Medical Association* 68:570.
———. 1925. "Book Notices." *Journal of the American Medical Association* 85:540.
Bowditch, M.; Drinker, C. K.; Drinker, P.; Haggard, H. H.; and Hamilton, A. 1940. "Code for Safe Concentrations of Certain Toxic Substances Used in Industry." *Journal of Industrial Hygiene* 22:251.
Brody, D. 1965. *Labor in Crisis: The Steel Strike of 1919.* Philadelphia: Lippincott.
Castleman, B., and Ziem, G. 1988. "Corporate Influence on Threshold Limit Values." *American Journal of Industrial Medicine* 13:531–559.
Cherniak, M. 1986. *The Hawk's Nest Incident: America's Worst Industrial Disaster.* New Haven, Conn., and London: Yale University Press.
Clark, S. A., and Wyatt, E. 1910–11. "Women Laundry Workers in New York." *McClure's Magazine* 36:401–414.
Committee on Occupational Hygiene. 1914. "Occupational Hygiene." *American Labor Legislation Review* 6, no. 4:528.
Committee on Medical Questions. 1923. "Committee on Medical Questions." *New York State Journal of Medicine* 23:35–41.
Connecticut. State Department of Health. 1925. *Annual Report, 1925.* Hartford.
———. 1929. *Annual Report, 1928.* Hartford.
———. 1930. *Annual Report, 1930.* Hartford.
———. 1931. *Annual Report, 1931.* Hartford.
———. "Controversy Obscures Facts in Compensation Decisions." 1922. *Nation's Health* 4:25.
Curran, J. A. 1970. *Founders of the Harvard School of Public Health, with Biographical Notes, 1909–1946.* New York: Josiah Macy, Jr., Foundation.
Davis, A. 1967. *Spearheads for Reform: The Social Settlements and the Progressive Movement, 1890–1914.* New York: Oxford University Press.

Derickson, A. 1988. *Worker's Health, Worker's Democracy: The Western Miners' Struggle, 1891–1925.* Ithaca, N.Y., and London: Cornell University Press.

Dreessen, W.; Dallavalle, J.; Edwards, T.; Miller, J.; and Sayers, R. 1938. "A Study of Asbestosis in the Asbestos Textile Industry." *Public Health Bulletin,* no. 241.

Dreessen, W.; Edwards, T.; Reinhart, W.; Page, R.; Webster, S.; Armstrong, D.; and Sayers, R. 1941. "The Control of the Lead Hazard in the Storage Battery Industry." *Public Health Bulletin,* no. 262.

Edsal, D. 1909. "Some of the Relations of Occupations to Medicine." *Journal of the American Medical Association* 53:1873–1881.

Edsal, D.; Wilbur, F. P.; and Drinker, C. 1919–20. "The Occurrence, Cause, and Prevention of Chronic Manganese Poisoning." *Journal of Industrial Hygiene* 1:183–194.

Fee, E. 1987. *Disease and Discovery: A History of the Johns Hopkins School of Hygiene and Public Health.* Baltimore and London: Johns Hopkins University Press.

Flexner, J. 1939. "The Work of an Industrial Hygiene Division in a State Department of Labor." *U.S. Department of Labor Bulletin,* no. 31.

Galishoff, S. 1975. *Safeguarding the Public Health: Newark, 1895–1918.* Westport, Conn., and London: Greenwood Press.

"Garment Workers' Union Tackling Tuberculosis." 1913. *Survey* 31:313.

Gompers, S. 1914. Remarks. *Transactions of the Tenth Annual Meeting of the National Association for the Study and Prevention of Tuberculosis: Washington, D.C. May 7–8,* 54–58.

Greenburg, L. 1926. "Benzol Poisoning as an Industrial Hazard." *Public Health Reports* 41:1516–1535.

Haber, S. 1964. *Efficiency and Uplift: Scientific Management in the Progressive Era, 1890–1920.* Chicago: University of Chicago Press.

Hamilton, A. 1912. "Lead Poisoning in Potteries, Tile Works, and Porcelain Enameled Sanitary Ware Factories." *Bulletin of the U.S. Bureau of Labor,* no. 104.

———. 1913. "Hygiene of the Painters' Trade." *Bulletin of the U.S. Brueau of Labor Statistics,* no. 120.

———. 1914. "Lead Poisoning in the Manufacture of Storage Batteries." *Bulletin of the U.S. Bureau of Labor Statistics,* no. 165.

———. 1925. *Industrial Poisons in the United States.* New York: Macmillan.

———. [1943] 1985. *Exploring the Dangerous Trades: The Autobiography of Alice Hamilton, M.D.* Reprint. Boston: Northeastern University Press.

Hatch, I. W. 1923. "Industrial Medicine in Its Relation to Workmen's Compensation." *Industrial Doctor* 1:209.

Hayhurst, E. 1925. "Industrial Poisons in the United States." *American Journal of Public Health* 15:907–908.

Hays, S. 1969. *Conservation and the Gospel of Efficiency: The Progressive Conservation Movement, 1890–1920.* New York: Atheneum.

Hazlett, T. L. and Hummel, W. 1957. *Industrial Medicine in Western Pennsylvania: 1850–1950.* Pittsburgh: University of Pittsburgh Press.

Ireland, G. H. 1886. "Preventable Causes of Disease and Death in American Manufactories and Workshops, and the Best Means and Appliances

260 C. C. SELLERS

for Preventing and Avoiding Them." In *Public Health: The Lomb Prize Essays of the American Public Health Association, Washington, D.C., 1885,* 139–153. Concord, N.H.: Republican Press Association.

Jasanoff, S. 1987. "Contested Boundaries in Policy-Relevant Science." *Social Studies of Science* 17:195–230.

Kerr, J. W.; McCurdy, S.; and Geier, O. 1916. "The Scope of Industrial Hygiene." *Journal of the American Medical Association* 77:1821–1822.

Kessler, H. 1929. "Some Medicolegal Aspects of Occupational Disease." *Archives of Internal Medicine* 43:874–877.

Kober, G. 1921. "History of Industrial Hygiene and Its Effect on Public Health." In *A Half Century of Public Health,* ed. M. Ravenel, 361–411. New York: American Public Health Association.

Kober, G., and Hanson, W., eds. 1916. *Diseases of Occupational and Vocational Hygiene.* Philadelphia: Blakiston's.

Leake, J.; Kolb, L.; Schwartz, L.; Lake, G.; Armstrong, C.; Harrison, W.; Mitchell, C.; Clark, W.; Elvove, E.; Remsburg, C.; Kinyoun, C.; Bloomfield, J.; Hall, W.; and Simkins, N. 1926. "The Use of Tetraethyl Lead Gasoline in Its Relation to Public Health." *Public Health Bulletin,* no. 163.

Legge, T., and Goadby, K. 1912. *Lead Poisoning and Lead Absorption.* London: Edward Arnold.

Lehmann, K. B. 1886. "Experimentelle Studien über den Einfluss technisch und hygienisch wichtiger Gase und Dämpfe auf den Organismus (Theil I und II: Ammoniak und Salzsaurgas)." *Archiv für Hygiene* 5:1–126.

Maclean, A. M. 1908–9. "Life in the Pennsylvania Coal Fields with Particular Reference to Women." *American Journal of Sociology* 14:329–351.

MacNutt, J. S. 1915. *A Manual for Health Officers.* New York: Wiley.

McBurney, R. 1927. "Industrial Hygiene Practice: Typical Case Illustrating Aid Rendered to Manufacturers." *Industrial Hygiene Bulletin* 3:41–44.

McCready, B. [1837] 1972. *On the Influence of Trades, Professions and Occupations in the United States, in the Production of Disease.* Reprint. New York: Arno Press and New York Times.

McFarlane, A. E. 1911. "Fire and the Skyscraper: The Problem of Protecting the Workers in New York's Tower Factories." *McClure's Magazine* 37:467–482.

Mock, H. 1919a. *Industrial Medicine and Surgery.* Philadelphia and London: Saunders.

———. 1919b. "Industrial Medicine and Surgery: A Resume of Its Development and Scope." *Journal of Industrial Hygiene* 1:1–7.

Montgomery, D. 1979. *Workers' Control in America: Studies in the History of Work, Technology, and Labor Struggles.* New York: Cambridge University Press.

Mowry, G. 1946. *Theodore Roosevelt and the Progressive Movement.* Madison: University of Wisconsin Press.

Nash, R. 1973. *Wilderness and the American Mind.* New Haven, Conn.: Yale University Press.

National Industrial Conference Board. 1917. *Workmen's Compensation Acts in the United States: The Legal Phase.* Boston: National Industrial Conference Board.

———. 1923. *Workmen's Compensation Acts in the United States: The Medical Aspect.* New York: National Industrial Conference Board.

———. 1926. *Medical Care of Industrial Workers.* New York: National Industrial Conference Board.

Neal, P.; Jones, R.; Bloomfield, J.; Dallavalle, J.; Edwards, T. 1937. "A Study of Chronic Mercurialism in the Hatters' Fur-Cutting Industry." *Public Health Bulletin,* no. 234.

New York. Bureau of Factory Inspection. 1913a. "Bureau of Factory Inspection." In *Annual Reports of Department Bureaus for the Twelve Months Ended September 30, 1911.* Albany, N.Y.: State Department of Labor.

New York. Bureau of Factory Inspection. 1913b. "General Report of Bureau of Factory Inspection." In *Annual Reports of the Commissioner of Labor for the Twelve Months Ended September 30, 1912.* Albany, N.Y.: State Department of Labor.

New York. Industrial Commissioner. 1922. *Annual Report for the Twelve Months Ended June 30, 1921: New York State Department of Labor.* Albany, N.Y.: State Department of Labor.

———. 1923. *Annual Report for the Twelve Months Ended June 30, 1922: New York State Department of Labor.* Albany, N.Y.: J. B. Lyon.

———. 1925. *Annual Report for the Twelve Months Ended June 30, 1924: New York State Department of Labor.* Albany, N.Y.: J. B. Lyon.

———. 1932. *Annual Report for the Twelve Months Ended December 31, 1931: New York State Department of Labor.* Albany, N.Y.: J. B. Lyon.

Nugent, A. 1983. "Fit for Work: The Introduction of Physical Examination in Industry." *Bulletin of the History of Medicine* 57:578–595.

Osler, W., and McCrae, T. 1915. *The Principles and Practice of Medicine.* New York and London: Appleton.

P. 1925. Review of *Industrial Poisons in the United States* by Alice Hamilton. *American Journal of Medical Sciences,* n.s., 170:595–596.

Palmer, W. B. 1911. "Women and Child Workers in Cotton Mills." *Publications of the American Statistical Association* 12:588–617.

Paull, J. M. 1984. "The Origin and Basis of Threshold Limit Values." *American Journal of Industrial Medicine* 5:227–238.

Price, G. 1915. "Medical Supervision in Dangerous Trades." *Journal of Sociologic Medicine* 16, no. 3: 96.

———. 1919. "Factory Inspection and Factory Inspectors." *Journal of Industrial Hygiene* 1:165–176.

Proceedings of the Conference of State and Provincial Health Authorities of North America, Washington, D.C., May 14, 16. 1927. Washington, D.C.

Proceedings of the Conference of State and Provincial Health Authorities of North America, Washington, D.C., June 18, 19, 20. 1930. Washington, D.C.

Proceedings· of the Conference of State and Provincial Health Authorities of North America, Washington, D.C., May 8, 10, 11. 1940. Washington, D.C.

"Protection for Compressed Air Workers." 1914. *American Labor Legislation Review* 6, no. 4:549.

Rohe, G. H. 1885. "The Hygiene of Occupations." *Public Health Papers and Reports, American Public Health Association* 10:165–173.

Rosen, G. 1958. *A History of Public Health.* New York: MD Publications.

————. 1988. "Urbanization, Occupation and Disease in the United States, 1870–1920: The Case of New York City." *Journal of the History of Medicine and Allied Sciences* 4:391–425.

Rosner, D., and Markowitz, G. 1985. "The Early Movement for Occupational Safety and Health, 1900–1917." In *Sickness and Health in America: Readings in the History of Medicine and Public Health*, ed. J. W. Leavitt and R. Numbers, 507–524. Madison: University of Wisconsin Press.

Rosner, D., and Markowitz, G. 1991. *Deadly Dust: Silicosis and the Politics of Occupational Disease in Twentieth-Century America*. Princeton, N.J.: Princeton University Press.

Russell, A.; Jones, R.; Bloomfield, J.; Britten, R.; and Thompson, L. 1933. "Lead Poisoning in a Storage Battery Plant." *Public Health Bulletin*, no. 205.

Sachs, T. 1914. "The Campaign in Chicago for Medical Examinations of Employees." *Transactions of the Tenth Annual Meeting of the National Association for the Study and Prevention of Tuberculosis: Washington, DC, May 7–8*, 35–38.

Salter, L. 1988. *Mandated Science: Science and Scientists in the Making of Standards*. Dordrecht, Holland: Kluwer Academic Publishers.

Sanville, F. L. 1910. "A Woman in the Pennsylvania Silk-mills." *Harper's Monthly Magazine* 120:615–662.

Sayer, H. 1923. "Report of the Committee on Medical Questions." *Industrial Doctor* 1:13.

Sayers, R.; Bloomfield, J.; Dallavalle, J.; Jones, R.; Dreessen, W.; Brundage, D.; Britten, R.; Miller, J.; and Goldman, F. 1935. "Anthraco-Silicosis Among Hard Coal Miners." *Public Health Bulletin*, no. 221.

Selby, C. D. 1919a. "Modern Industrial Medicine." *Modern Medicine* 1, no. 1:35.

————. 1919b. "Studies of the Medical and Surgical Care of Industrial Workers." *Public Health Bulletin*, no. 9.

Selleck, H., and Whittaker, A. 1962. *Occupational Health in America*. Detroit, Mich.: Wayne State University.

Sellers, C. 1991. "The Public Health Service's Office of Industrial Hygiene and the Transformation of Industrial Medicine." *Bulletin of the History of Medicine* 65:42–73.

Sicherman, B. 1984. *Alice Hamilton: A Life in Letters*. Cambridge, Mass., and London: Harvard University Press.

"Standards for Workmen's Compensation Laws." 1914. *American Labor Legislation Review* 6:585.

Subcommittee on Threshold Limits. 1946. In *Proceedings of the Eighth Annual Meeting of the American Conference of Governmental Industrial Hygienists: April 7–13, Chicago*, 54–55. Washington, D.C.

Teleky, L. 1948. *History of Factory and Mine Hygiene*. New York: Columbia University Press.

Tesh, S. 1988. *Hidden Arguments: Political Ideology and Disease Prevention Policy*. New Brunswick, N.J., and London: Rutgers University Press.

Thompson, W. G. 1914. *The Occupational Diseases: Their Causation, Symptoms, Treatment and Prevention*. New York: Appleton.

Toyama, T. 1985. "Permissible and Control Limits at Places of Work in Japan." *American Journal of Industrial Medicine* 8:87–89.

Transactions of the College of Physicians of Philadelphia after 1917 esp. 1917 (vol. 39), 1920 (vol. 42), and 1923 (vol. 45).

University of Pennsylvania. 1920. *University of Pennsylvania Bulletin, School of Public Hygiene: Announcement for 1920–21.*

Utley, F. B. 1922. "Anthrax." *Pennsylvania Medical Journal* 25:831.

Vigliani, E., et al. 1977. *Methods Used in Western European Countries for Establishing Maximum Permissible Levels of Harmful Agents in the Working Environment.* Milan: Fondazione Carlo Erba.

Vogel, M., and Rosenberg, C., eds. 1979. *The Therapeutic Revolution: Essays in the Social History of Medicine.* Philadelphia: University of Pennsylvania Press.

Warner, J. H. 1985. "Science in Medicine." In *Historical Writing on American Science: Perspectives and Prospects,* ed. S. G. Kohlstedt and M. Rossiter, 37–58. Baltimore and London: Johns Hopkins University Press.

Yale University School of Medicine. 1917. *Bulletin of Yale University School of Medicine, 1917–18.*

Young, A. N. 1982. "Interpreting the Dangerous Trades: Workers' Health in America and the Career of Alice Hamilton, 1910–35." Ph.D. diss., Brown University.

Zielger, L. 1921. "The Peril of Wood Alcohol and the Remedy." *Pennsylvania Medical Journal* 25:177–181.

• Afterword •

History, Occupational Health and Medical Education

FRANCIS P. CHINARD, M.D.

Notwithstanding the notorious rigors of a medical education, occupational hazards appear to be among the most difficult lessons for physicians to learn. The medical specialty devoted to primary care and diagnosis, internal medicine, has remained implacably indifferent to both occupational medicine and environmental health for most of this century. Francis P. Chinard, M.D., research professor of medicine at the University of Medicine and Dentistry of New Jersey, New Jersey Medical School; and first chairman of the school's Department of Medicine, offers insights into the implications of occupational and environmental medicine for medical education and for the role of the physician in our society. Steeped in medical history and its critical role in medical education, Dr. Chinard's vision is for a future in which physicians learn from the past as well as from tomorrow's molecular biology, in which social responsibility is an integral component of professional advancement. This vision is unusual but by no means unique in American medicine. While examining the case studies of industrial pollution in New Jersey, we have noted the influence of Drs. Bernardino Ramazzini, Charles Turner Thackrah, Edwin Chadwick, and John Simon in the European tradition. Drs. Benjamin W. McCready, John H. Griscom, Ezra M. Hunt, Alice Hamilton, Harrison S. Martland, and Irving J. Selikoff promoted social responsibility in American medical circles. These physicians, outside the mainstream, set a pattern of values for the future. But in this country, the medical profession is still catching up with concerned citizens such as Mrs. Lindon W. Bates, and Lawrence T. Fell, who pioneered the prevention of occupational diseases when most physicians had a more limited view of the role of their profession in society.

• • •

SINCE the days of Hippocrates, the traditional role of medicine has been the care of the sick. This role is emphasized today in medical schools and in residency training programs and is the role that society expects of physicians. This tradition is incarnated in the focus on the hospital as the place to treat the seriously ill and on the physician's office as the place for the recognition and management of minor problems and the detection of the early stages of potentially major ones. Unfortunately, relatively little attention is usually given to disorders arising from occupational or environmental exposures.

Such focus and emphasis are reflected in the contents of the curricula of American medical schools and in residency training programs. Medical school curricula are molded to a major degree by the examinations of the National Board of Medical Examiners and by various state boards. However, the granting of the degree of doctor of medicine signifies only the completion of an educational process. To become a physician licensed to practice medicine, additional postgraduate training, education, and experience are required. In the specialty of internal medicine this training is provided in hospital centers, almost without exception affiliated with a medical school. The content of the educational portion of the programs and the training aspects is determined, de facto, by the American Board of Internal Medicine, which reviews the programs and sets the certifying examinations. A residency program that gives too much time to a subject not, or only minimally, represented in board examinations would probably have fewer applicants and might be disapproved. In brief, if a subject is not included in these examinations, it is not likely to have significant representation in the curricula of medical schools or in the content of residency training programs.

Disorders and diseases related to occupations and to environmental factors are not represented in medical curricula or in residency training programs proportionate to their importance to the affected social, economic, and health domains. This relative neglect, which is certainly not benign, results in part from the evolution of medicine and its focus on disease and the sick patient, in part from the manner in which medical education is directed, and in part from the difficulties encountered in causally relating particular disorders or diseases to particular environmental or occupational exposure where a significant time period separates exposure and the manifestation of injury. The temporal relationship of challenge to response is of considerable importance to the recognition of a causal relationship.

Thus, the immediacy of a traumatic injury to the object inflicting the injury can leave little doubt about the cause, a relationship clearly understood since the beginnings of recorded history. By the end of the fifteenth century, sexual contacts were causally related to the development of the lesions of syphilis within a week or two of contact. So, too, at the same period, were the tremors occurring in miners of mercury and in workers involved in its distillation. To protect against battle trauma, shields, helmets, and body armor were developed. To protect against venereal disease, sheaths of animal origin and later of latex were used. To protect against mercury poisoning, the duration of the exposure was limited. Preventive measures were adopted. But when the time lapse between exposure and clinically recognizable symptoms is large, as in HIV infection and AIDS, recognition of the relationship may be delayed.

This delay between contact or exposure and the development of a clinically evident disorder has been of major importance in delaying the recognition of the causal relationship between exposure to asbestos and its associated lung diseases, and between ionizing radiation and cancer and leukemia. These delays in recognition have made already bad problems worse. Industries, cities, even nations will not readily take steps that may require an immediate outlay of funds for results that are to become evident only ten or twenty years later. Public pressure, often expressed by workers themselves, is required to achieve that end. This pressure is even more important when there is denial that a causal relationship exists, when relevant information is hidden, when facts are misrepresented, or when the data bearing on this relationship are falsified. Responsibility for the effects is rejected, and the effects themselves are attributed to other, remote causes. Another factor that may underlie such reactions is that managers and owners are driven by the need for a margin of profit that allows them to maintain and to expand their business. Jobs are involved. On occasion, even those who may eventually suffer are led to deny the existence of a risk. Blaming the victims is another way that responsibility can be evaded. The problem quite evidently enters into the domain of politics and the influencing of legislatures to pass appropriate regulations, not only for the prevention of future problems but also for the care of those who have already suffered illness or injury. A major educational effort is required, not only of industry and legislators but also of the general public and, very importantly, of the medical profession itself.

Such an effort can be considered to have come into being at the beginning of the eighteenth century with the publication of Bernardino Ramazzini's remarkable *De Morbis Artificium* (1713), a cornerstone of the education of physicians in occupational risks and diseases and in the development of preventive measures and of some appropriate therapeutic interventions. It has also served as a model to others seeking to relate occupations and diseases. Since its publication, much progress has been made in the identification and prevention of older problems. Progress has also been made in meeting the challenges and risks associated with the development of new industries, new products, and new environments. But there has always been a lag in the education of the medical profession. Its members practicing in industrial areas or in areas with special environments may be quickly made aware of these special problems, although responses to these problems may be delayed. Others may have obtained their knowledge and understanding from their own experiences. Still others may have obtained a measure of specific training in occupational and environmental medicine. But few will have heard much of such matters in their medical schools or in their residency training programs.

Fortunately, several positive factors that may help in the correction of these deficiencies have recently appeared. The general public is more aware of the problems posed by environmental pollution and of its delayed effects. There is the recognition that the ill effects of cigarette smoking are remote in time and that the destructive effects of ionizing radiation are similarly delayed. Of particular importance is the recent report of the Institute of Medicine (Warren 1988) identifying the need for physicians to be familiar with at least the major aspects of occupational and environmental medicine and the potential role of primary care physicians in filling that need. Finally, there is the report of Joseph S. Castorina and Linda Rosenstock (1990) on the shortage of physicians knowledgeable and involved in occupational and environmental medicine and, importantly, a position paper of the American College of Physicians (Kilbourne and Weiner, 1990), the de facto parent of the American Board of Internal Medicine. This position recommends an increased emphasis at all levels of medical education on topics related to occupational and environmental medicine. It also provides a list of hazardous occupations and possible resultant diseases, and an outline of an occupational medicine history. Recommendations of the American College of Physicians are generally quickly implemented in clinical training programs and can be expected to have, eventually, a significant impact at the level of the third and fourth medical school years.

The publication of the collection of reviews in this volume takes place at a particularly apposite time. The need for more education in this area, directed to the general public as well as to the medical profession, is being addressed, the complexity of the issues involved is being recognized, and the greater involvement of physicians in environmental and occupational issues has become a rational goal. The contributions presented here will serve greatly in focusing on the problems at hand and in meeting the needs of the future.

References

Castorina, J. S., and Rosenstock, L. 1990. "Physician Shortage in Occupational and Environmental Medicine." *Annals of Internal Medicine* 113, no. 12:983–986.

Kilbourne, E. M., and Weiner, J. 1990. "Occupational and Environmental Medicine: The Internist's Role." Position paper of the American College of Physicians. *Annals of Internal Medicine* 113, no. 12:974–982.

Ramazzini, B. [1713] 1964. *Diseases of Workers*. Translated from the Latin text of 1713 by W. C. Wright. *De Morbis Artificium*. 2d ed. New York: Hafner.

Warren, J., ed. 1988. *The Role of the Primary Care Physician in Occupational and Environmental Medicine*. Washington, D.C.: Institute of Medicine, National Academy of Medicine.

Index